Fiscal Sustainability of Health Systems

BRIDGING HEALTH AND FINANCE PERSPECTIVES

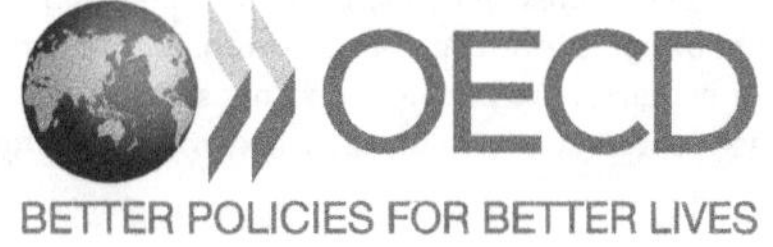

Please cite this publication as:
OECD (2015), *Fiscal Sustainability of Health Systems: Bridging Health and Finance Perspectives*, OECD Publishing, Paris.
DOI: http://dx.doi.org/10.1787/9789264233386-en

ISBN 978-92-64-23337-9 (print)
ISBN 978-92-64-23338-6 (PDF)

Photo credits: © *pogonici/Fotolia.com*

Corrigenda to OECD publications may be found on line at: *www.oecd.org/publishing/corrigenda*.

Foreword

The health systems we enjoy today and expected medical advances in the future will be difficult to finance from public resources without major reform. Such reforms require effective co-operation between Health and Finance Ministries. Public health spending in OECD countries has grown rapidly over most of the last half century. It represents on average about 6% of gross domestic product (GDP) in OECD countries, and is projected to consume an additional 2 percentage points of GDP over the next 20 years. These spending increases have contributed to important progress in population health: life expectancy at birth has increased, rising on average by ten years since 1970. The challenge is to sustain and enhance these achievements in a context of tight fiscal constraints in many countries, upward pressures on health spending from factors such as new technological advances and demographic change.

Finding policies that can make health spending more sustainable without compromising important achievements in access and quality requires joint efforts between Ministries of Health and Ministries of Finance. Sound governance and co-ordination mechanisms are therefore essential to ensure effective policy choices. Fiscal Sustainability of Health Systems: Bridging Health and Finance Perspectives *provides a detailed overview of institutional frameworks for financing health care in OECD countries. One of the main features of this book is a comprehensive mapping of budgeting practices and governance structure in health across OECD countries.*

This book provides a synthesis of the work developed by the OECD Senior Budget and Health Officials Joint Network. Over the past four years, this joint network has been an important forum to promote the dialogue and mutual comprehension between Health and Finance Ministries. It has provided a platform for budget and health officials to discuss together possible solutions to fiscal sustainability challenges in health care. It describes a wide range of responses by countries to the crisis – some clearly beneficial, achieving better value for money, others less so, reducing services across-the-board and potentially leading to poorer health outcomes and financial hardship from increasing costs borne by patients. This book presents a strong case for timely reforms of health care systems, based on close collaboration between budget and health officials.

Implementing effective policies will not be easy, however, particularly as policies may not only take time to produce savings, but also entail transitional costs. It is therefore urgent for countries to articulate a vision and a clear sense of direction for their national reform efforts, and to develop sound governance and co-ordination tools to facilitate them in this endeavour.

Acknowledgements

This book is the result of work undertaken by the OECD Senior Budget Officials-Health Officials Joint Network (OECD SBO-Health Joint Network). It is the product of a truly concerted effort between two directorates of the OECD: Public Governance and Territorial Development under the direction of Rolf Alter and Employment, Labour and Social Affairs under the direction of Stefano Scarpetta and Mark Pearson.

This book was co-ordinated by Camila Vammalle from the OECD Budgeting and Public Expenditures Division, and Chris James from the OECD Health Division, under the supervision of Jón Blöndal and Francesca Colombo. In addition to their active participation in the SBO-Health Joint Network and their production of one or more chapters, Ankit Kumar (Harvard Kennedy School of Government), Mark Blecher (South African Treasury), Grégoire de Lagasnerie (Caisse nationale de l'assurance maladie des travailleurs salariés) and Joseph White (Case Western Reserve University) provided invaluable comments and suggestions on the report during all phases of its production. Gijs van der Vlugt (Ministry of Finance, Netherlands) actively contributed to this publication, among others by spending three months as a secondee at the OECD working for the SBO-Health Joint Network. Rodrigo Moreno-Serra (University of Sheffield), Chris Heady (University of Kent), Delphine Rouillault (Ecole nationale d'administration), Claudia Hulbert (Consultant), Anita Charlesworth (the Health Foundation), Patrick Jeurisen (Ministry of Health, Welfare and Sports, Netherlands), Stephan Thewissen (Leiden University) and Tobias Orishing (Federal Ministry of Finance, Austria) are warmly thanked for their contributions.

This project would not have been possible without Michael Borowitz (former OECD Health Division, now at the Global Fund) and Edwin Lau (now at Reform of the Public Sector Division) who created the OECD SBO-Health Joint Network in 2011, and are still active contributors.

The OECD SBO-Health Joint Network is also very grateful to Geert van Maanen (Former Secretary General of Ministry of Health, Welfare and Sports, and Former Secretary General of Ministry of Finance, Netherlands), who has actively chaired the network since its creation.

The OECD SBO-Health Joint Network and this project were supported by grants from the Netherlands and from Japan.

This project benefited from the active participation in meetings and comments on the different chapter drafts of governmental delegates form Ministries of Finance, Ministries of Health and Social Security/Insurance Institutions. The close involvement with the OECD SBO-Health Joint Network and active participation in meetings of the WHO in the persons of Hans Kluge, Tamas Evetovits, Joseph Kutzin and Sarah Thomson and the World Bank represented by Naoko Miake, Cheryl Cashin and Akiko Maeda and the European Union with Ana Xavier is greatly acknowledged. Many thanks also to Klaus Dirk Henke (Technical University of Berlin) and Mark Stabile (University of Toronto). Comments and support from Valérie Paris, Ronnie Downes, Luiz de Mello, Yuki Murakami, Ane Auraaen, Gaetan Lafortune, Lisa Von Trapp are also warmly recognised.

Hélène Leconte Lucas and Lyora Raab provided invaluable assistance, in particular in the organisation of the meetings and workshops of the OECD SBO-Health Joint Network. Andrew Imlach, Marlène Mohier, Frédéric Daniel and Bonifacio Agapin provided editorial support.

Table of contents

Tables

Figures

Acronyms and abbreviations

ADHD	Attention Deficit Hyperactivity Disorder
CADES	French *Caisse d'Amortissement de la Dette Sociale*
CBA	Central budget authority
CBO	US Congressional Budget Office
CCG	Clinical Commissioning Group
CEA	Cost-effectiveness analysis
CMU	French *Couverture Maladie Universelle*
CNAMTS	French *Caisse nationale de l'assurance maladie des travailleurs salariés*
CPAM	French *Caisse Primaire d'Assurance Maladie*
CRDS	French *Contribution pour le remboursement de la dette sociale*
CSG	French *Contribution Sociale Généralisée*
CWAI	Cost-Weighted Activity Index
DRG	Diagnosis-related group
DTC	Diagnostic and treatment category
EBM	Evidence-based medicine
EOPYY	National Organization for the Provision of Healthcare Services
EWS	Early-warning system
FFS	Fee-for-service
GAO	US Government Accountability Office
GDP	Gross domestic product
GP	General practitioner
HMO	Health maintenance organisation
HMT	Her Majesty's Treasury
HTA	Health technology assessment
ICT	Information and communication technology
IVF	In-vitro fertilisation
LFSS	French *Loi de Financement de la Sécurité Sociale*
MOH	Ministry of Health
NHS	UK National Health Service
NICE	English National Institute for Health and Care Excellence
ONDAM	French National Objective for Healthcare Expenditure (*Objectif national des dépenses d'assurance maladie*)

ONS	UK Office for National Statistics
OTC	Ocver-the-counter
P4P	Pay-for-Performance
PbR	Payment by result
PCT	Primary care trust
PLFSS	French *Projet de Loi de Financement de la Sécurité Sociale*
QALY	Quality-adjusted life year
QIPP	Quality, Innovation, Productivity and Prevention
RHE	Regional health enterprise
SBC	Social Budget Committee
SBO	Senior Budget Official
SHI	Social health insurance
SNG	Sub-national government
THE	Total health expenditure
UHI	Universal Health Insurance
UNCAM	French *Union Nationale des Caisses d'Assurance Maladie*
VAT	Value added tax
WHO	World Health Organization

Preface

Spending on health has outpaced economic growth in most OECD countries for many decades. The question of the fiscal sustainability of health systems has been brought to the top of many political agendas. Government bureaucracies are struggling with how to meet such large fiscal challenges. Both Ministries of Health and Finance are at the forefront of these challenges. Ministries of Finance strive to create effective budgetary discipline and manage budgetary envelopes. Ministries of Health face the huge task of keeping their ageing populations healthy whilst improving the efficiency of their healthcare delivery systems.

Because the ecosystem of modern health care is complex, with multiple stakeholders, this is no easy task. In the case of Ministries of Finance and Health, better understanding each other's priorities and constraints, and subsequent co-ordinated action can help. For these reasons the OECD Senior Budget and Health Officials Joint Network was initiated, where we try to learn from each other, share ideas, and explore how OECD countries can address the fiscal sustainability challenge health systems face. Since 2011, representatives of Ministries of Health and Ministries of Finance have worked together with experts from the World Health Organization, World Bank and other international organizations, universities and think tanks.

Results of these discussions are synthesised in this publication. We cover the main issues at stake, such as: the meaning and impact of fiscal sustainability, the political economy of budgeting for health, the effects of aging on funding models, fiscal decentralisation, cost containment strategies and country responses to the recent financial crisis.

A key focus of the publication is on the institutional arrangements that structure countries' health financing systems. Fiscal sustainability starts with a thorough procedural framework that is able to guide the effective functioning of budgetary institutions. Important factors for such a framework include long-term forecasts, medium-term projections, timely information on spending, adequate and stable revenues, and expenditure management tools. But this publication shows that most health systems do not always naturally fit with many of these "classic" scholarly preconditions of public budgeting. Further, such institutions are more effective if they are underpinned by political agreement on budgetary targets and co-ordination mechanisms, a precondition that cannot be taken for granted given the highly politicised nature of modern health care systems.

Nevertheless, the main message from this work is that good institutions are essential for governments to control health spending and to stimulate value-for-money in this field. Chapter 3 covers – for the first time – how institutions for health budgeting function in 27 OECD member states. This forms an exciting starting point for future learning. However, we also need in-depth comparative case studies that provide a picture of the more intricate details of how budgetary institutions for health work. In this book country case studies are provided for France, the United Kingdom and the Netherlands. I hope this will be a first step in a process of searching for best practices.

Over the past decades, improved population health has been a significant accomplishment of all OECD member states. However, health spending has grown to become a major budgetary commitment in most countries. Our task ahead is to continue improving the health of our populations while at the same time keeping control of public spending. This report is the first contribution of the members of the joint network and the OECD secretariat. I am proud of what has been accomplished and I am sure it is a major step forward for our understanding of how to accomplish fiscal sustainability of our healthcare systems.

Geert van Maanen

Chair of the Joint Network on
Fiscal Sustainability of Health Systems
September 2015

Fiscal Sustainability of Health Systems
Bridging Health and Finance Perspectives

Executive summary

Over the last 20 years, the average annual growth rate of public health spending exceeded GDP growth in all OECD countries. While such spending has improved health outcomes, there are concerns on the fiscal sustainability of this upward trend. Indeed, in the absence of effective cost-containment policies, OECD projections show public spending on health and long-term care is on course to reach almost 9% of GDP by 2030, and as much as 14% by 2060. Pressures on health expenditure are mainly due to new technologies, which extend the scope, range and quality of medical services; rising incomes, which engender higher expectations on the quality and scope of care; and population ageing.

Across the OECD, health care is one of the most complex expenditure areas, and is considered by most budget officials as the hardest area in which to contain costs. Indeed, health care is perceived by citizens as a very high priority, and government policies in this area are closely watched. In addition, there are many stakeholders who intervene between the beneficiary of health care (the citizen/patient) and the public resources that finance it. These include purchasers (Ministries of Health, social security institutions, social insurance funds or sub-national governments); a wide range of service providers (clinicians with different specialities, operating within hospitals and other health facilities); providers of medicines, tests and equipment (pharmaceutical companies and laboratories); and other bureaucratic and administrative intermediaries.

Health is also one of the public policy areas with the greatest institutional variations across countries, whether in terms of financial sources (general taxation vs. social contributions), management (by government vs. independent social security institutions or sub-national governments) or service provision (public or private).

Today, budget and health officials face the shared challenge of ensuring that any increase in health spending respect fiscal sustainability constraints, while delivering the best value for money. To achieve this, countries need to create or strengthen appropriate governance frameworks and policy tools to:

1. *"Diagnose"* fiscal sustainability challenges

Governments need information about health care spending and funding sources. This includes long-term forecasts, taking into account demographic and economic factors; short-term spending requirements that governments can use to set/shape/establish their budgets; timely information on actual spending; and an evaluation of the evolution of possible revenue sources (taxes and/or contributions).

- Population ageing will affect how governments finance health services, particularly in countries that are more reliant on social security contributions, as population ageing will reduce the revenue-raising potential of social security contributions over time.

- "Early warning systems" have proven effective in several countries to allow corrective measures. However, such systems need timely information, and, in some countries, information on actual spending can take up to two years to be reported to the Ministry of Finance.
- Some countries have also used spending reviews to identify potential savings in health expenditure.

2. Identify the "*risk factors*" to the fiscal sustainability of health systems

Political and institutional factors can play a major role in promoting the intrinsic sustainability of health systems. These factors include: political agreement on the need to control health expenditure growth and on specific targets; effective co-ordination mechanisms among the different stakeholders; the degree of decentralisation of health services (in terms of functions and revenues); and the boundaries between public and private spending on health. While these supportive factors can be influenced in the medium to long term, they are more difficult to change in the short term, and their absence can be interpreted as risks to the fiscal sustainability of health systems.

- The survey of budget practices in health shows that most countries have targets or ceilings for health spending over several years. These are determined by economic rather than health-specific factors. Nonetheless, over-spending in health (i.e. spending more than the budgeted amount) remains endemic in many OECD countries.
- In most OECD countries, sub-national governments play a role in health spending. On average, they are responsible for 30% of public health expenditure, but this share exceeds 90% in federal, quasi-federal and northern European countries. Key challenges for decentralised systems include soft budget constraints (with central government implicitly responsible for bailouts), and geographical inequalities.

3. Develop "*treatments*" to ensure greater sustainability of health spending

There are a number of policy levers and tools which can be put in place to promote greater sustainability of health care spending without compromising important achievements in access and quality of health care. These include *supply-side policies*, such as provider payment methods, provider competition, generic substitution and joint purchasing; *demand-side tools*, such as gatekeeping or preferred drug list; *public management, co-ordination and financing policies*, such as direct controls on pharmaceutical prices/profits, health technology assessment or monitoring and evaluation; and *revenue policy*.

- On the supply side, provider payments that create the right incentives, provider monitoring and competition, and pharmaceutical generic and purchasing policies have helped contain costs across a range of countries. Insurer competition and workforce legislation have had more mixed results. Automatic cuts in health budgets have also been introduced in many countries. These have helped reduce growth in health spending, but are a rather blunt policy tool. Finally, some countries reduced spending on prevention following the crisis. While this leads to short-term savings, it may have harmful effects both on costs and on health outcomes in the longer term.
- On the demand side, expanded cost-sharing has helped contain costs but with adverse impacts on access to care. There is some evidence that physician gatekeeping and preferred drug lists have contained costs without adverse effects on patients; encouraging

private health insurance, however, has not been effective in relieving public budgeting pressures.

- Public management, co-ordination and financing reforms have had varying degrees of success. Direct control of pharmaceutical prices and profits has proved effective in containing costs, but the long-term effects remain controversial. Health technology assessments that include cost-effectiveness analysis can promote more informed, realistic decisions on public health care provision, but there are few studies of their impact on public health expenditure to date.
- On the revenue side, care needs to be exercised in advocating ever-increasing revenues as a response to rising expenditure pressures – not least given the distortionary economic effects of high marginal tax rates. Where additional revenues are required, a move towards broader-based models would appear appropriate, especially in countries with health insurance systems that are more reliant on payroll taxes. "Sin taxes" have important public health effects but play only a modest role in financing health services.

No matter the degree of success of governments in improving value for money in health spending and containing public health expenditure growth, future support for government spending on health will be shaped by politics as much as by economics. Indeed, publicly financed health systems entail a high degree of redistribution, not only from the healthy to the sick, but also from the wealthier to the less affluent. Citizen support for publicly financed health spending will therefore ultimately be a decision about the degree of redistribution they are willing to accept. Improved governance and co-ordination systems, which make clear the policy choices and trade-offs that arise in this context, will help citizens and policy makers arrive at a balanced dispensation that reflects national preferences.

Fiscal Sustainability of Health Systems
Bridging Health and Finance Perspectives

Chapter 1

Fiscal sustainability of health systems – Why is it an issue, what can be done?

OECD*

This chapter describes the fiscal sustainability challenge faced by OECD country health systems, and how it can be addressed. It analyses trends in health expenditure, showing that health spending has typically outpaced economic growth in the past. Although the global financial crisis of 2008 moderated health spending growth, projections forecast health spending to continue to rise as a share of GDP. Evidence on the key drivers of health spending are then presented, showing that it has been largely driven by new technologies and rising incomes, with demographic change (ageing) and institutional characteristics of health systems also important in some countries. Three general policy options for ensuring the fiscal sustainability of health systems are then discussed: raising more money for health, improving the efficiency of government health spending, and reassessing the boundaries between public and private spending.

* The main authors of this chapter are Mark Blecher (South African Treasury) and Chris James (OECD Health Division), with important contributions from Grégoire De Lagasnerie (OECD Health Division), Ankit Kumar (OECD Health Division) and Camila Vammalle (OECD Budgeting and Public Expenditures Division).

The statistical data for Israel are supplied by and under the responsibility of the relevant Israeli authorities. The use of such data by the OECD is without prejudice to the status of the Golan Heights, East Jerusalem and Israeli settlements in the West Bank under the terms of international law.

1.1. Introduction and main messages

Throughout the OECD, health care is often mentioned by countries as the most substantial challenge facing government budgets. Even prior to the global financial crisis it was widely noted that global health expenditure was rising at levels significantly above inflation. Rapid spending growth has widely been understood to have been driven primarily by technology and rising incomes, with demography and institutional characteristics relevant but less important factors.

After years of continuous growth of over 4% a year, average health spending slowed down throughout the OECD, growing at only 0.3% since 2009. Total health spending fell in 11 out of the 34 OECD countries between 2009 and 2011 (*OECD Health Statistics*). As the global financial crisis of 2008 continues to have after-effects in most countries, questions of sustainability and efficiency of public finances have moved more strongly to the forefront. Fiscal sustainability of public spending has important implications for health sector funding, while health expenditure is a key element of fiscal sustainability.

This chapter provides an overview of the fiscal sustainability of health systems challenge faced by OECD countries and how it can be addressed. After discussing the different ways in which the term fiscal sustainability can be defined (Section 1.2), trends in health spending are analysed (Section 1.3). This analysis outlines trends in health spending growth over the past thirty years, the extent to which the recent financial crisis has affected spending patterns, and projections for the coming decades. Section 1.4 then summarises what is known about the determinants of health spending growth. This is followed in Section 1.5 with an overview of the main policy options that can help ensure the fiscal sustainability of health systems. Section 1.6 concludes.

The main messages from this chapter are summarised below:

- Fiscal sustainability requires governments to manage public finances credibly. Health systems are a key challenge to fiscal sustainability, since rising costs, new treatment possibilities and demand for continued improvements to the quality of care will exert pressure on public finances.
- Health expenditure has typically outpaced economic growth. Whilst the global economic crisis moderated rapid growth in health spending, this is expected to be temporary. Indeed, projections forecast health expenditures to rise as a share of GDP.
- Spending on health has been largely driven by new technologies and rising incomes, with demographic change and institutional characteristics of health systems relevant but less important factors in most countries.
- The implications of rising costs are particularly important for public finances, since health care is predominantly funded from public sources. Moreover, ageing may lead to shortfalls in payroll taxes to finance health.

- Policy makers have three broad ways to ensure fiscal sustainability of health systems: raise more money for health, improve the efficiency of government health spending, and reassess the boundaries between public and private spending. Simpler blanket spending cuts can also evidently address fiscal constraints, but are more likely to have adverse effects.
- Health care is highly valued by populations and is a major contributor to countries' economies. Therefore spending more on health is not automatically a problem, particularly if citizens are willing to pay for this through higher taxes or cuts in other areas of government spending. The challenge is to ensure any increase in spending respects fiscal sustainability constraints, and delivers good value for money.

1.2. How can fiscal sustainability be defined in relation to health systems?

The OECD defines fiscal sustainability as the ability of a government to maintain public finances at a credible and serviceable position over the long term (OECD, 2013). Fiscal sustainability implies governments are able to maintain policies and expenditure into the future, without major adjustments and excessive debt burdens for future generations. The term refers to overall government spending, revenues, assets and liabilities that reflect past commitments and adapt to future trends such as socio-economic trends and environmental factors. Table 1.1 below provides further definitions from the European Commission and the International Monetary Fund.

Table 1.1. **Fiscal sustainability definitions from the European Commission and the International Monetary Fund**

European Commission	International Monetary Fund
The ability to continue now and in the future current policies (with no changes regarding public services and taxation) without causing public debt to rise continuously as a share of GDP (European Commission, 2014).	A set of policies is sustainable if a borrower is expected to be able to continue servicing its debt without an unrealistically large future correction to the balance of income and expenditure (IMF, 2007).

Source: European Commission (2014), "Identifying Fiscal Sustainability Challenges in the Areas of Pension, Health Care and Long-term Care Policies"; IMF (2007), *Manual on Fiscal Transparency*, IMF, Washington, DC.

For the health sector, fiscal sustainability is perhaps best understood as a constraint that needs to be respected, rather than an objective in itself (Thomson et al., 2009). This implies that *how* governments achieve fiscal sustainability matters, rather than it becoming a simple cost-cutting exercise. For example, as Thomson et al. note, increasing user charges for health services might seem an administratively simple way to reduce the budget deficit, but it also undermines health system goals of financial protection and health gain. A better solution would be to cut cost-ineffective interventions.

Ministries of Finance tend to focus their attention on finding a sustainable fiscal path whereby debt levels are kept under control. Typically they have macro-economists modelling growth projections; tax policy specialists modelling revenue estimates; and of most relevance to health officials, budget office and expenditure teams who work with line ministries. In the OECD countries, an ongoing debate is taking place as to whether fiscal policies of austerity are appropriate – noting revenue reductions and high deficits following the recession – or are too tight, and aggravating low growth. While macroeconomists may agree that debt levels should be sustainable, they often disagree on specifying thresholds at which national debt poses a threat to the economy.

Moreover, fiscal sustainability does not automatically preclude substantive increases to government spending on health. Societies often express greater willingness to contribute more for health care than other areas of government spending, reflecting the value placed on health and its contribution to human capital (OECD, 1998). The health sector is also a major and rapidly growing source of employment. A recent OECD study, reviewing expenditures from 17 countries for the period 1970-2008, found that if total government spending is kept unchanged, increased expenditure on health, education and transport were the key areas to raising long-term GDP growth (Barbiero et al., 2013). Consequently, from a growth perspective it may be preferable for health to crowd out less efficient forms of government spending. A related point is the adverse effects of ill-health on the labour market. For example, various studies have shown that smokers, heavy alcohol users, the obese and people with mental health disorders have a lower probability of being employed, earn less and/or are more likely to be absent from work (see, for example, Lundborg et al., 2010; OECD, 2012; Vahtera et al., 2002; Weng et al., 2012).

In this sense, the fiscal sustainability of health also becomes a question of political economy. Future support for government spending on health will be shaped by views on redistribution as much as economic drivers of future revenues, since publicly financed systems redistribute not only from the healthy to the sick, but also from the wealthier to the less affluent (see Chapter 2 for a further discussion). It will also depend on priority decisions between health and other competing areas of government spending.

Nonetheless, if it is not possible to find the support and means for raising sufficient funds, fiscal sustainability requires that even socially desired expenditures may have to be reduced.[1] Countries with high levels of debt and/or large public sector deficits are most likely to face fiscal sustainability constraints, as are countries where health spending is a large share of government spending, or where overall government spending comprises a large share of GDP (Oxley and Morgan, 2009).

1.3. Health care spending: Past, present and future

Health spending has typically outpaced economic growth

Health care poses an important budgetary challenge because spending on health has typically outpaced economic growth in most OECD countries (Figure 1.1). In some countries, notably the Slovak Republic, Turkey, Chile and Korea, relatively high health spending growth may in part reflect increased coverage that expanded access to publicly financed health care to a broader share of their population over time. However, for most OECD countries universal health care pre-dates this period, implying therefore that incrementally greater shares of incomes are being directed towards health care spending. This is of particular interest from a fiscal sustainability perspective, as public funds account for around three-quarters of total spending on health across the OECD, a share that has been broadly unchanged in the last couple of decades.

The economic crisis has slowed health spending growth

The recent global economic crisis has slowed health spending growth. After an average annual growth rate of just over 4% throughout the OECD[2] for the period 2000-08, health spending grew at an average of 2.6% in 2009, -0.4% in 2010, 0.3% in 2011 and 1% in 2012. This reflects both a general slowdown across most OECD countries and substantial reductions in some countries (Figure 1.2). In some countries, notably Greece, Ireland, Italy, Portugal and

Spain, health spending cuts reflect explicit austerity policies on public spending (Morgan, 2014). But these countries were joined by the Czech Republic, Denmark, Estonia, Iceland, Luxembourg and the United Kingdom, which have registered falls in real health spending since 2009.

Figure 1.1. **Average annual growth rate of real health spending and GDP per capita, 1990-2012 (or closest years)**

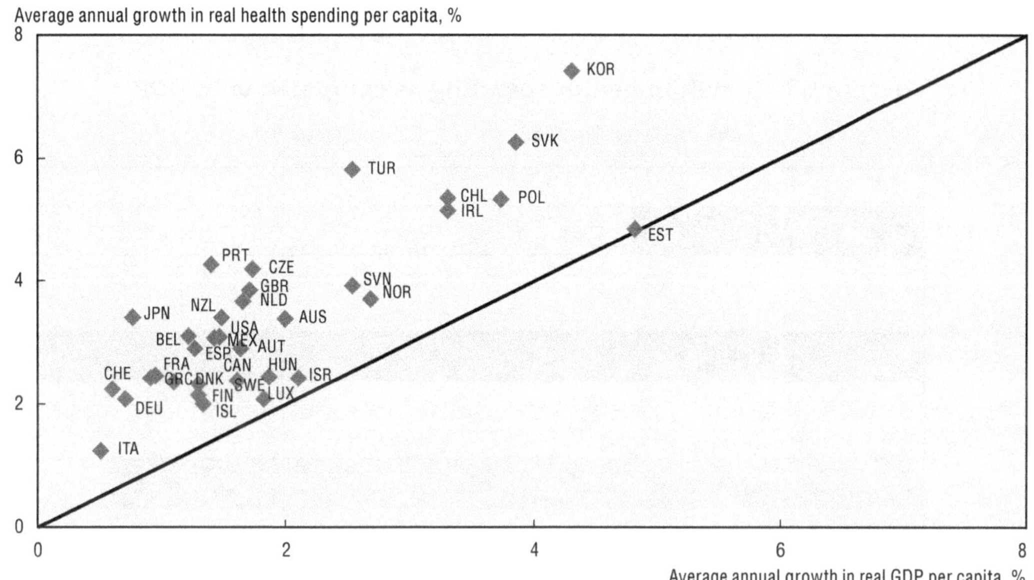

Source: *OECD Health Statistics, http://dx.doi.org/10.1787/health-data-en.*

StatLink http://dx.doi.org/10.1787/888933218560

Figure 1.2. **Average annual growth rates in real health spending per capita, from 2000 to the latest year**

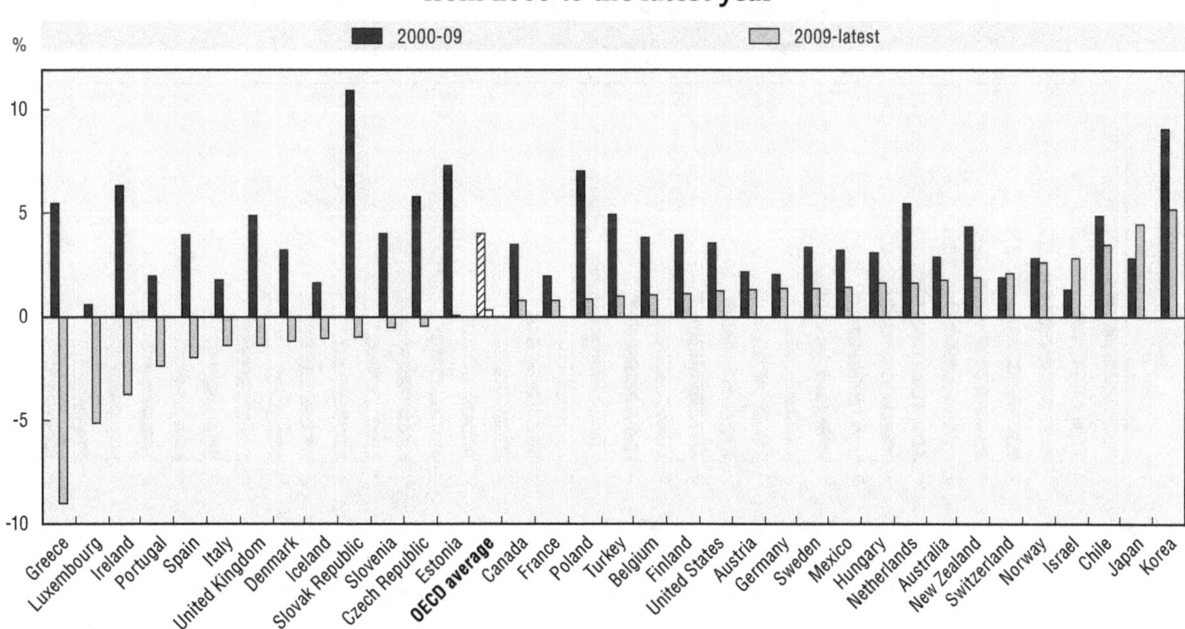

Source: *OECD Health Statistics, http://dx.doi.org/10.1787/health-data-en.*

StatLink http://dx.doi.org/10.1787/888933218572

Whilst the slowdown in health spending was to a large extent mirrored by reduced GDP growth rates or recession, health systems were often particularly affected by the economic downturn. Across the OECD as a whole, health spending accounted for 9.16% of GDP on average in 2012, slightly lower than 9.25% in 2011 and 9.36% in 2010. Moreover, growth in health spending has been slower than GDP growth in a majority of OECD countries in recent years. This is in marked contrast to the situation pre-crisis (Figure 1.3). Nevertheless, government spending on health continues to outweigh private spending in all OECD countries except the United States and Chile (Figure 1.4).

Figure 1.3. **Growth in health spending as compared with GDP**

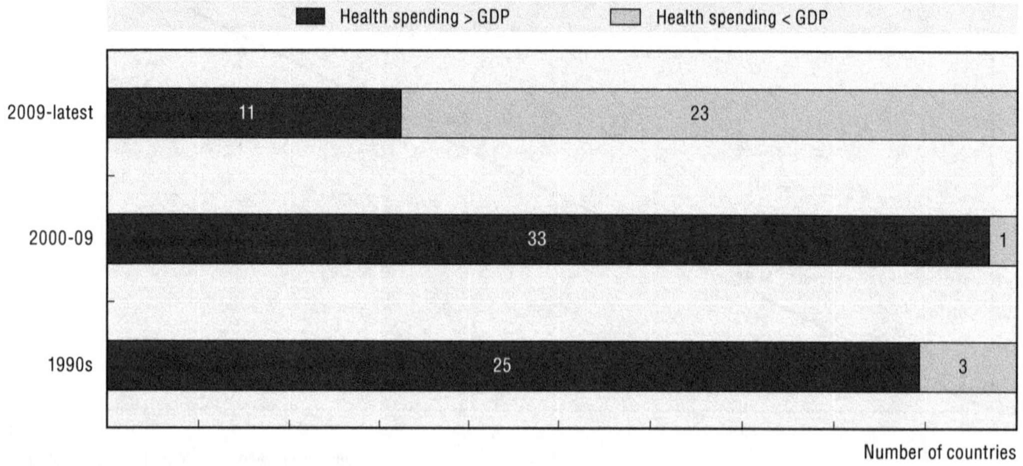

Health spending > GDP
Health spending < GDP
2009-latest 11 23
2000-09 33 1
1990s 25 3
Number of countries

Note: The 11 countries in which health spending growth outpaced GDP since 2009 are Australia, Belgium, Finland, France, Hungary, Israel, Japan, Korea, Netherlands, New Zealand and Switzerland.

Source: *OECD Health Statistics, http://dx.doi.org/10.1787/health-data-en.*

StatLink http://dx.doi.org/10.1787/888933218588

Figure 1.4. **Health spending as a share of GDP, 2012 or latest year**

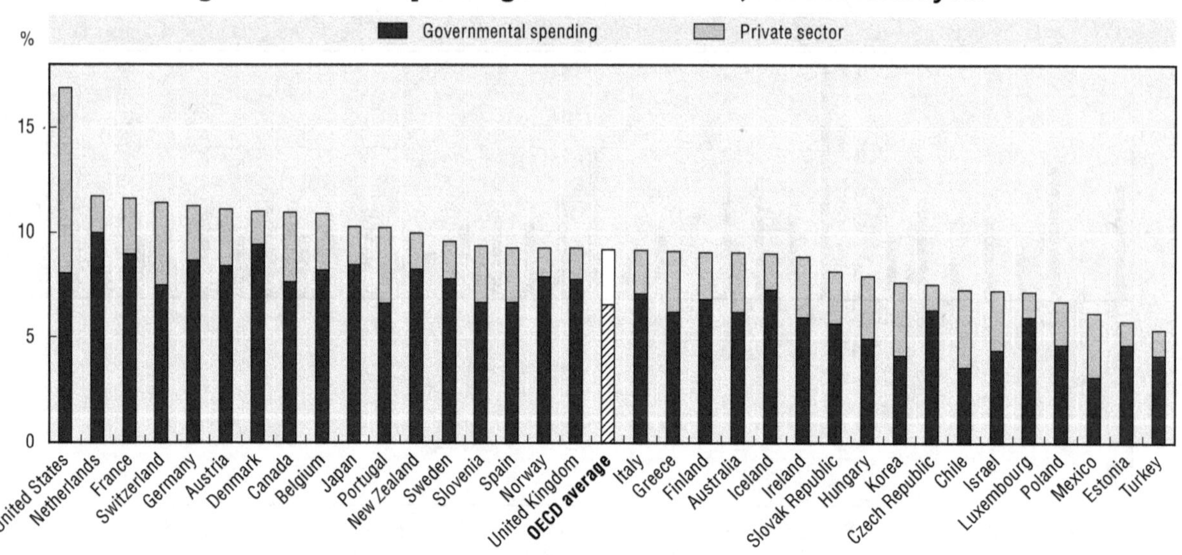

Note: Portugal, New Zealand and Australia latest data were from 2011. For Netherlands, data are for current health expenditure.

Source: *OECD Health Statistics, http://dx.doi.org/10.1787/health-data-en.*

StatLink http://dx.doi.org/10.1787/888933218595

Countries with higher rates of health spending growth before the economic crisis tended to have bigger falls after the crisis, with every 1% of additional growth before the crisis associated with a 0.9% drop after the crisis (Van Gool and Pearson, 2014). Public spending on health was more likely than private spending to be affected by the crisis. Across the OECD as a whole, average annual growth in public spending on health has been stagnant since 2009 (in real terms). During the same period, private spending continued to grow, albeit at a modest rate of about 1%.

Despite the recent slowdown, government health spending is expected to consume an additional 2% of GDP over the next 20 years

Although health spending growth has been markedly slower since the global financial crisis, a range of national and international projections suggest that health spending will continue to rise in the medium to long-term. This can pose fiscal sustainability challenges. For example, the European Commission found that 13 EU countries – Austria, the Czech Republic, Finland, France, Germany, Ireland, Malta, Netherlands, Poland, Portugal, Slovenia, Spain and the Slovak Republic – are at risk of substantive fiscal sustainability challenges because of health care spending (note that many of these countries also face fiscal sustainability concerns because of pensions and long-term care spending). This analysis was based on composite indicators reflecting projections of health care, other age-related expenditures and debt levels (EC, 2014).

OECD projections estimate public spending on health and long-term care across OECD countries will increase from around 6% of GDP today to 8.2% in 2030 and 9.5% of GDP in 2060, based on a scenario where governments are able to contain costs (de la Maisonneuve and Martins, 2013). Conversely, should governments be less successful at cost containment (referred to as a "cost-pressure" scenario), spending is projected to increase to 8.8% of GDP in 2030 and as much as 14% of GDP by 2060 (Figure 1.5).

Figure 1.5. **Projected public health and long-term care expenditure as a percentage of GDP in 2060**

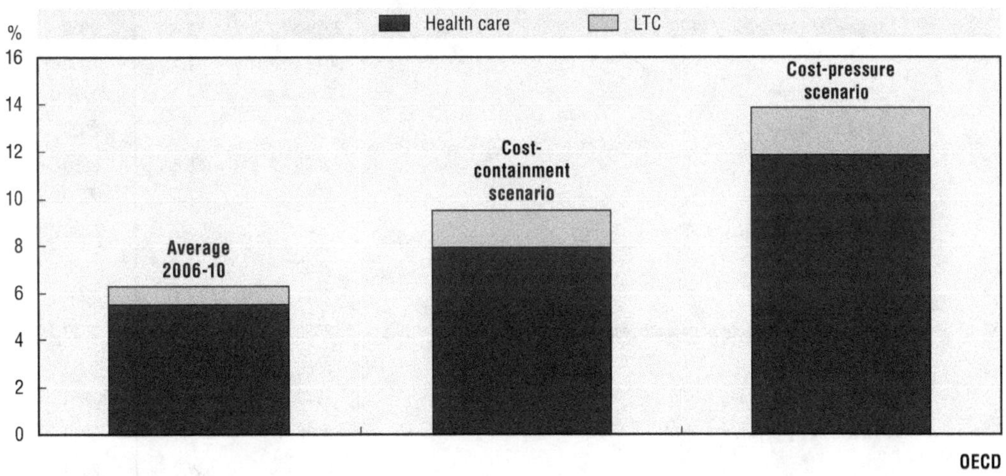

Source: De La Maisonneuve, C. and J. Oliveira Martins (2013), "Public Spending on Health and Long-term Care: A New Set of Projections", *OECD Economic Policy Papers* No. 06, OECD Publishing, Paris, *http://dx.doi.org/10.1787/5k44t7jwwr9x-en.*

StatLink *http://dx.doi.org/10.1787/888933218607*

Whilst methodological differences exist (Box 1.1), the OECD cost-containment projection is broadly consistent with estimates published by the European Union, and the cost-pressure scenario with IMF estimates (EC, 2012; IMF, 2010). They are also broadly in line with estimates undertaken by fiscal authorities of various OECD countries, notwithstanding methodological differences on how to model the impact of ageing (Table 1.2).

Box 1.1. **Modelling future health care expenditures: a brief summary of approaches**

A recent OECD paper reviewed models used for forecasting health care expenditures (OECD, 2012). They noted that models could be grouped into three main classes: micro models that simulate entire populations; component-based models drawing from the actuarial disciplines; and broader macro models that forecast on the basis of time-series or cross-sectional data on aggregate indicators. Essential to all model classes are realistic assumptions, particularly on the effects of ageing. A pessimistic assumption corresponds to an "expansion of morbidity" hypothesis (Gruenberg, 1977) whereby all gains in longevity translate into years spent in poor health. This reflects in part the likelihood that elderly people are more prone to costly chronic conditions. Conversely, evidence shows proximity to death to be a key driver of higher spending. Based on this "death-related costs" hypothesis alternative more optimistic assumptions are a "healthy ageing" hypothesis whereby gains in longevity translate one-to-one into years in good health (Manton 1982); and the "compression of morbidity" hypothesis whereby gains in longevity compress the time spent in morbidity (Fries, 1980). See OECD (2012) and EC (2012) for a further discussion.

Table 1.2. **Health spending projections by national fiscal authorities and the OECD**

Country	Government projection			OECD projection[1]	
	Health expenditure component, Reference	Year	% GDP	Year	% GDP
Australia	Public expenditure	2009-10	4.0	2006-10	5.6
	Intergenerational Report, 2010	2029-30	4.8	2030	.7.1
		2049-50	7.1	2060	8.1
Austria	Public expenditure	2011	7.1	2006-10	6.6
	Federal Ministry of Finance, 2012	-	-	2030	8.3
		2060	8.8	2060	9.0
Canada	Public expenditure	2012	7.5	2006-10	5.8
	Fiscal Sustainability Report, 2014	-	-	2030	7.6
		2060	11.7	2060	8.3
France	Public expenditure	2011	8.1	2006-10	7.4
	High Council for the Future of Health Insurance, 2013	2030	9.4	2030	8.8
		2060	10.4	2060	9.6
Germany	Statutory health insurance	2010	7.3	2006-10	7.3
	Federal Ministry of Finance, 2014	2030	8.0/.2	2030	8.9
		2060	8.2/.9	2060	9.6
Italy	Public expenditure	2010	7.3	2006-10	6.1
	Ministry of Finance, 2014	2030	7.3	2030	7.7
		2060	8.1	2060	8.7
Korea	National health insurance expenditure	2012	3.2	2006-10	3.3
	National Assembly Budget Office, 2012	-	-	2030	5.4
		2060	6.2	2060	7.0

Table 1.2. **Health spending projections by national fiscal authorities and the OECD** *(cont.)*

Country	Government projection			OECD projection[1]	
	Health expenditure component, Reference	Year	% GDP	Year	% GDP
Netherlands	Public expenditure	2011	9.8	2006-10	6.4
	Bureau for Economic Policy Analysis, 2010	2040	14.3	2030	8.2
		-	-	2060	8.8
New Zealand	Public expenditure	2011	6.9	2006-10	6.4
	Treasury, 2013	-	-	2030	8.0
		2060	10.8	2060	8.8
Slovak Republic	Public expenditure	2013	5.2	2006-10	5.4
	Council for Budget Responsibility, 2014	2030	6.0	2030	6.9
		2063	6.7	2060	8.0
Spain	Public expenditure	2008	6.0	2006-10	5.6
	Fiscal Studies Institute, 2011	-	-	2030	7.2
		2060	7.1	2060	8.4
Sweden	Total expenditure	2010	9.7	2006-10	6.6
	Government Office, 2010	-	-	2030	7.9
		2050	12.0	2060	8.6
Switzerland	Total expenditure	2009	9.5	2006-10	5.7
	Federal Finance Administration, 2012	-	-	2030	7.3
		2060	11.4	2060	8.3
United Kingdom	Public expenditure	2013-14	7.9	2006-10	6.5
	Fiscal Sustainability Report, 2014	2018-19	6.4	2030	7.9
		2063-64	8.4	2060	8.5
United States	Major public health care programmes	2014	4.8	2006-10	5.8
	Long-Term Budget Outlook report, 2014	2039	8.0	2030	7.6
		-	-	2060	8.3

1. OECD projections are for public spending on health care, and reflect the "cost-containment" scenario.

1.4. Why is spending on health increasing in OECD countries?

Technology, income, demography and institutional characteristics influence health spending

For low and middle income countries, it is fairly easy to understand why health spending is rising, as unmet needs are met and progress is made towards universal coverage of health services. However, researchers and policy makers have struggled to understand why in even the most economically developed OECD countries, health expenditure has continued to exceed inflation levels for decades. Four broad factors are commonly cited as determinants of health expenditure: new health technologies, changing demography, rising incomes and institutional characteristics of health systems (Gerdtham and Jonsson, 2000; Oxley and Morgan, 2009; Smith et al., 2009; IMF, 2010; Chernew and Newhouse, 2011; EC, 2012; De La Maisonneuve and Oliveira Martins, 2013a).

New health technologies extend the scope, range and quality of medical services. This increases health care costs, by offering better but more expensive care for complex illnesses, including those that may not have been previously treatable. The range of health interventions is extended and deepened, thereby increasing the use of health services overall. Conversely, new technologies can reduce costs through shortened morbidities or less costly treatment inputs.

Changing demography, particularly ageing populations, is another potentially important cost-driver. This assumes that the elderly are more likely to develop chronic conditions with multiple morbidities, which are more costly to treat. However, a challenge to this notion is found in research based on the 'compression of morbidity' hypothesis, where the onset of chronic illness is postponed more than the age of death is extended (Fries, 1980, 2011). The impact of demographic changes on health care costs therefore depends on how they change the *disease burden* in populations.

Rising incomes can also contribute to higher costs. Whilst at the individual level health care is often a necessity (and therefore income inelastic), expectations on the quality and scope of care rise as countries grow richer. Studies using national-level longitudinal data typically find income elasticities greater than one, as health spending exceeds economic growth (Chernew and Newhouse, 2011).

Institutional characteristics of health systems have also been shown to be important. For example, there is some evidence that primary care gatekeepers and regulations on the overall supply of providers have helped contain costs, whereas unregulated fee-for-service payment systems push up costs (Gosden et al., 2000). Across all health systems, the "Baumol effect" posits that health service productivity growth is lower (and price inflation higher) than other less labour-intensive sectors of the economy (Baumol, 1967), although the evidence for this effect is debated.

New technologies and rising incomes are major drivers of health spending growth

A range of econometric models have been developed to assess the relative importance of different factors on health spending growth. Notwithstanding significant methodological challenges (Box 1.2), technology and rising incomes have been widely understood to be the key drivers behind health spending growth, with demography and institutional characteristics much less important.

Box 1.2. **Methodological approaches to quantifying the impact of medical technology**

The impact of medical technology on health has traditionally been analysed using a residual approach. This approach is based on the assumption that technology is responsible for all changes not accounted for by other quantifiable factors (mainly ageing and income). That is, technical progress is taken to be exogenous, in a similar way to the traditional economic growth models pioneered by Solow. A challenge with such models is defining variables that reflect known factors behind health spending growth. Other approaches try to capture forces that drive technological progress. Referred to as affirmative or case study approaches, these assess the extent to which a specific technology has contributed to rising expenditures for a specific disease. For example, using this approach, Cutler and McClellan (1996) found that growth in treatment costs for heart attacks in the United States was driven entirely by the diffusion of innovative procedures. See Chernew and Newhouse (2011) for a further discussion.

A challenge common to all approaches is how to model interactions between demographic and non-demographic factors (for example, an older population may change community expectations on appropriate levels of care). A number of OECD countries are exploring the development of models based on "micro-simulations" of individual behaviours across the population, but these remain some way from having predictive capacity for health spending as a whole.

The seminal paper by Newhouse in 1992 concluded that advances in medical technologies were likely to explain at least half of health expenditure growth in the previous 50 years, and perhaps as much as 75% in the United States. Smith et al. (2009), updating these estimates with new data and a refined methodology, found that medical technology advances explained 27%-48% of health spending growth since 1960. Income accounted for a similar amount (29%-43%), with these two factors reinforcing each other. In contrast, medical price inflation explained 5%-19% of the increase in health spending, with demographic effects explaining 7%.

Results for other countries were broadly consistent with Smith's estimates for the United States. Looking back over 1995-2009, the most recent OECD projections found that income explained 42% of health spending growth and demography 12%, with technology accounting for much of the 46% residual across OECD countries as a whole (de la Maisonneuve and Martins, 2013). Chernew and Newhouse (2011), in an extensive review of the empirical evidence, note the consistent finding of technology as the primary determinant of spending growth in a range of high-income countries.

An important counterpoint to these findings, though, comes from Dormont et al. (2006; 2012). Whilst they found that technological innovation drove the vast majority of health spending growth in France for 1992-2000, for 2000-08 ageing explained 45% of spending growth, a similar explanatory share to technology. Similarly, the Japanese government estimated that ageing explained 41% and 84% of spending growth for 1992-2000 and 2000-08 respectively (Japan Ministry of Health, Labour and Social Welfare).

1.5. Ensuring the fiscal sustainability of health systems: what are the main policy options?

In addition to blanket spending cuts, policy makers have three broad ways to ensure fiscal sustainability of health systems: raise more money for health, improve the efficiency of government health spending, and reassess the boundaries between public and private spending. Policy efforts to date have been rather different across these options, with less policy attention given to reassessing public-private boundaries. Further, whilst improving efficiency in principle offers cost-savings without adverse effects on quality or access, policies often require a long time to implement. This is especially the case if such policies require behaviour change.

Reallocate spending, find new sources of revenue

Revenue-raising is mainly the responsibility of Ministries of Finance rather than Ministries of Health. Nevertheless, in several countries these parties have worked together to find solutions, particularly after the recent economic crisis. A first option is to explore reallocation possibilities within existing government budgets. Figure 1.6 shows that most countries in the OECD allocate close to the OECD average of 15% of government spending to health. However, four countries allocated 20% or more (Japan, Netherlands, Switzerland, United States) and four countries allocated less than 12% (Hungary, Israel, Poland, Turkey). It is also interesting to note that many countries have allowed health to become a bigger share of their budgets: across the OECD, health's share of government expenditure rose by 1.4 percentage points from 2000 to 2012.

Figure 1.6. **Health spending as a share of total government spending, 2012**

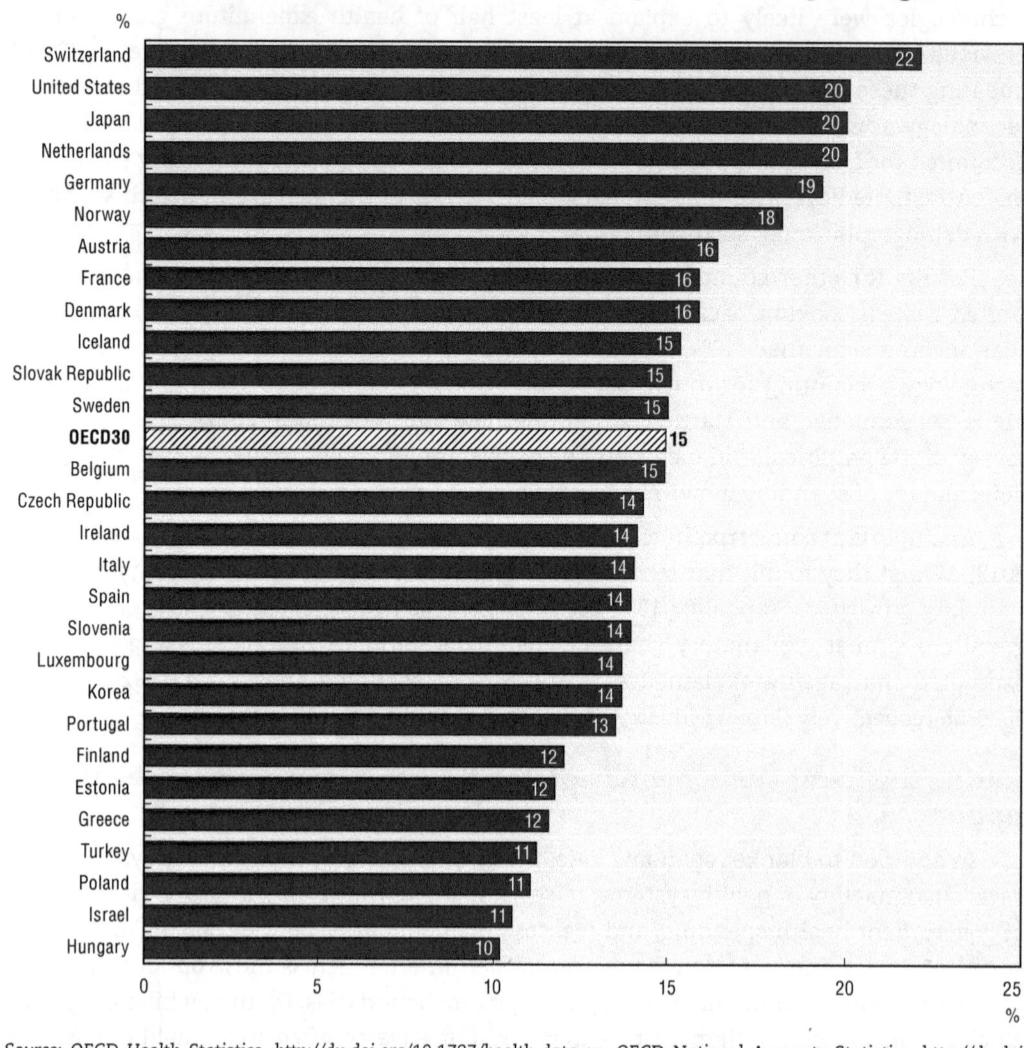

Source: *OECD Health Statistics, http://dx.doi.org/10.1787/health-data-en; OECD National Accounts Statistics, http://dx.doi.org/10.1787/na-data-en.*

StatLink http://dx.doi.org/10.1787/888933218616

Beyond allocation decisions, governments can look to raise general taxes or health insurance contributions, or broaden the revenue base through new or extended taxes. In France, Germany and Hungary, governments have in recent years diversified revenues to reduce reliance on payroll taxes (see Chapter 8; Morgan and Astolfi, 2014). Further, Thomson et al. (2014) report a broadening of the revenue base through extending contributions to non-wage income such as dividends (Slovak Republic), pensions (Croatia, for wealthier pensioners) or the self-employed (Slovenia). Other countries introduced new taxes earmarked for social security (Denmark, France, Hungary). So-called "sin taxes" or "public health taxes" are especially attractive, as they have the additional benefit of reducing consumption of products harmful to health, particularly tobacco products and alcohol but also unhealthy foods.

Such diversification of revenues is particularly important because of the revenue consequences of ageing populations (see Chapter 7 for a detailed discussion). The different models used to project the evolution of health care spending incorporate estimates of how an ageing population will increase utilisation and expenditure on health services, but not their revenue impact. Population ageing will reduce revenues generated from certain types of taxes, making it more difficult for countries to maintain or increase government spending on health. Indeed, the old-age dependency ratio[3] in OECD countries is forecast to increase by 20 percentage points over the next 30 years, reaching 45% by 2040. Yet many OECD countries have a high reliance on payroll taxes (Figure 1.7). For instance, in Austria, the Czech Republic, Germany, Korea, Poland, the Slovak Republic and Slovenia, more than 70% of revenues came from payroll contributions. Further, other than in France, "sin taxes" account for only a tiny fraction of government financing for health.

Figure 1.7. **Revenue sources for funding government health expenditures, 2010 or latest year**

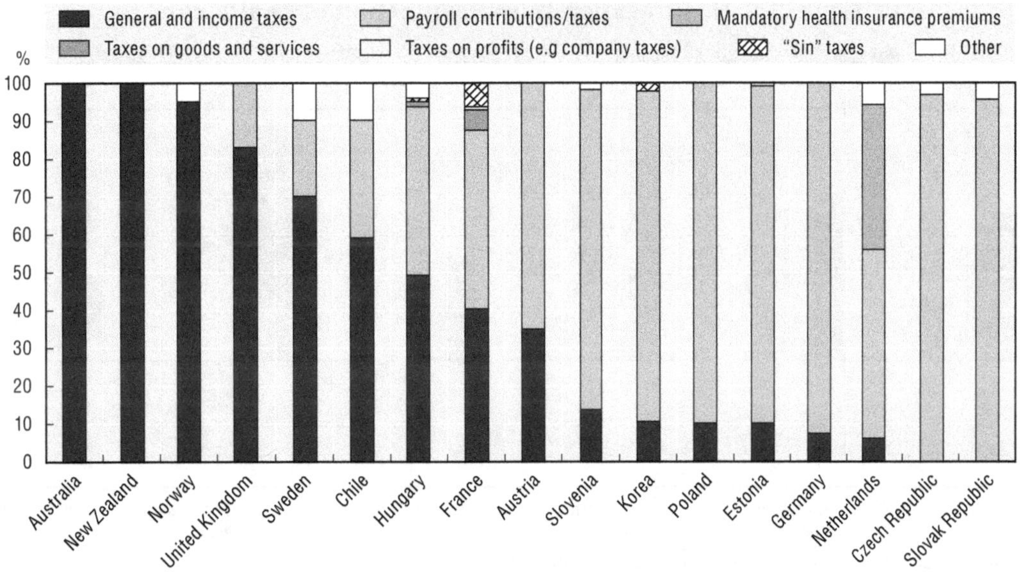

Source: OECD Survey of Budget Officials on Budgeting Practices for Health, 2013.

StatLink http://dx.doi.org/10.1787/888933218624

Improve efficiency of public spending

Eliminating inappropriate care and inefficient processes are at the heart of value-for-money reforms in health. A diverse literature details a range of policy options (see for example Chapter 5; OECD, 2009, 2010a, 2010b; and WHO, 2010). This section focuses on some policies that can offer substantive efficiency gains, rather than providing an exhaustive list of measures. Note that these policies are often longer-term in nature, and can entail their own transactional costs, only saving money in the longer term. Such policies contrast with some of the short-term measures introduced following the financial crisis. Box 1.3 illustrates which functions of health care were most affected by the crisis.

Contain pharmaceutical expenditure growth

Better pricing and reimbursement policies, in particular fuller exploitation of off-patent markets for generics and improved procurement procedures, are important ways to contain pharmaceutical spending. Product-specific agreements between manufacturers and public payers are an important way of sharing the risk of low or uncertain clinical effectiveness for new drugs (Paris, 2010).

Box 1.3. Which functions of health spending were most affected by the economic crisis?

Following the global financial crisis that began in 2008, most OECD countries put in place interventions to control health costs. Whilst some of these appear to be sensible strategies to achieve greater technical and allocative efficiency, particularly in the area of pharmaceuticals, other policies are likely to have more detrimental impacts, such as cuts in prevention spending. Figure 1.8 illustrates real expenditure growth by function of health care since 2007. It shows that spending on pharmaceuticals and prevention were particularly affected, though these are more likely to exhibit volatility as they constitute a relatively low share of health spending. Growth rates of public spending on outpatient care also slowed, and given the importance of the outpatient sector this was a major contributor to the overall decrease in public health spending growth rates.

Figure 1.8. **Health expenditure by function of health care**

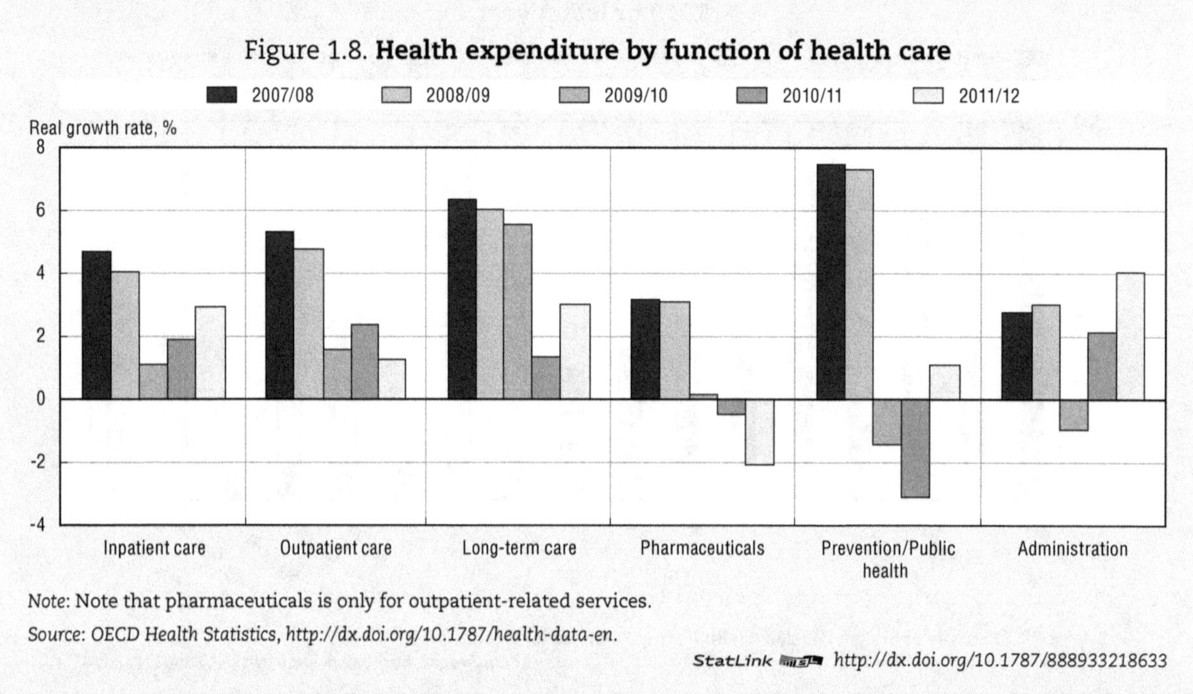

Note: Note that pharmaceuticals is only for outpatient-related services.

Source: OECD Health Statistics, http://dx.doi.org/10.1787/health-data-en.

StatLink http://dx.doi.org/10.1787/888933218633

Policy makers in OECD countries have attempted to contain expenditure growth through a mix of price and volume controls. Since the economic crisis, there has been a general move in many countries towards increasing the share of generic drugs – the value of generics in the total pharmaceutical market increased by 18% between 2008 and 2012, while in volume terms the share increased by 23%. Other important pharmaceutical policies include centralising procurement or adopting a tougher negotiating stance on prices. In the OECD as a whole, pharmaceutical spending fell in 2010 and 2011 (Box 1.3). Portugal, Greece and Spain were particularly active reformers, resulting in reduced spending on prescription pharmaceuticals by 20%, 13% and 8% respectively. In Greece, a EUR 1.2 billion decrease in the public pharmaceutical bill through negotiated prices and other cost-cutting measures contributed to around a third of the reduction in the public health budget between 2009 and 2011. This helped reducing the overall Greek public deficit by the equivalent of 1% of GDP. Higher co-payments for drugs have also been used to cut costs, particularly in Greece and Ireland (Remler and Greene, 2009). In contrast to policies on generics and procurement, higher co-payments are less obviously efficiency-enhancing, and are likely to worsen access to and financial protection for health.

Reduce variation in medical practice

Large medical practice variations, both across and within countries, raise concerns about the equity and efficiency of health systems. Whilst some variation may reflect differences in patient needs and preferences, others may reflect unnecessary or insufficient care. Figure 1.9 illustrates the extent of this variation, showing that hospital medical admission rates vary twofold or more across and within 13 OECD countries. Clinical guidelines, provider-level reporting and feedback, publication of variations, careful target-setting, and decision aids for patients can all help limit inappropriate practices (OECD, 2014) (Box 1.4).

Figure 1.9. **Hospital medical admission rates across and within selected OECD countries, 2011 or latest year**

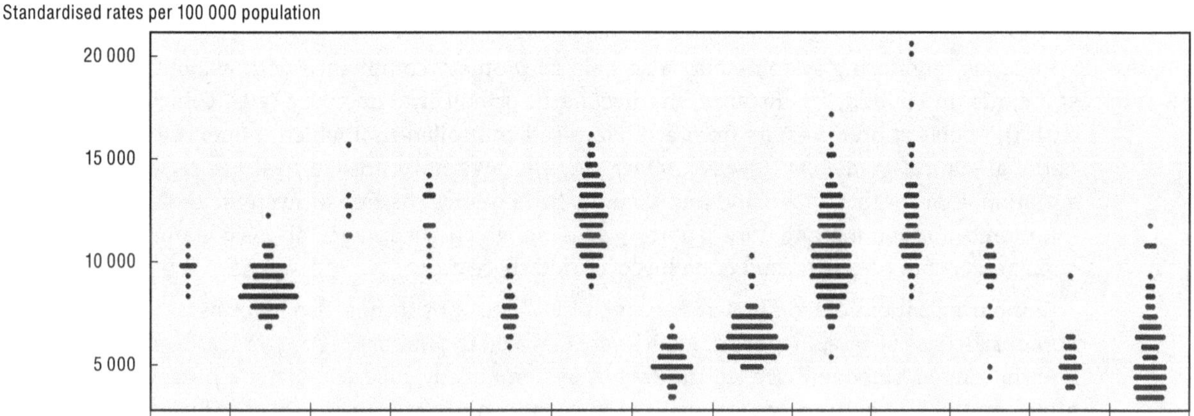

Standardised rates per 100 000 population

	Belgium	France	Israel	Germany[1]	Switzerland	Germany[2]	Spain	Italy	England	Australia	Finland	Portugal	Canada
Crude rate	10 337	8 802	11 878	13 342	7 047	13 342	5 244	7 403	10 276	10 986	8 168	5 277	4 376
Std rate	9 723	8 805	12 755	12 102	7 662	12 267	5 121	6 370	10 585	12 033	8 962	5 245	5 717
Coeff. of variation	0.08	0.11	0.12	0.12	0.13	0.14	0.14	0.15	0.19	0.20	0.20	0.21	0.34

Note: Each dot represents a territorial unit. Rates are standardised using OECD population > 15 years. Countries are ordered from the lowest to highest coefficient of variation within countries. Germany 1 and 2 correspond respectively to Länder and Spatial Planning Regions. Canadian data do not include mental hospital admissions in general hospitals leading to a relatively small under-estimation. Data for Portugal and Spain only include public hospitals. For Spain, the rates are reported based on the province where the hospital is located.

Source: OECD (2014), *Geographic Variations in Health Care: What Do We Know and What Can Be Done to Improve Health System Performance*, OECD Publishing, Paris, *http://dx.doi.org/10.1787/9789264216594-en*.

Improve co-ordination of care

A greater burden of chronic illnesses has resulted in more complex interactions between hospitals and primary care providers. Whilst co-ordination mechanisms can be costly, without them care becomes fragmented, resulting not only in low clinical quality but also in costly duplication of effort or ineffective referrals. Innovative reforms include integrating primary care and hospitals or assigning care co-ordinators for complex disease management programmes (Borowitz and Hofmarcher, 2009).

Reform provider payments

Central to provider payment reform are creating the right incentives. It is well known that fee-for-service payment systems have often been associated with too many health services being provided, thereby exacerbating cost-containment efforts (WHO, 2010). At the same time, there are concerns that salary and capitation payment systems have in some cases led to under-treatment or inappropriate referral behaviour (Iversen and Luras, 2006). Consequently, many OECD countries have in the last decade placed greater emphasis on case-based payment systems, notably diagnosis-related groups (DRGs) payments.

Box 1.4. **Examples of provider reporting and monitoring systems in OECD countries**

A number of initiatives can have an impact on addressing unwarranted variations in health care use. The development and monitoring of clinical guidelines is a key policy lever to standardise clinical practices. In almost all the 13 countries studied in the OECD 2014 report, physician societies and/or health authorities produced clinical guidelines for many of the procedures examined. The public expenditure constraints that have recently affected health systems have given an additional impetus to the development of such guidelines.

Rigorous monitoring systems may also help to promote compliance with established standards. In Finland, for instance, the decline in overall hysterectomy rates coincided with the publication of results from a randomised controlled trial which influenced the national clinical guideline. However, lower surgery rates have not led to lower regional variation, for example, in Finland and Canada. In Germany, the rate of hysterectomies is monitored through a mandatory reporting scheme which encourages discussion among stakeholders but no particular action has occurred thereafter.

Comparing patient outcomes across geographic areas or over time also helps assess the appropriateness of care. Overuse of health care can lead to diminishing outcomes. Sweden and the United Kingdom have led the way by systematically collecting patient outcomes after certain surgical procedures such as knee and hip replacement. The diffusion of decision aids for patients can help patient preferences to be taken into account. The United States and the United Kingdom publish decision aids for a range of procedures (e.g., knee replacement). These tools complement information provided by physicians and help patients assess the potential benefits and risks of different treatment options. In some cases, they can reduce the use of resource-intensive interventions.

Source: OECD (2014), *Geographic Variations in Health Care: What Do We Know and What Can Be Done to Improve Health System Performance*, OECD Publishing, Paris, *http://dx.doi.org/10.1787/9789264216594-en.*

Further, a growing number of new provider payment models are emerging that explicitly align payment incentives with health system objectives, often referred to as pay-for-performance (P4P) reforms. However, a review of several P4P programmes in OECD countries showed only modest impacts on quality, mixed results for equity, and ineffective impacts on efficiency (Cashin et al., 2014). Bundled payments have also been considered as a way of improving co-ordination of care. More generally, blended payment systems such as capitation with fee-for-service for priority activities, or fee-for-service with global budgets, can contain costs whilst maintaining quality. The challenge, though, is in avoiding administrative complexity (see McClellan, 2011 for an in-depth discussion).

Invest in health promotion and disease prevention

There is a growing body of evidence that investing in health promotion and disease prevention can improve health outcomes at relatively low cost (see McDaid et al., 2015 for an in-depth analysis). Yet prevention was one of the areas of government spending particularly hit since the beginning of the crisis. Such investments are particularly pertinent for OECD countries, where chronic diseases represent the main cause of death and disability. Tackling specific behavioural risk factors, such as tobacco smoking, harmful alcohol use, physical activity and unhealthy diets, are challenging but worthwhile investments, as they are often more cost-effective than waiting to treat poor health associated with these behaviours. Similarly, there are strong economic cases for mental health promotion and disorder activities, and policies related to the environment and road safety.

Efficiency savings: How substantial could they be?

The WHO estimated that between 20% and 40% of total health spending is consumed in ways that do little to improve people's health (WHO, 2010). This is equivalent to potential efficiency savings of USD 1 204 per capita in high-income countries, a relatively conservative figure compared with other estimates. For example, Berwick et al. (2012) estimate that six main sources of waste (failures of care delivery, care co-ordination, overtreatment, administrative complexity, pricing failures, fraud and abuse) equate to at least 21% (USD 558 billion) of total health expenditures in the United States in 2011, and up to 47% (USD 1 263 billion). The European Health Care Fraud and Corruption Network estimate that globally about USD 300 billion is lost annually to mistakes or corruption alone.

Extracting greater value-for-money from health spending is not only important from a financial perspective. Life expectancy at birth could also be raised by more than two years throughout the OECD – whilst holding health spending steady – if all countries were to become as efficient as the best performers (Joumard et al., 2008; OECD, 2010c).

Reassess the boundaries between public and private spending

In OECD countries, private health expenditures have in recent years grown more rapidly than government health expenditures. Private financing of health is particularly prominent in Chile, Mexico, the United States and Korea, where it accounts for around half of all spending, though it should be noted in most other OECD countries, the share of private spending in total spending remains relatively small (Figure 1.10).

Figure 1.10. **Relative share of public and private spending, 2012 (or nearest year)**

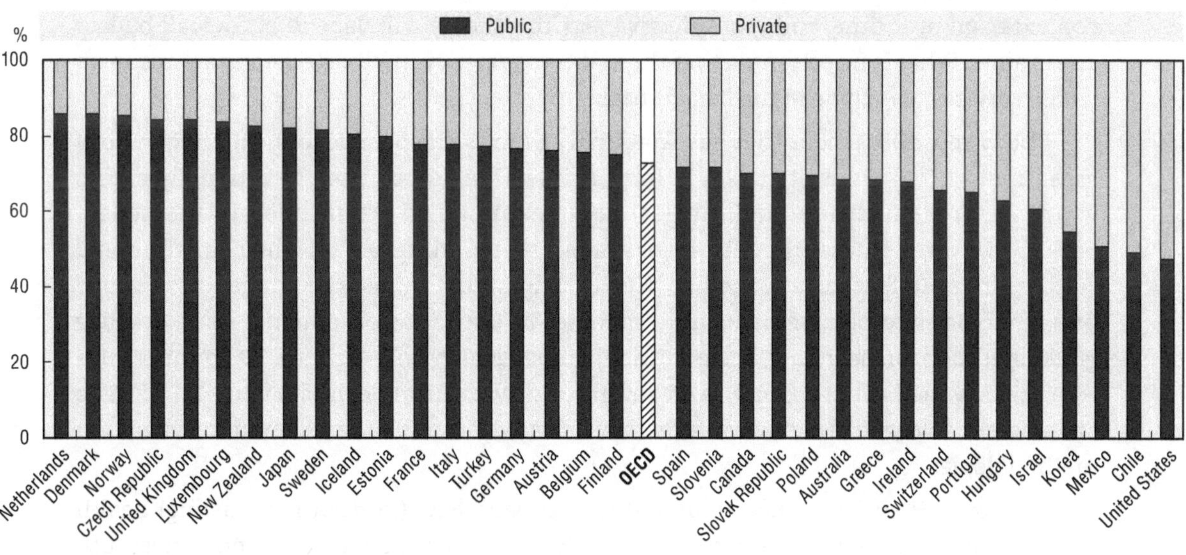

Source: *OECD Health Statistics, http://dx.doi.org/10.1787/health-data-en.*

StatLink http://dx.doi.org/10.1787/888933218645

From a purely fiscal perspective, letting private spending on health replace some government expenditures seems a relatively straightforward proposition. Covering fewer people through government funds (*population coverage*), increasing cost-sharing (*cost coverage*) or excluding certain health services (*service coverage*) can all reduce fiscal pressures. The challenge is to reconcile fiscal constraints whilst limiting any adverse equity or efficiency impacts from reduced coverage.

Do not reduce population coverage, avoid across-the-board increases in cost-sharing

Looking first at population coverage, leaving certain population groups to be voluntarily covered by *private health insurance* appears to be a logical policy option from a fiscal perspective. Indeed, the theoretical advantages of private health insurance are an expansion of individual choice, greater innovation and flexibility, as well as reduced public cost pressures. However, in practice the risks associated with private health insurance are numerous, including higher administrative costs, less bargaining power for insurers, pressure for tax incentives, and risk selection leading to inequitable coverage gaps (OECD, 2004; Pearson and Martin, 2005).

Given these issues, and coupled with strong social justice arguments, universality of population coverage should be maintained. In terms of cost coverage, blanket increases in cost-sharing and other forms of *out-of-pocket payments* is also undesirable, since they can deter health-seeking behaviour and can lead to people facing financial hardship (WHO, 2010). Small, targeted co-payments that include exemptions could be considered, but are unlikely to generate substantive revenues.

Be more specific and selective when defining the benefit basket

In order to bypass these drawbacks of private financing of health care, a better way to consider the role of private financing is to be more specific and selective in *defining the basket of services covered* by public prepayment systems. A first step is to define what services need to be accessible to all without any financial barrier. These should include all essential and cost-effective care. However, what is defined as "essential" may differ according to national contexts and over time, and cost-effectiveness thresholds will depend on overall budget constraints. What is important is that there is transparency in how decisions are made on which services to include in the benefit basket.

Today, most OECD countries have national agencies responsible for health technology assessment (HTA) (Paris et al., 2014). In principle, HTA can be used to rationally assess which services, medicines and medical equipment should be included in the benefit basket. However, these HTA agencies vary greatly in terms of their institutional setting (independent or attached to Health Ministries or insurance agencies), scope (in technologies to be assessed), and mandate (inform decision making, issue practice guidelines, horizon scanning, accreditation). In particular, only eight OECD countries use HTA for new medical procedures and seven for new medical devices (Figure 1.11). HTAs are also not always based on cost-effectiveness analysis and other economic evaluation methodologies.

Moreover, HTAs are typically limited to assessing new (rather than existing) health interventions. Decision-makers too often rely on health providers to no longer use interventions which are obsolete or no longer cost-effective. More active strategies to dynamically adjust the benefit basket should be considered, with disinvestment in cost-ineffective interventions or strong recommendations for professionals to not provide these services (Paris et al., 2014). Such policies may be politically difficult to implement, since citizens never like to lose benefits. Governments therefore need to inform citizens of the opportunity costs of providing such cost-ineffective care.

Figure 1.11. **Number of countries using HTA to make coverage decisions or set reimbursements**

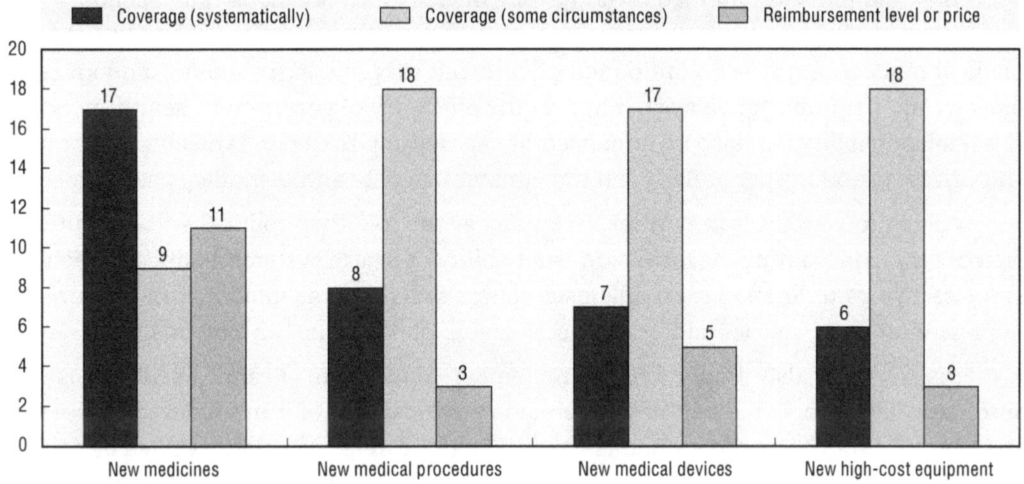

HTA: Health technology assessment.

Source: OECD Health Systems Characteristics Survey, 2012.

StatLink http://dx.doi.org/10.1787/888933218655

Use HTA for more nuanced cost-sharing policies

HTA can be used to inform cost-sharing policies, often referred to as "value-based benefit design". That is, as well as basing yes/no coverage decisions on HTA, it can be used to set reimbursement levels and the extent of cost-sharing. An important example is reference pricing. This involves covering the cost of the most therapeutic option, whilst letting patients choose alternative less cost-effective options as long as they pay the difference in cost. Evidence suggests reference pricing has induced a switch to using less expensive drugs with no adverse health effects (Kosters et al., 2006; Morgan et al., 2009). Other value-based policies include exempting poorer patients and those with chronic and severe conditions from co-payments for all treatments related to this condition; not reimbursing drugs if purchased over-the-counter; and higher co-payments for patients who bypass gatekeeping arrangements.

1.6. Conclusion

Fiscal sustainability is an important issue for health systems today and in the future, because of the rapid growth of health spending. Historically, health spending has typically outpaced economic growth, with spending largely driven by new technologies and rising incomes. Despite a recent slowdown following the economic crisis, government health spending is forecast to consume an additional 2% of GDP over the next 20 years. The implications of rising health care costs are particularly important for public finances, since health care is predominantly funded from public sources in most OECD countries. Moreover, ageing may lead to shortfalls in certain revenue-raising mechanisms, particularly payroll taxes.

Policy makers should therefore regularly monitor the fiscal sustainability of their health systems. This involves forecasting health expenditures based on known determinants of health spending, whilst accounting for forecasts of the revenues available for health. Developing a core set of fiscal sustainability indicators could also be a useful monitoring tool.

This chapter also outlined a range of policies that can constrain spending and enhance value. Policies to contain pharmaceutical expenditure growth, reduce variation in medical practice, improve co-ordination of care, reform provider payments, and invest in prevention offer important ways to improve the efficiency of government health spending. Fiscal sustainability can also be enhanced by reassessing the boundaries between public and private spending, particularly through greater use of health technology assessment.

Looking forward, it is important to remember the role that political and institutional factors play in promoting the intrinsic sustainability of health systems. Political agreement and effective co-ordination mechanisms amongst different stakeholders can improve the implementation of policies addressing fiscal sustainability of health systems.

Finally, it is also important to remember that more health spending is not automatically a problem. Good health remains a critical part of human development and an important contributor to economic growth. Health care is also highly valued by society. Accommodating greater health spending as a share of government budgets is therefore not automatically a problem. The challenge is to ensure that any increase in spending respects fiscal sustainability constraints, and that the money is effectively spent.

Notes

1. That is, there may be a disconnection between desiring more spending on health, and willingness to accept more taxes or contributions to finance it.
2. This and all subsequent OECD averages are unweighted, unless otherwise stated.
3. Old age defined as 65 years or older, as a share of those aged 20-64 years.

References

Balabanova, D., M. McKee and A. Mills (eds.) (2011), "Good Health at Low Cost' 25 Years On. What Makes a Successful Health System?", London School of Hygiene and Tropical Medicine.

Barbiero, O. and B. Cournède (2013), "New Econometric Estimates of Long-term Growth Effects of Different Areas of Public Spending", *OECD Economics Department Working Paper* No. 1100, OECD, Paris, *http://dx.doi.org/10.1787/5k3txn15b59t-en.*

Baumol, W. (1967), "Macroeconomics of Unbalanced Growth", *American Economic Review*, Vol. 57, No. 3, pp. 415-426.

Berwick, D. and A. Hackbarth (2012), "Eliminating Waste in US Health Care", *Journal of American Medical Association*, Vol. 307, No. 14, pp. 1513-1516.

Blecher, M. (2014), "Country Experience of Dealing with Fiscal Constraint Following the 2008 Recession", *Fiscal Sustainability of Health Systems*, OECD Publishing, Paris.

Borowitz, M. and M. Hofmarcher (2010), "Improving Co-ordination of Care for Chronic Diseases to Achieve Better Value for Money", Chapter 5 in *Value for Money in Health Spending*, OECD Publishing, Paris, *http://dx.doi.org/10.1787/9789264088818-en.*

Cashin, C., Y-Ling Chi, P. Smith, M. Borowitz and S. Thomson (2014), *Paying for Performance in Healthcare: Implications for Health System Performance and Accountability*, Open University Press.

Cecchini, M., F. Sassi, J. Lauer, Y. Lee, V. Guajardo-Barron and D. Chisholm (2010), "Tackling of Unhealthy Diets, Physical Activity and Obesity: Health Effects and Cost-effectiveness", *The Lancet*, Vol. 376, pp. 1775-1784.

Chernew, M. and J. Newhouse (2011), "Health Care Spending Growth", Chapter 1 in M. Pauly, T. McGuire and P. Barros (eds.), *Handbook of Health Economics*, Vol. 2.

De La Maisonneuve, C. and J. Oliveira Martins (2013a), "Public Spending on Health and Long-term Care: A New Set of Projections", *OECD Economic Policy Papers* No. 06, OECD Publishing, Paris, *http://dx.doi.org/10.1787/5k44t7jwwr9x-en*.

De La Maisonneuve, C. and J. Oliveira Martins (2013b), "A Projection Method for Public Health and Long-term Care Expenditures", *OECD Economics Department Working Papers* No. 1048, OECD Publishing, Paris, *http://dx.doi.org/10.1787/5k44v53w5w47-en*.

Dormont, B. and H. Huber (2012), "Vieillissement de la population et croissance des dépenses de santé", Rapport pour l'Institut Montaigne, *www.institut-montparnasse.fr/wpcontent/files/Collection_recherches_n_2.pdf*.

Dormont, B., M. Grignon and H. Huber (2006), "Health Expenditure Growth: Reassessing the Threatof Ageing", *Health Economics*, Vol. 15, No. 9.

EC – European Commission (2014), "Identifying Fiscal Sustainability Challenges in the Areas of Pension, Health Care and Long-term Care Policies", *Occasional Papers* No. 201, Brussels.

EC (2012), "Aging Report: Economic and Budgetary Projections for the 27 EU Member States, 2010-2060", *European Economy* 2|2012.

European Healthcare Fraud and Corruption Network (2010), *The Financial Cost of Healthcare Fraud*.

Fries, J.F. (1980), "Ageing, Natural Death, and the Compression of Morbidity", *New England Journal of Medicine*, Vol. 303, No. 3, pp. 130-135.

Fries, J.F., B. Bruce and E. Chakravarty (2011), "Compression of Morbidity 1980-2011: A Focused Review of Paradigms and Progress", *Journal of Aging Resources*.

Gerdtham, U. and B. Jonsson (2000), "International Comparisons of Health Expenditure: Theory, Data and Econometric Analysis", Chapter 1 in A. Culyer and J. Newhouse (eds.), *Handbook of Health Economics*.

Gosden, T., F. Forland, I.S. Kristiansen, M. Sutton, B. Leese, A. Giuffrida, M. Sergison and L. Pedersen (2000), "Capitation, Salary, Fee-for-Service and Mixed Systems of Payment: Effects on the Behaviour of Primary Care Physicians", *The Cochrane Database of Systematic Reviews* 2000, No. 3.

Gruenberg, E. (1977), "The Failure of Success", *Milbank Memorial Fund Quarterly*, Vol. 55, pp. 3-24.

IMF – International Monetary Fund (2010), *Macro-Fiscal Implications of Health Care Reform in Advanced and Emerging Economies*, Washington, DC.

IMF (2007), *Manual on Fiscal Transparency*, IMF, Washington, DC.

Iversen, T. and Luras, H. (2006), "Capitation and Incentives in Primary Care", Chapter 26 in *The Elgar Companion To Health Economics, Second Edition*, Edward Elgar Publishing, pp. 280-288.

Joumard, I., C. André, C. Nicq and O. Chatal (2008), "Health Status Determinants: Lifestyle, Environment, Health Care Resources and Efficiency", *OECD Economics Department Working Paper*, No. 627, OECD Publishing, Paris, *http://dx.doi.org/10.1787/240858500130*.

Lundborg, P., P. Nystedt and D. Rooth (2010), "No Country for Fat Men? Obesity, Earnings, Skills, and Health among 450000 Swedish Men", *IZA Discussion Paper* No. 4775, Institute for the Study of Labour (IZA), Bonn.

Manton, K. (1982), "Changing Concepts of Morbidity and Mortality in the Elderly Population", *Milbank Memorial Fund Quarterly*, Vol. 60, pp. 183-244.

McClellan, M. (2011), "Reforming Payments to Healthcare Providers: The Key to Slowing Healthcare Cost Growth While Improving Quality?", *Journal of Economic Perspectives*, Vol. 25, No. 2, pp. 69-92.

McDaid, D., F. Sassi, and S. Merkur (2015), "Promoting Health, Preventing Disease: The Economic Case", European Observatory on Health Systems and Policies.

Ministry of Health, Labour and Social Welfare, Japan (2015), "The Estimates of National Medical Care Expenditure", *www.mhlw.go.jp/toukei/list/37-21.html*.

Morgan, D. and R. Astolfi (2014), "Health Spending Continues to Stagnate in Many OECD Countries", *OECD Health Working Paper* No. 68, OECD Publishing, Paris, *http://dx.doi.org/10.1787/5jz5sq5qnwf5-en.*

Newhouse, J.P. (1992), "Medical Care Costs: How Much Welfare Loss?", *Journal of Economic Perspectives*, Vol. 6, No. 3, pp. 3-21.

OECD (2014), *Geographic Variations in Health Care: What Do We Know and What Can Be Done to Improve Health System Performance*, OECD Publishing, Paris, *http://dx.doi.org/10.1787/9789264216594-en.*

OECD (2013), *Health at a Glance 2013: OECD Indicators*, OECD Publishing, Paris, *http://dx.doi.org/10.1787/health_glance-2013-en.*

OECD (2012), *Sick on the Job? Myths and Realities about Mental Health and Work*, OECD Publishing, Paris, *http://dx.doi.org/10.1787/9789264124523-en.*

OECD (2010a), *Value for Money in Health Spending*, OECD Publishing, Paris, *http://dx.doi.org/10.1787/9789264088818-en.*

OECD (2010b), "Health Care Systems: Getting More Value for Money", OECD Economics Department Policy Notes, No. 2, *www.oecd.org/eco/growth/46508904.pdf.*

OECD (2010c), *Health Care Systems: Efficiency and Policy Settings*, OECD Publishing, Paris, *http://dx.doi.org/10.1787/9789264094901-en.*

OECD (2009), *Achieving Better Value for Money in Health Care*, OECD Publishing, Paris, *http://dx.doi.org/10.1787/9789264074231-en.*

OECD (2004). *Private Health Insurance in OECD Countries*, OECD Publishing, Paris, *http://dx.doi.org/10.1787/9789264007451-en.*

OECD (1998), "Public Opinion Surveys as Input to Administrative Reform", *SIGMA Papers*, No. 25, OECD Publishing, Paris, *http://dx.doi.org/10.1787/5kml611pccxq-en.*

Oxley, H. and D. Morgan (2009), "Patterns of Health Care Spending Growth", Chapter 1 in *Achieving Better Value for Money in Health Care*, OECD Publishing, Paris, *http://dx.doi.org/10.1787/9789264074231-en.*

Paris, V. (2010), "Drawing All the Benefits from Pharmaceutical Spending", Chapter 6 in *Value for Money in Health Spending*, OECD Publishing, Paris, *http://dx.doi.org/10.1787/9789264088818-en.*

Paris, V. G., G. De Lagasnerie, R. Fujisawa et al. (2014). "How Do OECD Countries Define the Basket of Goods and Services Financed Collectively?", OECD unpublished document.

Pearson, M. and J.P. Martin (2005), "Should We Extend the Role of Private Social Expenditure?", *IZA Discussion Papers* No. 1544, Institute for the Study of Labour (IZA), Bonn.

Remler, D.K. and J. Greene (2009), "Cost-Sharing: A Blunt Instrument", *Annual Review of Public Health*, Vol. 30, pp. 293-311.

Thailand Health Insurance System Research Office (2012), "Thailand's Universal Coverage Scheme: Achievements and Challenges. An Independent Assessment of the First 10 Years (2001-2010)".

Thomson, S., T. Foubister, J. Figueras, J. Kutzin, G. Permanand and L. Bryndova (2009b), "Addressing Financial Sustainability in Health Systems", WHO on behalf of the European Observatory on Health Systems and Policies, Copenhagen.

Thomson, S., J. Figueras, T. Evetovits, M. Jowett, P. Mladovsky, A. Maresso, J. Cylus, M. Karanikolos and H. Kluge (2014), "Economic Crisis, Health Systems and Health in Europe: Impact and Implications for Policy", WHO/European Observatory on Health Systems and Policies, Copenhagen.

Vahtera, J., K. Poikolainen, M. Kivimaki, L. Ala-Mursula and J. Pentti (2002), "Alcohol Intake and Sickness Absence: A Curvilinear Relation", *American Journal of Epidemiology*, Vol. 156, No. 10, pp. 969-976.

Van Gool, K. and M. Pearson (2014), "Health, Austerity and the Economic Crisis: Assessing the Short-term Impact in OECD Countries", *OECD Health Working Papers* No. 76, OECD Publishing, Paris, *http://dx.doi.org/10.1787/5jxx71lt1zg6-en.*

Weng, S., S. Ali and J. Leonardi-Bee (2013), "Smoking and Absence from Work: Systematic Review and Meta-analysis of Occupational Studies", *Addiction*, Vol. 108, pp. 307-319.

WHO – World Health Organization (2010), *Health Systems Financing: The Path to Universal Coverage*, Geneva.

Fiscal Sustainability of Health Systems
Bridging Health and Finance Perspectives

Chapter 2

The challenge of budgeting for health care programmes

by
Joseph White*

This chapter provides a more political economy perspective on budgeting practices, questioning conventional views in some ways. It challenges the usual understanding of how health care programmes can be "unsustainable", making the point that sustainability ultimately depends on the tolerance of political systems for redistribution. The chapter also revisits common explanations of spending growth, stressing the importance of social processes that define and expand notions of "necessary" care. It shows how budget making is made more difficult by a uniquely confusing proliferation of ideas about how to control spending. The impact of two structural features is then considered: whether services are delivered by a bureau or as an entitlement, and whether they are funded by dedicated revenues.

* Joseph White is Luxenberg Family Professor of Public Policy and Chair of the Department of Political Science at Case Western Reserve University, Cleveland, United States.

2.1. Introduction

Since governments directly or indirectly assumed responsibility for citizens' access to health care, that commitment has created particular problems for government budgeting. Total health care spending is already a large part of any modern economy, and spending tends to grow more quickly than per capita GDP. Therefore, if governments finance care, that spending will be a large part of budgets and take up a large part of any available increments.

Recent experience within the OECD might suggest that many of these conditions have become less important. As budget processes caught up with the change in economic conditions from the financial crisis that began in 2008, the long-term pattern of health care spending increases suddenly stopped. Average spending growth of 5% from 2000 to 2009 was succeeded by "sluggish growth of 0.5% in 2010 and 2011". Average spending across the OECD declined from 9.5% of GDP to 9.3%. Governments that faced the most severe economic crises made substantial spending cuts, but many others reduced the trend to plus or minus 1 or 2%.[1]

Yet one should not base policy and projections on conditions created by the worst economic crisis since the Great Depression. We can only hope that at some point those conditions fade. What then?

In this chapter, Section 2.2 discusses the particular challenge of health care compared to other policy areas, and the meaning of "fiscal sustainability" in the health care spending context. Section 2.3 reviews how health care spending, as an independent variable, may influence the economy. Section 2.4 considers why the demand for health care spending appears to be especially strong and difficult to resist. To the extent this demand comes from the mass of citizens, it might be moderated by making the delivery of care more efficient. Section 2.5 therefore reviews why the pursuit of efficiency is so challenging. Section 2.6 is an overview of how systemic design differences – such as between systems that are more or less "Beveridge" (where health care is provided and financed by government) than "Bismarck" (social health insurance systems) in design – might influence the challenge of budgeting for health care.

This chapter provides a more political economy perspective on budgeting practices, questioning conventional views in some ways, most notably by challenging the usual understanding of how health care programmes can be "unsustainable". The core observations and implications for policy choice identified in this chapter are:

1. Health care programmes are not "unsustainable" in an economic sense, as long as governments are willing to accept health expenditure making up a growing share of GDP.
2. The sustainability of programmes in a political sense, however, is open to question. This involves the tolerance of political systems for redistribution.
3. Health care spending is so hard to control in part because citizens (voters) deeply value health care services. Political demand is strong and real. It is a demand for care and rescue, not "health".

4. The intensity of demand does not explain its scope. That involves social processes which define "necessary care". Provider-induced demand does not occur only in physicians' offices. Budget makers should seek ways to counter the processes that seek medical solutions for larger parts of individual and social life.
5. The pursuit of efficiency involves relating inputs to outputs and outputs to outcomes. Improving the ratio of outputs to inputs is difficult, but less problematic than trying to adjust outputs to achieve outcomes more efficiently. The latter approach faces much the same obstacles as programme budgeting. The search for a better mix of outputs is worthwhile – but should be done very carefully.
6. The diagnosis of "Baumol's disease" (or, more neutrally, the Baumol effect), in which health service productivity growth ostensibly is lower, and therefore price inflation higher, than for other sectors of the economy because health care is more labor-intensive, is not a useful observation even if correct, and the evidence for the diagnosis is less than compelling.
7. Ageing makes an independent contribution to spending increases in all countries. However, the effect has in most countries been significantly smaller than the effects of other policy choices and demand influences. For ageing to be the major challenge, a country has had to be relatively successful in addressing other factors and have an especially high proportion of seniors within its population.
8. The effects of "technology" depend largely on policy choices, and "technology" is often an inaccurate name for the social process that expands ideas about need. Policy makers should focus on choices such as prices, purchase of equipment and defining the bounds of social sharing.
9. Pursuit of efficiency is made more difficult by the amazing variety of alternative proposals. Budget makers must guard not only against policy being captured by interest group claimants, but against capture by enthusiastic tribes of experts. Good budget analysis, based on independence and hard-headed scepticism, is especially important.
10. The budgetary challenge is affected by whether programmes are organised as bureaus or entitlements. There is some reason to believe spending for bureau programmes is somewhat easier to limit.
11. The challenge is also influenced by whether programmes have dedicated funding. This is especially important because the intensity of demand for care means dedicated funding is likely to be possible. Although there are many qualifications to this claim, dedicated funding probably helps meet budgetary challenges.

2.2. Health care spending and fiscal sustainability

Health care and other policies

We can see how health care is especially challenging by comparing spending patterns for health care with education and pensions among a set of very roughly comparable OECD members.[2]

In 2010 total health care spending ranged from 9.1% of GDP in Australia to 12% in the Netherlands; the United States, then, was an extreme outlier at 17.6% of GDP. Public expenditure on health ranged from 6.1% of GDP in Greece to 9.5% in Denmark.[3] The health care spending share of GDP across these countries grew by nearly 2 percentage points between 2000 and 2010.[4]

Total spending on education is lower in each of these countries. In 2009 total spending ranged from 4.9% of GDP (Italy) to 8% of GDP (Iceland). Public spending ranged from 3.6% of GDP (Japan) to 7.5% (Iceland).[5] Spending growth has also been slower.[6] The dynamics that drive spending higher appear to be weaker for education than for health care.[7]

Pensions are a more comparable source of budgetary stress. Public expenditure on pensions in many countries is a larger share of GDP.[8] But government responsibility for the pension system appears to be much less broadly agreed in different countries. This can be seen in the greater dispersion of spending shares: in 2009, public expenditure on pensions was under 6% of GDP in seven countries (Australia, Canada, Iceland, Ireland, the Netherlands, New Zealand and Norway) and over 11% of GDP in six others (Austria, France, Germany, Greece, Italy and Portugal). Ageing populations could lead to increased spending for both pensions and health care, and more directly so for pensions. Pension spending did rise more quickly as a share of GDP in some countries, mainly those with higher proportions of elderly in the population.[9] However, health care spending as a share of GDP grew more quickly than pension spending in most countries.

Moreover, there were countries in which the pension spending share actually declined, or grew much more slowly than the health care share. Thus, governments may for political or historical reasons spend more on pensions than on health care, and history does constrain choices. Yet there appears to be more room to restrain pension spending, either because it is politically easier or it is easier to find effective policy instruments.

Due to the large and usually growing budgetary share for health care, many observers see these programmes as a threat to budgetary sustainability or fiscal stability.[10] Yet the fact that health care is a major challenge may not justify claims it is "unsustainable".

Meanings of "sustainability"

It is common for budget makers to worry about "fiscal space".[11] From a fiscal space perspective, long-term commitments are inherently unwise, whether they are for pensions or medical care security. Citizens, however, may strongly prioritise these guarantees. Fiscal space arguments can claim that health care commitments displace productive public investment. But voters in many countries may, with good reason, have more confidence that money will be spent well for health care than for public investments. If health care spending crowds out other spending, that could be viewed as the legitimate result of representative government. Voters may also be willing to pay extra revenues to maintain health care programmes, and extra revenues would reduce any "crowd out". If health care is a priority for citizens, budget makers who prefer lower taxes or other spending will risk imposing their own preferences in the guise of "maintaining fiscal space".

This is not to say any spending is justified. Spending can be excessive and have major negative effects on the budget. If health care spending per person in the United States resembled the levels in other countries, much of the projected US long-term deficit problem would disappear. But that means US health care should be managed more efficiently. It does not mean care guarantees themselves would drive the budget out of control.

Nor should we assume high health care spending must have "unsustainable" effects on national economies. That topic is addressed more fully below; but one reason for doubt should be mentioned here. The United States currently spends a share of its GDP on health care which would seem unthinkable and horrifying to policy makers in any other country. It seems unnecessary and wasteful to many Americans. Yet the US economy certainly has survived that level of spending. If the United States can survive its much higher spending, why would that level be "unsustainable" for other countries?

The most plausible way in which spending could be "unsustainable" would be if political support for the expense could not be sustained. Fundamentally, this means political support for redistribution. In all modern economies, the average cost of medical care is now unaffordable for a significant portion of the population. All health care finance systems accordingly redistribute not just from the healthy to the sick, but from those with higher incomes to those with lower incomes. Systems are funded roughly in proportion to ability to pay; if they are not, then some people are likely to receive much less care. Therefore the capacity to spend on health care for all citizens depends on the ability to collect the necessary funds from the higher income strata within the country.

As the United States is an extreme case that suggests doubts about economic unsustainability arguments, it provides the clearest evidence of the political sustainability problem. The United States faces the most extreme redistribution challenge both because spending is so high, making costs less affordable for individuals, and because incomes are especially unequal, making average costs even more daunting for the lower-income groups.[12] In the United States, limits on redistribution work not to make national health insurance unsustainable but to prevent its creation. The political struggle over health insurance expansion in 2009-10 showed both the importance and difficulty of redistribution. The major source of funding for expansion through the Affordable Care Act (as amended by the Reconciliation Act) was a tax increase on high-income taxpayers. Yet the reform as passed did not promise universal coverage, because President Obama set a limit on total spending that could not possibly cover everyone. He apparently judged that he could not enact enough redistribution to pay for full coverage.

Nations' political systems have different levels of tolerance for redistribution; and economic growth, as always, makes spending easier to support. Yet, in any given country, there may be a point at which the political system is no longer able to collect enough money from people with higher incomes to pay for care for those with lower incomes. From this perspective, "unsustainability" means that governments would have to break current promises to give relatively (never totally) equal access to necessary (however defined) medical (also however defined) care for all citizens. We can see this as a budgetary problem; but it is fundamentally a social challenge. The key consequence is worse health care and a perception of major inequities for a substantial portion of the population.

There are political forces in every country which do not see such inequalities as inequities. These citizens may see redistribution of income as more unfair than unequal access to health care. Whether budget makers agree with this view will depend on their own values or whom they think they should represent.

Defining sustainability in terms of redistribution has further implications. From a budgetary perspective, measures that reduce total spending by reducing the promised level of care might seem entirely reasonable because they meet the challenge of matching the funds collected to the funds spent. Budget makers are most concerned with national and budgetary aggregates. Voters, however, focus on their own budgets, which may be endangered by the same policies that improve government budgets. This difference largely explains why US policy experts hail a recent slowdown in the growth of health care costs, while opinion polls show that "almost 60% of the American people" say, "the cost of health care for the nation has been going up faster than usual in recent years" (Altman, 2014). The slowdown in total spending may be attributed in large part to individuals having to pay more for care and therefore doing without.

Second, controls on spending that do not reduce adequacy and equity of care would satisfy both budgetary and consumer perspectives. Yet that should draw attention to another form of redistribution: health care spending redistributes income towards the providers of care. If one country provides the same services as another for less money, then the former is redistributing less income to medical providers.

Third, as in all public finance, the ways in which revenue is collected will shape the ease of collection. In general, less visible taxes are more viable than more visible ones, and taxes dedicated to popular purposes may be easier to raise than general revenues.[13] Yet the advantages of less visible or more dedicated revenues would be true regardless of whether taxes are collected from higher-income citizens or others. In fact, less visible taxes (e.g. consumption levies) and dedicated payroll contributions tend to be regressive compared to income taxes (Warren, 2008). If health care is financed from less progressive sources it will redistribute less. Yet it still is fundamentally redistributive, compared to buying medical care in the market.

2.3. What is the effect of health care spending on a national economy?

Two concerns are especially prominent. The first presumes that higher spending on health care, usually through government budgets, will not be matched by higher revenues or offsetting cuts in other programmes. Thus health care will lead to growing deficits and (all other things being equal) to lower national savings. Lower savings in turn will lead to lower investment, and so less economic growth (see e.g. Gale and Orszag, 2003). The second concern applies when health care costs are paid largely out of the income flow of employers – either through social insurance payroll contributions (as in Germany, France and Japan) or when employers purchase insurance as part of employee compensation (as in the United States).[14] Health care therefore can raise the price of labour so employers hire fewer employees.

These concerns are widely shared. All things being equal, the effects likely run in the presumed negative direction. There is little evidence, however, that the effects are large enough to justify viewing health care spending as a major threat to economic performance.

Effects from budget deficits

The effect of health care spending on the economy through effects on the budget depends on how the budget balance affects the economy. That is a highly contested topic; fundamental issues such as the effects of deficits on interest rates and inflation evoke deep disagreement.[15]

Yet claims that health care spending reduces investment and so economic growth are less convincing than their ubiquity may suggest.

Analysis by the US Congressional Budget Office (CBO), for example, estimated during the 1990s that 20% to 50% of any deficit reduction would be offset by individuals reducing their own savings so as to maintain consumption. Then between 32% and 47% of net savings would be devoted to reducing net capital inflows. Moreover, growth from higher investment would stop once that level of investment was needed to replace the extra depreciation on a larger capital stock. Thus in the 1990s, mainline estimates of the overall effects of reducing the deficit by 3% of GDP ranged from GDP eventually being 1% to 6% larger; the CBO's analysis was about 3% (sources can be found in White, 2003). These estimated effects in 20 or 30 years would have been far smaller than other factors influencing per capita real income, including simple uncertainty about projections.[16]

An OECD analysis in 2004, based on 16 countries with data from 1970 to 2002, reiterated the slippage between budget savings and investment. It concluded that "the evidence of partial, yet substantial, direct, offsetting movements in private savings is strong. The aggregate initial offset is about half in the short term after allowing for income, interest rate and wealth effects (which have an important impact on saving), rising to around 70% in the long term." (OECD, 2014b) More recent CBO estimates of the effect of alternative fiscal scenarios in the United States show effects similar to the 1990s projections. Thus if deficits were "larger by 0.2% in 2012, 2.5% in 2013 and 4.0% on average over the 2014-2022 period", then "by the end of 2022 real GDP would be between 2.1% smaller and 0.2% larger".[17] The baseline would benefit whoever received the larger growth – but would hurt whoever lost the 4% of GDP in lower spending and higher taxes.

An economy without the modest extra growth associated with higher savings is not "unsustainable". Beliefs about "unsustainable" budgets therefore must be based on doomsday scenarios about spiralling interest costs. There are two versions, which we might call slow track and fast track.

In the United States during the 1990s, the Government Accountability Office (GAO) and the CBO developed models of the slow-track road to collapse. They projected that, over a long enough time and if left unchecked, deficits would become large enough to feed on themselves as interest costs burgeoned. Eventually, government borrowing would soak up all investment capital, there would be no way to offset depreciation, capital stock would decline, production fall and the economy totally collapse.[18] Given this assumption that nothing else would ever be done, many budget commentators argued that social insurance programmes were unsustainable.

The slow-track argument, however, had some weaknesses. First, the United States actually balanced its budget from 1997 to 2001 with barely noticeable reductions in entitlement spending. Second, the idea that programmes are "unsustainable" confuses programmes with deficits. It presumes voters would not choose to pay for programmes or make them more efficient if the alternative were cutting benefits. This presumption so far does not fit US experience.[19]

The fast-track argument involves market dynamics of interest costs. At some point, bond holders could become less willing to hold a nation's debt because of fears the government would "either default on ... or monetise the debt ... in a way that would result in rapidly increasing price inflation that reduces the existing debt's relative value" (Labonte, 2012, quotes p. 1). Some, however, would be willing to buy the debt at higher interest rates – raising deficits further in a fast version of the interest costs spiral to budgetary and maybe economic failure. Events since 2007 have heightened attention to this possibility.

Yet some of the nations that have suffered most from rising interest rates since the financial crisis, such as Portugal and Spain, had relatively conservative pre-crisis fiscal policies. Loss of confidence among bond holders could have had only a tenuous relationship to health care spending, and should have been more clearly related to the collapse of housing prices, attendant problems with private lending and the current account balance.[20] The United States and Japan have run very large deficits without attendant increases in interest rates.[21] In Greece, where a true sovereign debt crisis is strongly related to the pre-crisis trend of budget deficits, health care costs appear to be at best a minor cause.[22]

It seems fair to say that better control of health care spending, or policies which collect extra revenues to match extra health care spending, allows more conservative public finance; and more conservative public finance can reduce the risk of capital flight and/or spiralling interest rates. Yet there is little if any visible link between health care spending and the countries which have experienced the most severe debt and interest rate pressures in recent years.

None of these arguments that health care spending through government budgets will be economically "unsustainable" are convincing. Effective financing and control of spending are important for more traditional budgetary reasons, and political sustainability is still a major issue.

Effects on employment

Health care spending could directly affect employment in countries where it is funded largely by payroll contributions. This includes nations for which spending is not directly on-budget (the Social Health Insurance countries such as France and Germany) as well as those where an on-budget system has a dedicated payroll tax (US Medicare). The employer contribution then appears to be an extra cost for hiring each worker, raising the question in Germany of, as one article puts it, "how high can non-wage labour costs be raised without affecting international competiveness?" The authors reported that "non-wage labour costs are increasingly viewed as the main cause for worldwide industries' reluctance to invest in Germany and to create new jobs" (Stock et al., 2006). A later OECD study made the same assumption that "rising health care costs have also put a strain on employment" (Brandt, 2008). Similar concerns are raised about the costs of coverage provided by US employers.[23]

Payroll contributions can only raise the cost of labour, and so reduce hiring, if employers cannot reduce wages by the same amount. Therefore any effect on hiring requires that wages be "sticky".[24] If a wage is already close to a legislated minimum, employers will not be able to reduce it by as much as they are paying for health care. Wage cuts might also be prevented by union contracts or competition within the labour market. These effects may be common, yet we should normally expect any effects on employment to be offset somewhat by wage restraint. They might also be offset by employment of those who provide the funded health care.

There is very little research to address the net effect of these factors.[25] Two exceptions are from the United States and Germany. The US study addressed the underlying dynamic rather than the specific effects of mandated contributions. It asked if "industries where benefits were a larger share of total compensation were hit harder by rising health care costs", looking at trends from 1987-2005. It concluded that "industries with a higher share of benefits suffer greater employment and output loss due to rising medical prices". The report could not, however, measure possible offsetting increases in health-related employment.[26]

The German study was conducted in the 1990s by the official Advisory Council for Concerted Action in Health Care. It may provide the most thorough review of relevant factors. One is that labour productivity in health care tends to be low; in a closed economy then, "employment could be increased simply by shifting demand from more productive, but less labour-intensive industries to less productive, but more labour-intensive health care services" – so long as the extra demand does not raise prices instead (Advisory Council for Concerted Action in Health Care, 1996). In an open economy, industries open to foreign competition could lose more jobs due to higher payments for health care; at the same time health care, and especially its labour-intensive services, face less international competition than other industries. Effects at that time would have varied by industry also due to different levels of insurance contributions and shares of non-wage labour costs within total labour costs. The Advisory Council commissioned a simulation based on the business cycle model of the German Institute for Economic Research. It estimated that in Germany at that time, a 1-percentage point increase in the contribution rate, if used entirely for further consumption of health care, would result in a quite small increase in employment.[27]

As the Advisory Council emphasised, such estimates should be considered with a great deal of caution. Effects should depend further on the conditions of the labour market. Nonetheless, the Council noted in a subsequent report, even "unproductive health services do stimulate demand and, given underutilised resources, increase employment and economic growth" (Advisory Council for Concerted Action in Health Care, 1998).[28] The economic effects would be more positive if the services created better health among workers, who therefore could be more productive. From this perspective, health care spending can be an investment as well as consumption. At the first meeting of the Joint Network, Professor Dr. Klaus-Dirk Henke built on this research to argue that there "is no optimal health expenditure quota".[29]

As with the economic effects through budget deficits, the effect on employment from taxation of payroll to pay for health care should be complex and depend on many other factors. Yet rhetoric about unsustainability seems extreme. There are powerful reasons to worry about the prospects for employment in advanced industrial (or post-industrial?) economies. Globalisation likely means that, "the enormous growth in the global labour supply will affect the composition of employment, the distribution of wages and incomes, transitions into and out of employment and unemployment, job security, and other important aspects of the labour market" (Coe, 2007). It is less clear that the effects of health care charges on employers are either strong in relation to the underlying trends, or clearly reduce employment.[30]

A significant concern, but "unsustainable" only by assumption

A third argument is less amenable to analysis. It assumes that government spending or taxes inherently distorts economic activity so must be inefficient. For example, the George W. Bush Administration in the United States argued that spending for homeland security, unless offset by other spending cuts, would damage the national economy by reducing private investment. Moreover, raising taxes to pay for new homeland security would damage the economy further, for "every dollar collected in taxes results in distortions that reduce the efficiency of the economy and lower national income".[31]

By this logic any government spending, or taxes to pay for it, hurts the economy; and it would be difficult to justify the systems of health care finance in any OECD member state. It suggests that perhaps policy makers will have to live with existing inefficiencies; but any increase in spending or revenues should be resisted strongly, regardless of the cause served by the increase – whether it be health care or protection against terrorism. Policy makers who take this view need to know more: policy is determined by the underlying assumptions about macroeconomic cause and effect.

Evidence related to more mainstream economics does not support the idea that health care programmes are economically unsustainable. Policy makers still have good reason to worry about financing health care, because the programmes are a large share of budgets and the social and political stakes in budget decisions are so high.

2.4. Demand for public spending on health care

We have seen that pressure to spend more on health care is stronger than pressures on even the largest other categories of spending: education and pensions. There are two basic reasons.[32] First, public demand for the social definition of needed care is especially strong. Second, that social definition of need expands more quickly and continually than understandings of need for other expenditure, such as education or public investments. This process of "need" expansion may be mistaken for an increase in "technology".

Socialised risks and consumption

Medical care is a good consumed by individuals. It can also be viewed as an investment to improve health outcomes and productivity, or as having community benefits, but these benefits are neither its essential nature nor the main reason for political demand.

When needed, medical care is as important to people as food, shelter or clothing. Yet among those necessities of life, only medical care is generally provided, for everyone, through some socialisation of finance. Socialised finance is the norm, even in the United States, because costs are so high and incidence uncertain. It is not practical to pay from current income for the most important care. Yet it is also not practical to save, since many people could not save enough money without foregoing vital other consumption, and even those who arguably could save enough over many years might well need to pay for medical care before they had saved enough. Nor is borrowing practical for the most important care, because very sick people are not good credit risks.

Hence systems of private insurance, government insurance, government-mandated social health insurance (SHI) and government health care bureaus all redistribute from the healthy to the sick, and all but market insurance redistribute from higher to lower incomes. Only quite a small portion of citizens could imagine paying for all care they might need from their own funds; and many of those will have relatives and friends they want to be protected.

Public support for public or semi-public SHI health care systems is based on a mix of self-protective prudence and beliefs about equity. No system offers precisely equal care to everyone. In any given country there is some safety valve so that well-to-do patients can obtain better amenities and perhaps more personal service; in some countries this means they can avoid waiting lists by "jumping the queue". There is however, much more equality of health care consumption, for a given level of illness, than of housing or shelter or clothing. I do not know of survey data that explains why, but the simplest answer is most likely to be true. There appears to be something basic about health care that makes inequality less acceptable in any country with enough wealth to do something about it.

Death and fear of death, or pain and fear of pain, are likely to attract more empathy than differences in diet or clothing or shelter. Anyone can imagine getting sick and therefore what it would be like to be sick and have no hope of rescue. Above some level, differences in food or clothing or shelter can be viewed as wants rather than necessities. It is harder to view someone else's desire for the same chance to survive illness, or equal remission of pain, as simply a consumption choice. That is especially difficult if an economy clearly has the resources needed to offer everyone similar prospects for rescue. Therefore the standard for equality of chances is likely to be much closer to the maximum level of consumption for health care than for other necessities.

Equity here means equity of care, so relatively equal access to rescue, not equality of health. Outside of the public health community there seems to be little pressure for equal health in any country. It is doubtful that voters anywhere think government can or should equalise health. Government cannot be expected to eliminate the bad luck that allocates much of disease. Moreover, equalising the social determinants of health would involve massive restructuring of societies, in ways to which voters could object for many reasons unrelated to health. When a large portion of any society has access to life-saving rescue, however, it is logically possible to offer that to everyone without changing much else – except for collecting more money and training more caregivers. Inequality of rescue is both more frightening and less necessary than other inequalities.

Equality here means access to some social standard of necessary care – there will always be extras that are defined as consumption people might choose but not need. Countries define necessary care differently; there is wide variation in the terms of socialisation of dental care, mental health care, long-term care and even the costs of prescription drugs.[33] The bounds of necessity are important questions for policy, and decisions can either limit or expand sharing. Yet if there is a plausible argument that a category has become a larger part of normal care over time – as certainly has happened with pharmaceuticals – there will be strong pressure to expand coverage. This is partly due to changes in practice, yet there is also a process of idea formation. When the health policy world declares that chronic care is the new crisis, or that chronic care can save money and pain by preventing the need for acute care, then unequal access to "preventive" medicines becomes a grave inequality.

Economists may assume that any non-market subsidy for consumption creates excess demand.[34] That is not helpful because no country could have a politically (and arguably morally) acceptable health care system without such "excess". It also begs the question of why governments (or SHI systems) that are paying for care do not have sufficient incentive to control costs. For budgeting purposes, demand is political: how pressures to spend for health care compare to pressures to spend for other purposes or to restrain taxes. Support for health care spending appears to be unusually high.

Expanding "need": Outcomes, outputs and inputs

For the reasons given above, it is especially difficult for budget makers to resist need for health care. Yet intensity of demand is not the same as extent of demand. Intense demand to meet perceived need would only create the kind of spending increases that are common if perceived need grows relatively quickly. What, then, drives perceived need for health care?

Policies involve outcomes, outputs and inputs. In health care the outcome is recovery from, prevention, or amelioration of maladies. The outputs are services. The inputs are what is needed to produce the services and so (hopefully) outcomes. Therefore there are three basic ways the need for inputs (spending) can expand or decline: conditions may change, the production function may change or the definition of desirable outcomes and outputs may change.

If conditions become closer or further from a desired outcome level, that in turn will call for fewer or more outputs and so fewer or more inputs. If there is more crime, more police patrols become necessary. If there is an epidemic, more care is needed.

Here the basic question is how other factors shape health and so demand for health care. Increased wealth might reduce disease, but expanding inequality might increase it.[35] Economic development may increase wealth and so factors like nutrition and government spending on sanitation that improve health. Yet it also may be accompanied by overconsumption that leads to diabetes, or by pollution that makes people sick.[36] Immigration might bring into a country populations with greater medical needs because of previous poverty or lack of treatment; but it also may attract especially healthy people who can overcome the barriers to immigration (Domnich et al., 2012). There are many possibilities, yet there is little reason to believe that, when they are all combined, over the past few decades social factors have made the residents of rich democracies systematically less healthy.

The exception is population ageing. In any society, up until very advanced age, older people have on average higher health care costs than the rest of the population. As people live longer and have fewer children, both the average age of the population and the proportions that are old or very old rise. Thus many would expect an "ageing society" to raise health care costs. Yet while the direction of effect is likely right, numerous studies have projected that it is not large enough to cause a crisis. Cross-sectional studies have generally shown little or no correlation between a country's age profile and its health care costs.[37] Time series analyses also suggest significant but small effects. One OECD study estimated that "between 1981 and 2002 ... public health spending grew on average by 3.6% per year for OECD countries, of which 0.3% per year was accounted by pure demographic effects" (OECD, 2006). A 2013 update reported average growth in real health spending between 1995 and 2009 at 4.3% per year, of which 0.5% was ascribed to ageing (De la Maisonneuve, C. and J. Oliveira Martins, 2013).

As a recent overview reports, "there is a growing consensus that ageing does not have to be an inevitable drain on health care resources". Two "strands of research" explain why. First, much of the observed higher costs at higher ages are caused by the cost of dying. On average, more 85-year-olds die than 75-year-olds. Dying is expensive; "proximity of death is a more important predictor of health care expenditure than ageing itself", and so, "the high annual health care cost associated with older people is in large part the consequence of the fact that they are more likely to die within a year" (Rechel et al., 2009, p. 10). As people live longer there will be more 85-year-olds but that will be in part because fewer 75-year-olds die, which suggests that group will become less expensive. To put this another way, "if mortality falls over time, due to a permanent increase in longevity, fewer will be at the very end of life in each given year, mitigating health care costs" (OECD, 2006, p. 11).

This reduction in deaths at each age then would interact with another observation: that in any nation, past a certain age, the costs associated with dying tend to decline, as do rates of health care utilisation (see discussions in Rechel et al., 2009; OECD, 2006; White, 2004). There is also reason to believe that ageing is associated with "compression of morbidity" – that is, that most of the extra years are relatively healthy. The OECD 2013 report assumed a healthy ageing effect and that, "consistent with a large number of previous studies ... what matters for health spending is not ageing but rather the proximity to death" (De la Maisonneuve and Martins, 2013, p. 13). Overall, then, in these projections "the demographic effect only accounts for a small increase in [public] expenditure. In OECD countries and on its own, it pushes spending from 5.5% of GDP on average to 6.2% in 2060."[38]

On balance, ageing populations therefore should be expected to change objective conditions in a way that increases public health care spending. But that cannot explain the unusually high growth of health care spending compared to other public programmes, and justifies only modest worries about the future. Nevertheless, two other factors should be kept in mind. Population ageing could increase need to spend on long-term care by larger amounts, and much more proportionally, than the demand to spend on traditional health care.[39] Secondly, the most important effect of ageing on the ability to finance programmes may be on the revenue side. If healthy ageing is accompanied by a vibrant job market that allows extended working careers, there will be more revenue to pay for care for both working and non-working elderly. If healthy older workers cannot find employment, budget difficulties will be more severe. Hence analyses by OECD and the European Community have concluded that labour-market developments and policies greatly mediate any budgetary effect of ageing.[40]

Need or demand for spending may also change because of changes in the production function – the relationship of inputs to outputs and outputs to outcomes. The production function determines the efficiency of care. Usually we hope innovations will create efficiencies. So perhaps electronic surveillance can replace expensive human patrols; or a cheaper drug will replace an expensive surgical procedure. But the inputs required may change in the opposite direction: criminals may find new ways to evade detection, requiring more effort; or experience may show a treatment has risks that require replacement by more expensive inputs.

Hence one question is whether the relatively rapid increase in health care spending as a share of GDP might occur because the production function becomes *relatively* inefficient over time. This is hypothesised as the Baumol effect or "Baumol's disease", on the grounds that health care is labour-intensive and so cannot be made more efficient as quickly as the rest of the economy. Thus if output grew at the same rate as the rest of the economy, inputs would grow more quickly.[41]

The Baumol argument can be interpreted as reason not to worry so much about health care costs. If productivity of other goods and services is rising, then we are getting more even if health care consumes a larger share of income.[42] Yet this scenario is at the level of the entire economy. Given unequal incomes, pooling funds to pay for individuals' care still requires redistribution. If health care becomes a larger and larger share of total product, then ever more must be redistributed. The Baumol theory does not solve the budgetary challenge at all if the challenge is really about redistribution.

More important, is the theory actually true? There are many examples of technological change in medical care, including: creation of less invasive procedures, doing a much larger share of procedures outside hospitals, drugs replacing psychoanalysis, and what the vendors and physicians call major quality improvements in imaging. It is hard to measure outputs in a comparative way, and hard to measure outcomes. But one indicator of improved production of outcomes is the fact that, across 16 nations over the decade to 2006-07, death rates from "amenable mortality" – conditions that could be successfully treated – declined by at least 20% (Nolte and McKee, 2011).

If quality (outcomes) has improved substantially, that is not much help to budget makers. Yet it does redefine the problem as how to resist or pay for demand for quality, rather than inherent inefficiency. Long-term care is more evidently a domain in which quality would be less dynamic and changes in delivery less common. The recent OECD spending model projects a Baumol effect for long-term care, but not for other health care.[43]

On balance, the Baumol theory does not seem helpful for policy makers, and using it to explain previous spending growth requires too many assumptions. While the health care production function may be less amenable to efficiency improvements than other industries, the important questions for policy would be how it could be improved. The OECD and other organisations have done extensive evaluations of alternative policies to improve the health care production function.[44] Section 2.5 of this overview will identify some challenges to improving efficiency. For this section's discussion of forces that expand need, we might only note two factors.

First, both inputs and outputs are choices, at least potentially. Somebody chooses to pay for inputs and to approve payment for particular services (outputs). They do not happen automatically or naturally. Therefore it does not make sense to see either as a matter of expanding need. They are certainly a policy lever; but if choices lead to higher spending, that is not remotely exogenous to the policy process – unless those who pay for care choose to cede control.

Secondly, the relationship between outputs and outcomes is complicated by the fact that the processes of the outputs are part of the outcomes. At one level, open heart surgery is an intermediate good: its purpose is to help the patient live longer and feel better afterwards, and we might evaluate it according to this outcome. Yet the service is itself an experience, and an especially unpleasant one. The benefit to the patient is really the result net of the pain and discomfort from the procedure. This is a reason why creating less invasive procedures can lead to greater consumption of care. From the patient's perspective, getting to the same (or a better) end state with less pain or recuperation along the way is a better outcome. In this way "technology," meaning invention of new processes, could legitimately lead to greater demand for spending.[45]

Demand for spending may also grow because expectations for the desired outcome may change. Here the basic question is: what is this "health care" for which it is important to redistribute income so as to have a more equitable society?

In all policy areas, budgetary claimants work to increase the political priority of their programmes. One of their tactics is to highlight or redefine need. The military may redefine security to mean ability to deter more and more threats, education advocates may claim the job market requires more skills than it did 20 years ago, and environmental advocates will identify more and more threats.

This process may be more powerful for health care, however, because it involves far more than lobbying. It is a pervasive part of modern societies.

One way "need" expands is through the medicalising of social and individual conditions. Children are not doing well in school because they are not paying attention. This has always been common, but it is transformed into Attention Deficit Hyperactivity Disorder (ADHD). People are unhappy; it becomes a medical diagnosis, depression. A problem previously not discussed in polite company becomes medical (so ubiquitous in advertisements in the United States) as "erectile dysfunction". Alcoholism becomes not bad behaviour but a disease.

Some redefinitions are more easy to justify, and some less so. In all cases, however, they expand the concepts of disease and so of need. The incentives to do so range from desire to reduce blame on "victims", to individuals and institutions finding medical definitions less challenging than the alternatives (if the child is sick it's not the school's or parents' fault), to simple pursuit of profit by drug makers. Once a problem is officially medical, and a treatment is reimbursed by health care systems, there are strong incentives to diagnose and perhaps over-diagnose it.

Perceived need also expands due to increasing expectations of what is possible, so desirable. As people age, they have increasing aches, pains and mobility problems. That could be viewed as an inevitable consequence of ageing, or as something to be fixed. In the United States, Medicare spending for physical therapy burgeoned in the early 1990s. That could have been recognition of previously untreated need, redefinition of need, fraudulent services, or more likely a mix of all three (GAO, 1999). Yet clearly service volumes increased without obvious change in need or technology.

In other cases, improved technology has made care more desirable. Joint replacements made it possible to greatly relieve pain and immobility. That in turn would increase demand for care. Arthroscopic surgery made treatment of knee injuries much more attractive than it was in the early 1970s, when treatment was both much more invasive and seemingly less reliable. This dynamic should not be confused with, but can be combined with, a change in incentives for providers of care. If new technology makes providing a service more profitable (which means if payment rules do not recognise that change), providers are more likely to try to sell it to their patients.

This example points to a well-known pattern: demand by patients is largely induced by providers. We do not need to get into common health policy disputes about that process to recognise that this makes citizens' ideas of "need" for health care more easily manipulated by the sellers of care than is true for the "need" for defence or education.[46] Advocacy occurs in physician offices and other sites across every country every day.

Forces that expand demand further pervade societies in news coverage of new treatments described as advances and, in some countries, through advertisements. The idea that medical progress offers new miracles is deeply engrained in modern cultures, with some help from promotion by the medical industry. To a lesser extent in some countries than others, but probably everywhere, "new" is expected to be "better". This gives the benefit of doubt to sellers who create new drugs and devices and treatments and expect buyers – governments or insurers – to pay more for those new products than for the products they might replace. The promise is that new outputs will yield better outcomes. And, if better outcomes are possible, they should be available to everyone due to the social desire for relative equality of rescue.

While it cannot be proved formally, it seems likely that a significant portion of the excess growth in health care costs over per capita income is due to this dynamic – expanded services due to the belief that they will produce better outcomes, and in many cases to a further expansion of the aspects of life that are viewed as amenable to medical correction. We certainly have seen a vast expansion over time in the range of medical services which are rationalised in these terms. Perhaps health care spending grows as a share of the economy in part because people view a larger part of life as a matter of health or medicine.

In this interpretation, if policy makers want to better control health care costs, they will need to find better ways to resist the pressures to do more good through medical care. That raises tough questions. After all, lives might be improved by ADHD drugs, or anti-depression medication. Should only rich people be able to resist depression with medications as a consumption choice? In practice, however, these choices are not new.

They were always present in the decisions about how much society should fund services such as long-term care and mental health care.

Given the analysis above, in what sense can "technology" be a major cause of either past or projected growth in health care spending? In this framework "technology" *per se* does not tell us enough to mean much. Yet we can use the foregoing discussion to understand how technological developments can influence costs.

We should first distinguish new methods for delivering care (i.e. medical technologies such as new surgical processes, drugs and equipment) from management technologies (such as information systems that could reduce administrative personnel in hospitals). Management technology is rarely if ever described as a reason costs rise quickly.[47] Instead, "technology" generally means medical technology, and tends to be a residual after other variables are included in a model (for one overview see Kaiser Family Foundation, 2007). Even when measured, the variables can seem quite indirect – the 2013 OECD study uses information about patents and research and development expenditures (De la Maisonneuve and Martins, 2013, p. 42).

The "effects of technology", therefore, can easily be the effects of unmeasured policy choices. For example, new technology might be priced poorly. In fact, the expenses associated with any service, whether new technology or not, depend on its price. They do not occur at all without a decision to purchase it. Therefore the effects of technology on spending must be mediated through policy decisions. Sellers of any technology will claim it has a "cost" that must be paid if it is to be provided. Yet in many cases, such as drugs and devices, this includes substantial development costs. These can be spread over more or fewer years, and because they are sunk costs the seller has incentives not to risk receiving no payment at all. In other cases, the "cost" includes expectations of income for sellers such as physicians and hospitals; again, there is unlikely to be an objective level.

Any claim that new technology "causes" a specific increase in spending makes sense only if we assume the pricing and purchase decisions could not be different. Yet we know these choices must vary, because the technology that could be used is the same in all rich democracies, yet both levels of spending and increases vary substantially. At best, the argument that technology "causes" spending increases must involve some minimum increase that, over time, no nation's policy makers have been able to resist.

The discussion above suggests some ways that minimum increase could occur, but also shows why "technology" may not be the best way to think about it. Increased medicalisation of social and individual problems appears to be a common trend. It has been termed "technology" because it is a residual in models of cost growth. Yet that does not mean the explanation is correct. The increase in physical therapy in US Medicare was not due to technical advances. Invention of ADHD drugs, or of new drugs for depression, probably encouraged more diagnoses, and success stories (accurate or not) probably encouraged worried parents and individuals to seek treatment. In these cases, the availability of technology likely did induce demand. Yet even in these cases social factors other than technology, such as teachers' (in)ability to maintain order in classrooms, shape the extent to which these services spread.

Thus new technology can create pressures for more spending, but the independent effect of technology from this dynamic is not likely to resemble the claims that simply define technology as a residual encompassing all other policy weaknesses and pressures for extra services. And there is a further puzzle about technology as a "cause" of increased spending.

As the "Baumol disease" argument suggests, in many industries technological advance reduces the input costs of services. By standard economic logic, competition among sellers then should reduce prices. To take a health care example, as it became less expensive to do cataract surgery, prices should have fallen such that the incomes of ophthalmic surgeons did not increase much: in a competitive market, the benefits of efficiency-enhancing technology should mainly accrue to consumers.

This market logic may not work so well in many cases, but it clearly does not apply in health care. Consumers are: very poorly informed compared to providers, in no condition to shop, not interested in shopping, not sufficiently interested in shopping because the insurer is paying most of the charge or all of the above. Normally payment rates are set or negotiated by large payers such as the government or cartels of insurers. Yet there is reason to doubt that these payers adjust prices enough in response to technological change. The common claim that "proceduralist" physicians see their incomes rise more quickly than "evaluative" physicians[48] shows the reason for doubt. If proceduralists are able to do more and more procedures, that means they have more output for their input. Yet the system is not capturing this efficiency; they are.

One of the puzzles in health policy discussion is how the "Baumol disease" argument and the "technology causes cost increases" argument could both be believed. There has to be technology for it to cause cost increases. The question is why it would cause cost increases rather than greater efficiency. The answers can tell us something about the reasons health care spending has generally increased faster than GDP. First, some increases in spending are caused by increased demand that is created not by "technology" but by social processes of medicalisation and expansions of the standard for health care outcomes. Second, policy choices may overpay for or allow overuse of new technology; that is a failure of other policies, not an effect of technology. Last, health care policies in some countries mean that the efficiencies created by new technology are not fully captured for the system.[49] As a result, prices do not go down as much as they should when new technology creates efficiencies. This too is not an effect of technology, but of other choices.

2.5. The challenge of efficiency

Regardless of the pressures that increase demand, the discussion above might only confirm that increasing efficiency – the ratio of inputs to outputs or positive outcomes – is the best way to resolve the tension between budget makers' need to restrain spending and public demand for care.[50]

Common methods to limit the input for a given amount of output include: limiting the prices (inputs) paid for individual services, limiting the capital stock available to produce services and reducing overhead costs by simplifying insurance. National differences in spending and spending growth are largely due to differences in these policy choices. They certainly explain most of the difference between the United States and other countries (Pearson, 2009). Efficiency in this sense is also related to how institutions are managed. For example, the ways physicians are paid and managed can shape the productivity of hospital physical plant.[51] Hospital managers can be given incentives to meet targets for output improvement – though they may reduce what isn't measured.[52] The staffing of a general practice can be more or less efficient, and the organisation of specialty care involves myriad opportunities for greater efficiency.

Yet improving efficiency in producing specific outputs faces a series of obstacles, ranging from resistance by the affected interests to measurement issues. Doctors and drug companies prefer and fight for higher prices. Hospitals are very complex organisations so hard to manage well, and they have so much overhead that cost allocations to specific services are quite arbitrary. Moreover, shifting a service from one venue to another does not eliminate all the costs in the first venue, because the overhead still exists. If the seller (particularly a hospital) can do so, it will shift the charges for overhead costs to other services. This is why "improvements in efficiency" that are almost universally endorsed among health policy analysts and budgeters may not save money. The primary example is shifting patients from inpatient surgery to outpatient surgery. Budget makers must be very careful to avoid false efficiencies caused by flawed accounting (Reinhardt, 1996).

Producing hospital services more efficiently, either within or outside the hospital, involves producing the same output more efficiently. Many efficiency ideas, however, seek to improve outcomes by changing outputs. For example, increasing primary care might provide better management of chronic conditions such as diabetes. If the new service (such as primary care) is less expensive than the old service (acute hospital care) then better outcomes will result from fewer inputs. This is the promise of many ideas, such as that evidence-based medicine (EBM) with cost-effectiveness analysis (CEA) both save money by keeping patients out of the hospital and improve patients' outcomes. The promise is seductive; achieving it is rather difficult.

One problem is political. The providers who profit from selling the service that is to be replaced may challenge the analysis and exert political pressure against change. They may frighten patients with claims that "bureaucrats" are limiting their care, or form alliances with politicians who are opposed to the agency that sponsors change for some other reason. Policy makers might make change less threatening to patients by making new services available first, hoping they are chosen by patients, and then (if the theory is correct) benefiting from savings on the other services. But then the policy begins with a new expense and only promises of later reductions, and so requires a leap of faith from budget makers. Often, policy makers should not be so confident that spending and outcomes will change in the desired ways.

In the most ambitious versions of theories about changing outputs, all activities should be compared and a package chosen that would maximise the overall output of "health". This involves not just comparing different kinds of care for diabetics, but comparing care for diabetes with care for cancers or dementia. These ambitions are analogous, in principle, to budgeting for performance. Efforts to budget for performance, or results, occur in many countries, recur in many countries (especially the United States), and do not work very well.[53] A short list of why performance budgeting rarely succeeds would include the following:

1. Performance is very hard to measure even for a single activity, especially because logically it requires measuring a beginning state and end state, and then distinguishing the effect of the activity from other factors.
2. Results for different activities involve different outcomes, and any metric that seeks to compare them may seem (or be) arbitrary.
3. Different activities may serve different people with different utilities, and again any interpersonal utility metric may be questioned.

4. Not only citizens but policy makers may evaluate different programmes differently, so performance budgeting means one set of policy makers' preferences must prevail over others' preferences.
5. The level of performance does not actually say much about what funding is appropriate. Poor performance may be due to insufficient funds, so suggest more funding is needed so as to attain an important goal. Good performance could mean no more funding is necessary, and perhaps satisfactory results could be achieved with a little less.

The health policy equivalents may seem more plausible because it is easier to imagine comparing the outcomes of joint replacements and statin therapy than comparing the outcomes of defence spending and early childhood education. In theory, all health outputs can be compared in terms of their effects on quality-adjusted life years (QALYs) for patients. Yet even if it is easier to imagine a shared metric, that does not eliminate the other difficulties with performance comparisons. Moreover, hardly anyone in most political systems other than some health policy analysts accepts that QALYs are a reliable and objective metric.[54] Whether to spend a certain amount on asthma screening or joint replacements is a distributional question, so in that sense political.[55] Although it is possible to assess individual procedures or treatments (whether observers agree or not) in principle, there are far more services than could possibly be evaluated. Thus organisations such as the English National Institute for Health and Care Excellence (NICE) leave the vast majority of services unassessed – and NICE's judgements can still be very controversial. When the focus turns to the funding of alternative organisations, such as individual hospitals, there are continual disagreements over whether seemingly worse outcomes are due to having sicker patients (the risk-adjustment problem).

The obstacles to providing credible evidence that some services produce more health for the money than others do are aggravated by the timing issues mentioned above. Providing more primary care to the chronically ill first requires training and equipping more primary care providers. Extra spending on preventive care might (though it usually does not[56]) lead to larger savings on acute care; but policy makers who discount for uncertainty and have to worry more about short-term than long-term deficits may rationally want rather better proof of the return to investment than they usually will be able to obtain. This tension between long-term and short-term cost/benefit equations is common in many policy areas, but especially significant for most ideas about shifting the mix of health care services. Many of the most widely-promoted ideas at present (such as developing more evidence about treatments, investing in prevention and reorganising delivery) must cost more in the short run in return for uncertain benefits in the long run. In practice, politically rational budget makers might prefer more definite short-term savings, such as by underinvesting in the capacity to deliver hospital care, even if it might eventually blow up in political protest against a later government.

As the review above hints, there is one further challenge for policy makers: too many alternatives. Budget makers in any country should easily recognise this pattern, though they may not have defined it as a problem.

One only needs to browse the health policy journals, such as *Health Affairs* or *Health Policy*, to see a range of alternatives that could not possibly be matched in any other policy area, such as education or pensions.[57] The range can be bewildering: "get better evidence for care (EBM)", "select more cost-effective care (CEA)", "get people out of hospitals" (they're expensive places), "do more primary care", "replace physicians with other caregivers", "create medical homes", "integrate care through chronic care case management", "create accountable care organisations" (whatever that means), "pay for performance", "cut pay for non-performance" (e.g. hospital-acquired infections), "standardise care", "reduce prices through limiting patents", "prescribe generic instead of brand-name drugs", "create better electronic medical records", "gatekeeping for services", "put financial risk on primary care gatekeepers", "regulate prices", "do a better job of regulating prices", "create price competition by deregulating prices", "bundle payments to limit incentives for increased volume", "charge the patients more so they will only consume what they really need", "reduce litigation", "streamline administration", "create competition among insurers", "simplify insurance by standardising it", "integration", "decentralisation", "incentives".

Some of these ideas will save money; some won't. Some have been tried extensively and some are more like "policy unicorns" – pretty creatures that have not been observed in nature (Vladeck, (999. Many require technologies that have not been developed sufficiently for the ideas to work as promised – such as outcome measurements or risk adjustments. The flaws, however, have little or no influence on the advocates, and the advocates appear to be permanent parts of policy debate. "Managed competition", like communism, cannot fail. All disappointing results are blamed on insufficient implementation, not flaws in the basic theory.

Policy choices proliferate in part due to the immense division of labour in health care. Should policy target physicians' offices, hospitals or drugs? Can some functions be shifted to less expensive (and critics would say less skilled) labour, such as nurses instead of doctors or nurses' aides instead of licensed nurses? The division of labour creates interest groups which clamour for other groups' business, claiming that will save money for the system – or resist, claiming that supposed savings are false. Policy alternatives proliferate further because of the many different tribes of experts in the health care policy community. Economists of various leanings, public health specialists, health service researchers and other social scientists generate proposals which follow from their training and emphasise different problem definitions and policy instruments.[58]

Many decision processes require procedures to reduce many alternatives to a few, and then more carefully investigate those. The selection of policies to increase health care efficiency does not require as much reduction, because multiple approaches can be implemented together. There is also some merit in trial-and-error. Yet having so many alternatives creates a risk that policies will be chosen not based on evidence of success, but more based on which seems to face least political opposition. After all, virtually anything will have credentialed experts who say it will work.

One goal of this project is to better link the work of the health officials to budget makers. That work may help budget makers sort through alternatives. Yet there will be eminent experts in any country promoting virtually any idea, without regard for more neutral assessments. In the United States two of the world's leading health economists, David Cutler and Karen Davis, rejected estimates by the Congressional Budget Office and Medicare actuaries that the package of reforms in versions of the Affordable Care Act would do little to reduce spending. Rather than believe those estimates, they wrote that "it is imperative to cast a wider net than traditional evidence standards" (Cutler et al., 2009).

2.6. Effects of programme structure: Beyond "Bismarck" vs. "Beveridge"

Budgeting strategies often include a macropolitics of structure (Meyers, 1996). Health care systems vary substantially in the structure of financing, and moderately in how care is delivered.[59] The budgetary challenge is affected by these choices.

Bureaus vs. entitlements

The first involves the form of the promise to provide health care. Government spending programmes have two main forms: bureaus and entitlements (White, 1998a). In a bureau programme, government creates an organisation that will provide services – such as the national (or county) health services in many countries. Citizens are promised access to the bureau, which is responsible for providing care. In the entitlement approach, a government promises to pay cash benefits or reimburse for services according to some eligibility rules. In health care, that is the logic of social insurance or government insurance systems. Some providers in these systems might be owned by governments, but many will not be. The promise is that specific services will be paid for as needed.

In a bureau or health service programme, funds are allocated to the organisation, their amount is a direct budget allocation and the level of service that follows depends on how the organisation is managed. Budget control then follows from the original allocation – unless the budget is spent before the end of the year in a way that forces a supplemental appropriation. In an entitlement programme, spending depends on the rules of payment for services and the demand for services, so it is hard to enforce a total in advance – although there are examples of automatic fee adjustments that can be effective.[60]

Systems can involve mixes of the two principles. In many countries with entitlement systems governments own hospitals – though a different government may own the hospitals than operates the insurance system (Australia) or the insurance may be non-governmental (France, Germany). In a bureau system providers may not be officially employees of the state (as with general practitioners in the British national health services). The two approaches, however, clearly shape the budget challenge.

Bureau systems allow more direct management of providers – so greater ability to implement process efficiencies (e.g. "targets and terror") if political authorities know how to do so. Cost overruns can be made less likely by sanctioning managers. Control of physical capacity can be easier if it is financed entirely from capital budgets; if anything, normal budget behaviour is likely to lead to underfunding capital in order to maintain operational funding (Aaron and Schwartz, 2005). Scholars and managers of bureaucracy are likely to notice all the limits on hierarchical control of organisations, and they are right.[61] Nevertheless, the range of instruments available for controlling behaviour is much wider within hierarchies than for outsiders trying to influence organisations. It is probably no accident that the best-known implementations of a policy that requires extensive planning and co-ordination such as electronic medical records are within large bureaucracies, such as the US Veterans Health Administration. Organisations are created because of their power to co-ordinate activity – however much that may fall short of the ideal.

If budget makers are fortunate, they may in addition be able to displace blame for public disappointment with the level of service to the "bureaucrats", the agency managers who in theory could reduce waiting lists if they only managed better. If nothing else, policy makers can spend many years responding to complaints by implementing new management initiatives. Cost controls for entitlements generally have to be more specific: definitions of exactly which services will be discouraged and exactly which providers will be paid less.

From a budgetary perspective, the entitlement form has fewer advantages. One could be flexibility. Governments that do not own capacity have fewer sunk costs in it, so may have more ability to shift resources.[62] If entitlements include semi-public bodies responsible for management of the system as with the German sickness funds and their associations or the French CNAMTS (*Caisse nationale de l'assurance maladie des travailleurs salariés*), governments may sometimes be able to obscure or share the blame for cost controls. In the ideal case, those managers may be able to negotiate cost control with the providers, using the threat of government intervention to obtain agreements that might be as good as the government would have obtained, at less cost to the government. In the entitlement model, governments also may bear less responsibility for failures or scandals in the delivery system. If cost control might lead to delivery failures, it seems better to have bought the services from somewhat separate organisations than for the organisations to be part of the government.

Policy makers in many countries seem to be seeking some of the advantages of the bureau form within an entitlement design. They attempt to do this by bundling, which means paying not for individual services but for a package of services. When Dutch policy makers hope insurers will control costs, they are asking insurers to take on the management responsibilities of a bureau. When American policy makers have tried to move patients into health maintenance organisations (HMOs) and now accountable care organisations, the idea has been to make a lump-sum payment to these insurers and then have them manage costs – like a bureau. Attempts to pay all costs for an episode could only make sense if some organisation is created to manage across the different providers involved. In any of these cases, the potential advantage is that the bureau would get the blame for measures to limit costs, including any restrictions on output.

The risk is that organisations will try to do as little as possible for their lump payments so as to maximise their operating margins. The result could be worse outcomes and less value for money – at best, economy without efficiency. In the theory of managed competition, informed patients would recognise skimpy performance, risk adjustment would eliminate incentives to avoid sicker patients and market forces would prevent organisational shirking; but this has yet to be demonstrated in practice. Concerns about government oversight also seem ubiquitous. From a bundling perspective, the logical way to pay hospitals is by giving them budgets. Yet numerous countries have moved towards efforts to pay hospitals by case and diagnosis, on the grounds that this provides better incentives for productivity.[63]

In the terms of this chapter's previous discussion, the bureau form may be seen as a way to limit demand somewhat by directing it at the bureaus (in part) rather than the payers. The bureau form probably increases ability to make production of outputs more efficient. Neither form has a clear advantage for better linking outputs to outcomes, because that depends most on good theory about medical cause and effect. The entitlement form may have a slight advantage if policy makers want to change the mix of outputs.

Dedicated vs. general revenues

A second major choice is whether health care is financed by dedicated or general revenues. Social health insurance systems, like any social insurance system, are built on an assumption that entitlement to benefits is based on contributions towards the fund from which they are paid. Government programmes normally are funded from a pool of general revenues. So there is a historical association between the entitlement approach (as social insurance) and dedicated revenues, while bureau programmes are more likely to have general revenues. Yet there are numerous exceptions. Early social insurance systems often funded bureaus in the form of polyclinics. Canada's entitlement system is not traditional social insurance, for most provinces do not have dedicated contributions. Increasingly, the finance of entitlements in traditional SHI systems is being supplemented with general revenues.[64]

From a public finance perspective, dedicated revenues are problematic. As Alan Auerbach summarises: "We may end up relying too heavily on some taxes rather than others, thereby reducing the tax system's efficiency. Also, our mix and level of public spending may be distorted by the connections of particular types of spending to specific sources of funding. Money is fungible, in principle, so financing a particular type of spending in part with dedicated revenues ought to have no impact on overall spending of this type. But where dedicated revenues constitute a large share of the funding for a particular type of spending, the level of dedicated tax revenues can have a strong impact on the level of associated spending, with unattractive consequences" (Auerbach, 2009).

On the other hand, policy makers have many motives for adopting dedicated taxes. Dedicated funding may make raising taxes easier because "taxpayers might be more willing to pay taxes if they perceive that these taxes are spent on something that they value, even if there is no tax-benefit linkage at the individual level". A dedicated tax might be adopted also "either to protect or limit the amount of a particular type of spending". Advocates of a programme may seek the security of "a claim on a specific source of revenue .... On the other hand, one of the reasons advanced for providing a dedicated source of revenue such as the VAT for health care has been to try to force health spending growth to conform to the growth of VAT revenues. In either case, though, the influence of tax dedication on funding need not go in the right direction from a social perspective" (Auerbach, 2009, p. 21).

Choices about dedicated funding therefore could influence ability both to control spending and to raise revenues – but in which direction? Although the issues are analytically separate, they are hard to separate in practice, because if dedicated funding raises revenues, it may reduce the need to limit spending. In a bureau system with particularly strong budget controllers and fiscal pressures, such as the United Kingdom for most of the history of the NHS, relying on general revenues is likely to lead to lower spending. But that doesn't answer the question of whether budget makers are better off relying on general revenues than dedicated revenues, because there may have been more room to finance other programmes and control deficits in the United Kingdom if the NHS had had its own dedicated funds.

As a very provisional judgement, it appears that dedicated funds probably inhibit raising spending more quickly than that revenue stream. However, separate revenues make it difficult to cut spending below the amount of revenues.[65] On balance, if dedicated revenues allow collection of more money, they are likely to reduce budgetary pressures. Dedicated funding also clarifies budgetary consequences. When programmes are funded from general revenues, it is easy for virtually everyone to demand that their spending be protected, yet refuse to pay more because they want other people's spending to be cut.[66] If spending is financed from dedicated funds, it is more plausible to say the level accurately reflects public preferences.

As always, there are complications. The income on which most dedicated revenues have been based – wages – becomes steadily less adequate as costs increase and the labour share of GDP falls in most countries (OECD, 2012). In systems built on dedicated funding, this creates pressure to redistribute further by financing a part of care from general revenues. Ironically, the fact that most of the money comes from dedicated funds may make a portion of general revenues seem a small price to pay for preserving a large and highly popular programme.

Nevertheless, on balance, dedicated funding appears to have budgetary advantages. From a budgetary perspective, the best structural combination may be a mostly bureau system financed mainly from dedicated revenues.

The scope of coverage

A third structural choice has been discussed in part earlier in this chapter. What health care will be financed socially and what will be treated as "wants" rather than "needs", so as a matter for personal consumption instead of redistribution? In addition to what will count as medical care, this choice involves issues such as the extent of cost-sharing within the system of coverage and the roles of gap and parallel insurance in health care systems.[67]

The scope of benefits can only be a value choice. There is no "right" answer. Budget makers, however, have good reason at least to insist that this be a choice – that expansions of the medical realm not continue without reflection. The extent of cost-sharing is almost a theological issue. It involves questions of fact – what the effects of cost-sharing are, for which types of people. Yet how people evaluate these facts, and even what facts they choose to accept, seems to vary greatly, partly with belief in equality in general and partly with faith in the merits of market forces. Budget makers can only seek the best and most comprehensive research and then decide based on their own values. Yet they should be aware that cost-sharing tends to be unpopular for the same reasons as demand for health care programmes is high.

2.7. Conclusion

Government support for citizens' medical care, whatever the form of the programme, has become a basic part of modern societies – even in the United States. In some cases (Canada, the United Kingdom) these programmes have become part of national identity. In others, such as Germany, they were part of creating the nation-state. These programmes have had major successes – in enhancing national solidarity and improving the populations' health.[68] Unfortunately, none of that eliminates the basic challenge of budgeting: how to reconcile preferences about spending and taxing, details and totals. Yet the basic message of this chapter should be that it is possible to find acceptable options. Taking a political economy perspective, the usual suspects for inevitable spending increases – the Baumol effect, ageing and technology – are not so important as to counsel despair. The Baumol argument is not convincing; technology is not self-executing; and the effects of ageing will only be pre-eminent if a country, as might be argued of Japan, both has especially high proportions of seniors and has implemented other cost control policies quite effectively.

Unlike with many programmes, dedicated funding is a real option. And there are many alternatives for spending control: the budgeting challenge is how to sort through them and distinguish wishful thinking from evidence.

Notes

1. The most substantial cuts were in Estonia, Greece, Iceland, Ireland and Portugal. "Health spending continues to stagnate, says OECD", OECD Health Policies and Data, 27 June 2013 at *www.oecd.org/newsroom/health-spending-continues-to-stagnate-says-oecd.htm*. For a discussion of measures taken for 2010-11, see Morgan, D. and R. Astolfi (2013), "Health Spending Growth at Zero: Which Countries,

Which Sectors Are Most Affected?", *OECD Health Working Papers*, No. 60, OECD Publishing, Paris, *http://dx.doi.org/10.1787/5k4dd1st95xv-en*.

2. Comparisons are based on 23 countries: European OECD members that were not part of the former Soviet bloc, Australia, Canada, Japan, New Zealand and the United States.

3. *OECD Factbook 2013: Economic, Environmental and Social Statistics*, available at *http://dx.doi.org/10.1787/factbook-2013-en*, p. 249. Note that no public/private breakdown for the Netherlands was provided for 2010; it can be difficult to determine what the classifications in the Netherlands should be.

4. Author's calculation from ibid., Table p. 249. This involves adding figures rounded to one decimal point and averaging over 23 countries, so is imprecise. The average came to 1.87 percentage points of GDP. Only one country, Iceland, saw a spending decrease as a share of GDP from 2000 to 2010, and that was only 0.2%.

5. Ibid., p. 195.

6. For an imprecise comparison see Table B4.2 from OECD (2013), *Education at a Glance – OECD Indicators*. The table shows public expenditure on education as a share of GDP for 1995, 2000, 2005 and 2010. The definition of education spending, however, is more extensive than in the *OECD Factbook* because it includes subsidies to households for student living costs (e.g. for scholarship students). Also, the change between 2000 and 2010 is affected by the general decline in the denominator (GDP) in 2010.

7. Much of the expansion of education "need" will involve longer periods of training and only a portion of the population will be eligible for such expansion of tertiary education, while nearly all citizens could be eligible for further medical services.

8. Examples as of 2009 were Austria, Belgium, Finland, France, Germany, Greece, Italy, Japan, Luxembourg, Portugal and Spain. Pension figures are in *OECD Factbook 2013*, op. cit., p. 215. For 2009, the public spending is roughly calculated from the tables, "Total expenditure on health as a percentage of gross domestic product" from OECD Health Statistics, downloaded from *http://dx.doi.org/10.1787/hlthxp-total-table-2013-2-en* and "Public expenditure on health as a percentage of total expenditure on health" from *OECD Health Statistics*, downloaded from *http://dx.doi.org/10.1787/hlthxp-pub-table-2013-2-en*.

9. The old-age support ratio is the number of people of working age (20-64) per person of pension age (65+). An Excel spreadsheet of data is available at *www.oecd.org/els/public-pensions/indicators.htm*, under subhead 4, "Demographic and economic context". The data part of the spreadsheet have been used to rank-order the countries in this analysis for 2008, from having the largest share of elderly (1) to the least (23). From the tables on health care and pension spending trends in the previous footnote, it appears that pension expenditure as a share of GDP grew more quickly than health care spending as a share of GDP in Finland, France, Ireland, Japan, the Netherlands, Portugal and Sweden. This is associated with the old-age support ratio by the fact that these countries ranked 1, 4, 7, 8, 11, 16 and 23. Ireland, at 23, is clearly an outlier.

10. For a typical discussion see Clements, B., D. Coady and S. Gupta (eds.) (2012), *The Economics of Public Healthcare Reform in Advanced and Emerging Economies*, International Monetary Fund, Washington, DC.

11. For a general discussion of the theme, see Schick, A. (2009), "Budgeting for Fiscal Space", *OECD Journal on Budgeting 2009/2*.

12. In 2010 the United States had the largest gap between incomes of the richest and poorest deciles of the population among the 23 countries compared. Among OECD nations, only Turkey, Mexico and Chile had greater inequality. See OECD (2014), *Society at a Glance – OECD Indicators*, Chapter 5, Table 5.1, as updated 4 December 2013.

13. For a discussion of visibility by one of the most prominent sources for this argument, see Wilensky, H.L. (2002), "Rich Democracies: Political Economy, Public Policy and Performance", University of California Press, Berkeley. For an overview of dedicated financing in the US context, see Patashnik, E. (2000), *Putting Trust in the US Budget: Federal Trust Funds and the Politics of Commitment*, Cambridge University Press, Cambridge.

14. This is simplifying greatly.

15. In addition, results of any analysis will depend on choices about modelling techniques and how to measure national savings, neither of which are straightforward. The discussion that follows cannot settle these issues, but offers some perspective. For an early example of analysis see Herd, R. (1989), "The Impact of Increased Government Saving on the Economy", *OECD Department of Economics and Statistics Working Paper*, No. 68, June.

16. Normal productivity growth would swamp the savings effect. In fact, technical adjustments in the consumer price index would at least seem to increase workers' real incomes over that period by substantially more. See White, J. (2003), "False Alarm", op cit., pp. 83-84.

17. CBO – Congressional Budget Office (2012), "The Budget and Economic Outlook: Fiscal Years 2012 to 2022", p. 29, January. CBO added that GNP would be a better measure, and at the end of 2022 "real GNP would be between 3.7% and 1.0% smaller". Still, the midpoint is half of the total deficit change.

18. See the discussion in White, J. (2003), "False Alarm", op. cit., pp. 84-88.

19. Voters clearly have chosen mainly to pay for rather than cut social security pensions, with continual contribution increases until 1983. Since then there has been no need. The solvency of the Medicare Hospital Insurance Trust Fund has been addressed by a combination of cuts to spending but not benefits (i.e. payment reforms) and higher contributions both through taxes and premiums paid by individuals with higher incomes. In short: by greater redistribution.

20. The eurozone southern tier has also not had the option of monetising their debt, though fears they might leave the Eurozone could affect potential bondholders.

21. In each case interest rates may be low because there is far more capital than safe places to put it and in spite of the deficits Japanese and US bonds appear safer than alternatives. But the Japanese case mainly appears to involve Japanese capital, while the US case involves the world's.

22. From 1999 to 2008 health care spending as a share of GDP did rise fairly quickly in Greece, from 8.7% of GDP to 10.1%. During the same time, however, spending rose as quickly in Canada, the Netherlands, New Zealand, Sweden, the United Kingdom and the United States – none of which faced the same kind of bondholder response. The Greek crisis can more reasonably be ascribed to indications of fraudulent accounting, "overstaffing and poor productivity in the public sector" across functions, pensions that are extremely generous compared to other countries and weak revenue collection – in part because the informal economy could exceed a quarter of Greek GDP. In other words, Greece is an exceptional case. For one summary see Nelson, R.M., P. Belkin and D.E. Mix (2010), "Greece's Debt Crisis: Overview, Policy Responses, and Implications", Report No. R-41167, United States Congress, Congressional Research Service, 14 May, available at *http://fpc.state.gov/documents/organization/142363.pdf*, p. 5.

23. For example, in 2004 the same US corporations would have paid nearly USD 1 300 extra in employee health care costs to build the same car in Michigan as in Ontario, which should inhibit hiring in Michigan. For a detailed review of the issues in the US context, see Office of the Assistant Secretary for Planning and Evaluation, United States Department of Health and Human Services (ASPE), "The Effect of Healthcare Cost Growth on the U.S. Economy", Final Report for Task Order #HP-06-12, at *aspe.hhs.gov/health/reports/o8/healthcarecost/report.pdf* cited hereinafter as ASPE (2008).

24. ASPE (2008) p. 13. This source provides a further review of the "range of factors including the legal or institutional environment under which a firm operates" (14) that would determine any effect on employment.

25. For example, the effect of health care costs on employment does not appear to be addressed in the series of *OECD Social, Employment and Migration Working Papers*.

26. See ASPE (2008), quotes pp. 29, 34. This report sought to measure effects on overall unemployment by comparing states, and found weak, statistically insignificant indications that greater expenditure was associated with higher unemployment.

27. Ibid., pp. 41-45; the point estimate was an increase of 35 000 jobs, see p. 44. Note that at a given point in time revenues might be increased to make up for deficits in a fund, so for past consumption expansions. If so, it would not be financing new consumption and might lead to a small decrease in employment.

28. Advisory Council for Concerted Action in Health Care (1998), "The Health Care System in Germany: Cost Factor and Branch of the Future", *Vol. II: Progress and Growth Markets, Finance and Remuneration*, Bonn, *www.svr-gesundheit.de/fileadmin/user_upload/Gutachten/1997/Kurzf-engl97.pdf*, p. 15. This second volume reported a slightly different model result, at p. 18.

29. See the PowerPoint presentation, "Improving value for money from a health economics perspective", from the conference. Downloadable from *www.oecd.org/gov/budgeting/49094979.pdf*. See also Henke, K.D. and K. Martin (2008), "Health as a Driving Economic Force", *Technische Universität Berlin Diskussionspapier 2008/2*, at *www.wm.tu-berlin.de/fileadmin/f8/wiwidok/diskussionspapiere_wiwidok/dp02-2008.pdf*. These possibilities are also noted in ASPE (2008).

30. There presumably would be situations where large differences in charges for comparable industries between comparable countries would be more significant, as in the Canada/US automobile industry comparison mentioned above.

31. US Government, White House Office of Homeland Security, National Strategy for Homeland Security (July, 2002), p. 65, at *http://permanent.access.gpo.gov/lps20641/nat_strat_hls.pdf*. The report estimated the "deadweight loss" of taxes as an extra USD 0.27 per dollar of revenue.

32. Arguably there is a third, but not much could be said about it. At any given time all citizens could need medical care – unlike education or pensions, though any citizen will need all three at some point in the lifecycle.

33. The classic review of the core policy reasons for such differences remains Glaser, W.A. (1991), *Health Insurance in Practice: International Variations in Financing, Benefits and Problems*, Jossey-Bass, San Francisco. See Chapters 12-15 for these four types of care.

34. For one discussion of disciplinary assumptions that may be hidden in plain sight, but determine conclusions in advance, see Rice, T.E. (2002), *The Economics of Health Reconsidered*, 2nd ed, Health Administration Press, Chicago.

35. The effect of inequality is controversial; for one sceptical review see Deaton, A. (2003), "Health, Income, and Inequality", NBER Reporter Research Summary, Spring 2003, at *www.nber.org/reporter/spring03/health.html*.

36. On pollution see Plumer, B. (2013), "Coal Pollution in China is Cutting Life Expectancy by 5.5 Years", *Washington Post Wonkblog*, 8 July 2013 at *www.washingtonpost.com/blogs/wonkblog/wp/2013/07/08/chinas-coal-pollution-is-much-deadlier-than-anyone-realized/*.

37. See the discussions in Rechel, B. et al. (2009), "How Can Health Systems Respond to Population Ageing?", *European Observatory on Health Systems and Policies Policy Brief* 10, at *www.euro.who.int/__data/assets/pdf_file/0004/64966/E92560.pdf*; and in White, J. (2004), "(How) Is Ageing a Health Policy Problem?", *Yale Journal of Health Policy, Law and Ethics*, Vol. 4, No. 1, Yale Schools of Law, Medicine, Epidemiology and Public Health, and Nursing, New Haven.

38. De la Maisonneuve and Martins (2013), p. 17. Note that these figures are lower than might otherwise be expected because they include the OECD countries that are at the lower end of health care expenditure as they are at earlier stages of economic development. For other studies with similar results see OECD (2006), op. cit., and also Gruber, J. and D. Wise, (2002), "An International Perspective on Policies for an Aging Society", in Stuart H. Altman and David I. Shactman (eds.), *Policies for an Ageing Society*, The Johns Hopkins University Press, Baltimore, pp. 34-62.

39. See the long-term care tables in OECD (2006), op. cit.; also Karlsson, M. and F. Klohn (2011), "Some Notes on How to Catch a Red Herring: Ageing, Time-to-Death and Care Costs for Older People in Sweden", University of Oslo Health Economics Research Programme, *Working Paper* No. 2011:6, *www.med.uio.no/helsam/forskning/nettverk/hero/publikasjoner/skriftserie/2011/2011+6.pdf*.

40. See for example European Community Economic Policy Commission, "Progress Report to the ECOFIN Council on the Impact of Ageing Populations on Public Pension Systems", 7 November 2000 at *www.consilium.europa.eu/uedocs/cmsUpload/Progress%20Report%20on%20the%20impact%20of%20ageing%20population.pdf*; OECD (1998), "Work Force Aging: Consequences and Policy Responses", *OECD Working Paper* No. AWP4.1, at *www.oecd.org/els/public-pensions/2429096.pdf*; Cotis, J.P. (2003), "Population Ageing: Facing the Challenge", *OECD Observer*, Vol. 26 September, at *http://www.oecdobserver.org/news/archivestory.php/aid/1081/Population_ageing:_Facing_the_challenge.html*.

41. For the most recent of a half century of these arguments, see Baumol, W.J. (2012), "The Cost Disease: Why Computers Get Cheaper and Health Care Doesn't", Yale University Press, New Haven. For a review that refers to many studies of the overall claim (not just limited to health care), and an argument that the basic dynamic exists, see Nordhaus, W.D. (2006), "Baumol's Diseases: A Macroeconomic Perspective", *NBER Working Paper* No. 12218, May, *www.nber.org/papers/w12218.pdf?new_window=1*.

42. See the interpretation in Wallace, A. (2012), "The Case for Calm over Rising Health Costs", *New York Times*, 6 October 2012 at *www.nytimes.com/2012/10/07/business/cost-disease-offers-a-case-for-healthcare-calm.html?_r=0*.

43. De la Maisonneuve and Martins, op. cit. They note that it might have been possible to make such estimates for individual sectors (p. 13); but this is questionable because part of any efficiency increases would be substitutions across sectors.

44. Docteur, E. and H. Oxley (2003), "Healthcare Systems: Lessons from the Reform Experience", *OECD Economics Department Working Papers*, No. 374, *http://dx.doi.org/10.1787/884504747522*. Joumard, I., C. André and C. Nicq (2010), "Healthcare Systems: Efficiency and Institutions", *OECD Economics Department Working Papers*, No. 769, *http://search.oecd.org/officialdocuments/displaydocumentpdf/?doclanguage=en&cote=eco/wkp%282010%2925*. Moreno-Serra, R. (2013), "The Impact of Cost-containment

Policies on Health Expenditure: Evidence from Recent OECD Experiences", Paper prepared for the second meeting of the Joint Network on Fiscal Sustainability of Health Systems, 25-26 March, OECD, Paris (unpublished). The OECD Health Division has numerous studies of specific approaches. An excellent review for the US context is CBO (2008), "Key Issues in Analysing Major Health Insurance Proposals", December, *http://cbo.gov/sites/default/files/cbofiles/ftpdocs/99ss/doc9924/12-18-keyissues.pdf.*

45. Assuming there are no policy choices to ensure spending does not burgeon as a result. "Technology" is discussed further below.

46. One common dispute is whether "induced demand" means that attempts to control prices do not work because providers will simply induce extra volume to compensate for the lost income. The answer, at least in the United States, is "no". For evidence see CBO (1998), "Major Issues", op. cit., p. 109; Medicare Actuaries (1998), "Memorandum: Physician Volume and Intensity Response", August. 2013, *www.cms.gov/Research-Statistics-Data-and-Systems/Research/ActuarialStudies/downloads/PhysicianResponse.pdf*; Technical Review Panel on the Medicare Trustees Reports (2000), "Review of the Medicare Trustees' Financial Projections", December, *www.cms.gov/Research-Statistics-Data-and-Systems/Statistics-Trends-and-Reports/ReportsTrustFunds/downloads/TechnicalPanelReport2000.pdf.* Another dispute is whether medical care providers know that what they advise is the right course of treatment for the patient. The answer appears to be "sometimes".

47. Various technology fads may waste large amounts of money in US hospitals and perhaps elsewhere. But it is questionable whether that makes hospitals different from other institutions, and at any rate arguments that technology causes rising costs focus on medical services.

48. Until the evaluators, in the United States, buy an imaging machine and start running a lot of tests. But that does not work for, say, endocrinologists. And it only works so long as policy allows them to buy the machines.

49. But not in Japan, which has a very flexible price-setting system. See Campbell, J.C. and N. Ikegami (1998), "The Art of Balance in Health Policy: Maintaining Japan's Low-Cost, Egalitarian System", Cambridge University Press, Cambridge.

50. The OECD and CBO studies cited earlier are very useful. My own analyses include "Cost of Health Care in Western Countries", in Warrell, D., A. Timothy, M. Cox and J.D. Firth (eds.), *Oxford Textbook of Medicine*, 5th edition, Vol. 1, pp. 112-116, Oxford University Press, Oxford; and "Targets and Systems of Healthcare Cost Control", *Journal of Health Politics, Policy and Law*, Vol. 24, No. 4, August 1999, Duke University Press, Durham.

51. One issue is how to get satisfactory productivity from salaried physicians. This involves all the issues that normally apply to salaried personnel – sense of mission, possible sanctions, oversight, culture, etc. But payment methods can be both more and less problematic than salary. At one end of the spectrum, if hospital physicians receive fees for each procedure, they have strong incentives to push hospital managers to maximise throughput. At the other end, if physicians are paid per session (e.g. four hours), and the time for a procedure does not divide neatly into that unit (perhaps it is normally three hours), then physicians might not work for all the time for which they are paid.

52. The English NHS regime, under the Blair government, of "Targets and Terror" to reduce waiting times has been described as an example of successful, if perhaps unpleasant, management. For one discussion with some citations see *www.kingsfund.org.uk/projects/general-election-2010/key-election-questions/performance-targets.* See also Propper, C., M. Sutton, C. Whitnall and F. Windmeijer (2007), "Did 'Targets and Terror' Reduce Waiting Times in England for Hospital Care?", *Centre for Market and Public Organisation Working Paper* No. 07/179, November 2007, at *www.bris.ac.uk/cmpo/publications/papers/2007/wp179.pdf.* But the comparative data used for these analyses is a bit shaky; see the discussion of data problems in Connolly, S., G. Bevan and N. Mays (2011), "Funding and Performance of Health Care Systems in the Four Countries of the UK Before and After Devolution", Nuffield Trust, London, at *www.kingsfund.org.uk/projects/general-election-2010/key-election-questions/performance-targets.*

53. For a discussion of the "long, if irregular history" of performance budgeting in the United States, see Schick, A. (2013), "The Metamorphoses of Performance Budgeting", *OECD Journal on Budgeting*, Vol. 2013/2, pp. 49-80. For an update on US experience with further commentary, see White, J. (2012), "Playing the Wrong PART: The Programme Assessment Rating Tool and the Functions of the President's Budget", *Public Administration Review*, Vol. 72, No. 1, January, pp. 112-120, John Wiley and Sons.

54. For a good discussion of doubts about the concept see Ashmore, M., M. Mulkay and T. Pinch (1989), *Health and Efficiency: A Sociology of Health Economics*, Open University Press, Milton Keynes and Philadelphia. For all their problems, QALYs are better than measures such as the US PART scores, which were pretty arbitrary. See an explanation in White, J. (2012), "Playing the Wrong Part", op. cit.

55. It also involves judgements about efficiency that can be questioned: How much asthma or asthma-related misery will be reduced by screening? What is the value of the mobility advances from joint replacements? How do we know to whom to give the screening or surgeries, and doesn't the result depend on who gets them and who does them?

56. For a short recent summary of the issues see (no author) "The Economics of Prevention" (2012), Academy Health Research Insights at *www.academyhealth.org/files/FileDownloads/RI_Econ_Prevention.pdf*.

57. The September/October 2009 and May 2013 issues of *Health Affairs* are good examples of the variety. A quick look at the Health Policy website on 11 April 11 2014 found articles on 14 different aspects of costs either published in 2014 or in press as of that date.

58. For one review see White, J. (1998), "Healthcare Reform: What is the Problem?", in T.R. Marmor and P.R. De Jong (eds.), *Ageing, Social Security and Affordability*, Aldershot, United Kingdom, and Brookfield, Ashgate, United States.

59. The most common distinction is between "Beveridge" (essentially health service) and "Bismarck" (social health insurance) systems. A good source on that distinction and how it is weakening is Rothgang, H. et al (2010), *The State and Health Care: Comparing OECD Countries*, Palgrave MacMillan, New York. For an alternative typology see Moran, M. (2000), "Understanding the Welfare State: The Case of Health Care", *British Journal of Politics and International Relations*, Vol. 2, No. 2, John Wiley and Sons, pp. 136-160.

60. The major example is how the Germans have paid for physician services for many years. In essence, fees for each service are defined not in euros but in points; then the number of points each quarter is added up and divided into the budget allocation to create what is essentially a retrospective fee for each service. A similar approach has been designed, though perhaps not totally implemented, for public hospital payments under the French version of a DRG system.

61. For a comprehensive explanation of the admittedly extreme circumstances of the United States, see Wilson, J.Q. (1989), *Bureaucracy: What Government Agencies Do and Why They Do It*, Basic Books, New York.

62. This is one rationale for replacing ownership by contracting in an "internal market". How well it works in practice, however, is not so clear.

63. For a discussion of this developments see Busse, R., A. Geissler, W. Quentin and M. Wiley (eds.) (2011), "Diagnosis-Related Groups in Europe: Moving Towards Transparency, Efficiency and Quality in Hospitals", Open University Press, Maidenhead, England. There is great variation in use of DRGs, and in many cases they are being used more as a measurement tool than a payment category; but the trend away from set hospital budgets is clear.

64. On the current transitions see Rothgang et al. (2013), "The State and Health Care", op cit., for the earlier history see Glaser (1991), "Health Insurance in Practice", op. cit.

65. This judgement is based on comparison of trends across countries as reported in Flood, C., M. Stabile and C. Tuohy (eds.) (2008), "Exploring Social Insurance: Can a Dose of Europe Cure Canadian Health Care Finance?", McGill-Queen's University Press, Montreal and Kingston. The main motivation for the conference is an example of calculations about possible effects. The organisers wanted to explore whether creating new social insurance for pharmaceutical benefits could both make coverage more adequate and equitable, and help provincial budgets by replacing general revenues that were being used for non-universal pharmaceutical benefits. In my chapter (pp. 233-249) I relied on both my own less systematic data and my interpretation of data reported in Sherry Glied's chapter, "Health Care financing, efficiency and equity".

66. For explanations of this dynamic see Downs, A. (1960), "Why the Government Budget Is too Small in a Democracy", *World Politics*, Vol. 12, No. 4, July 1960, pp. 541-563, Princeton Institute for International and Regional Affairs, Cambridge University Press; White, J. (1998), "Making 'Common Sense' of Federal Budgeting", *Public Administration Review*, Vol. 58, No. 2, March/April 1998.

67. The literature about cost-sharing is massive; a good review is Remler, D.K. and J. Greene (2009), "Cost-Sharing: A Blunt Instrument", *American Journal of Public Health*, Vol. 30, pp. 293-311. See also the discussions in the sources cited above in note 66. On the roles of private insurance, which sometimes is called "complementary" or "supplementary" but inconsistently across authors, see

White, J. (2009), "Gap and Parallel Insurance in Healthcare Systems With Mandatory Contributions to a Single Funding Pool for Core Medical and Hospital Benefits for All Citizens in Any Given Geographic Area", *Journal of Health Politics, Policy and Law*, Vol. 34, No. 4, pp. 543-583.

68. Recall the striking advances even over a recent decade in preventing avoidable mortality, as reported in Nolte and McKee (2011), "Variations in Amenable Mortality", op. cit.

References

Aaron, H.J. and W.B. Schwartz (2005), *Can We Say No? The Challenge of Rationing Health Care*, The Brookings Institution, Washington, DC.

AcademyHealth (2012), "The Economics of Prevention" (2012), *Academy Health Research Insights* at *www.academyhealth.org/files/FileDownloads/RI_Econ_Prevention.pdf.*

Advisory Council for Concerted Action in Health Care (1998), "The Health are System in Germany: Cost Factor and Branch of the Future", Vol. II: Progress and Growth Markets, Finance and Remuneration. Bonn, p. 15, *www.svr-gesundheit.de/fileadmin/user_upload/Gutachten/1997/Kurzf-engl97.pdf.*

Advisory Council for Concerted Action in Health Care (1996), "The Health Care System in Germany: Cost Factor and Branch of the Future", Vol. I: Demographics, Morbidity, Efficiency Reserves and Employment, Bonn, p. 41, *www.svr-gesundheit.de/fileadmin/user_upload/Gutachten/1996/Kurzf-engl96.pdf.*

Altman, D. (2014), "Healthcare Cost Growth Is Down, Or Not. It Depends Who You Ask", *http://kff.org/health-costs/perspective/health-cost-growth-is-down-or-not-it-depends-who-you-ask/.*

Ashmore, M. et al. (1989), *Health and Efficiency: A Sociology of Health Economics*, Open University Press, Milton Keynes and Philadelphia.

Auerbach, A. (2009), "Public Finance in Practice and Theory", Paper presented as the Richard Musgrave Lecture, CESifo, Munich, 25 May, p. 20, *www.iipf.org/Auerbach_Alan_Public_Finance.pdf.*

Baker, D. and D. Rosnick (2011), "7 Things You Need to Know about the National Debt, Deficits, and the Dollar", Center for Economic and Policy Research, Washington DC, *www.cepr.net/documents/publications/debt-2011-06.pdf.*

Baumol, W.J. (2012), *The Cost Disease: Why Computers Get Cheaper and Health Care Doesn't*, Yale University Press, New Haven.

Blöndal, J.R. et al. (2003), "Budgeting in the United States", *OECD Journal on Budgeting*, Vol. 3/2, pp. 31-39, OECD Publishing, Paris, *http://dx.doi.org/10.1787/16812336.*

Brandt, N. (2008), "Moving towards More Sustainable Healthcare Financing in Germany", *OECD Economics Department Working Papers*, No. 612, p. 5, *http://dx.doi.org/10.1787/242647737261.*

Busse, R. et al. (eds.) (2011), "Diagnosis-Related Groups in Europe: Moving towards Transparency, Efficiency and Quality in Hospitals", Open University Press, Maidenhead, United Kingdom.

Campbell, J.C. and N. Ikegami (1998), *The Art of Balance in Health Policy: Maintaining Japan's Low-Cost, Egalitarian System*, Cambridge University Press, Cambridge, United Kingdom.

CBO – United States Congressional Budget Office (2012), *The Budget and Economic Outlook: Fiscal Years 2012 to 2022*, Washington, DC, p. 29.

CBO (2008), "Key Issues in Analysing Major Health Insurance Proposals", Washington, DC, *http://cbo.gov/sites/default/files/cbofiles/ftpdocs/99ss/doc9924/12-18-keyissues.pdf.*

Clements, B., D. Coady and S. Gupta (eds.) (2012), *The Economics of Public Healthcare Reform in Advanced and Emerging Economies*, International Monetary Fund, Washington, DC.

Coe, D.T. (2007), "Globalisation and Labour Markets: Policy Issues Arising from the Emergence of China and India", *OECD Social, Employment and Migration Working Papers*, No. 63, p. 18, OECD Publishing, Paris, *http://dx.doi.org/10.1787/057638253043.*

Colleen, F., M. Stabile and C. Tuohy (eds.) (2008), *Exploring Social Insurance: Can a Dose of Europe Cure Canadian Healt-Care Finance?*, McGill-Queen's University Press, Montreal and Kingston.

Connolly, S., G. Bevan and N. Mays (2011), "Funding and Performance of Healthcare Systems in the Four Countries of the UK Before and After Devolution", Nuffield Trust, London, *www.kingsfund.org.uk/projects/general-election-2010/key-election-questions/performance-targets.*

Cotis, J.P. (2003), "Population Ageing: Facing the Challenge", *OECD Observer*, *www.oecdobserver.org/news/archivestory.php/aid/1081/Population_ageing:_Facing_the_challenge.html*.

Cutler, D.M., K. Davis and K. Stremikis (2009), "Why Health Reform Will Bend the Cost Curve", Commonwealth Fund Issue Brief, p. 10, *www.commonwealthfund.org/~/media/Files/Publications/Issue%20Brief/2009/Dec/1351_Cutler_Davis_Health_Reform_129_CAPAF.pdf*.

De la Maisonneuve, C. and J. Oliveira Martins (2013), "A Projection Method for Public Health and Long-Term Care Expenditures", *OECD Department Working Papers*, No. 1048, p. 9, OECD Publishing, Paris, *http://dx.doi.org/10.1787/5k44v53w5w47-en*.

Deaton, A. (2003), "Health, Income and Inequality", *NBER Reporter Research Summary*, Spring, *www.nber.org/reporter/spring03/health.html*.

Docteur, E. and H. Oxley (2003), "Healthcare Systems: Lessons from the Reform Experience", *OECD Economics Department Working Papers*, No. 374, OECD Publishing, Paris, *http://dx.doi.org/10.1787/884504747522*.

Domnich, A. et al. (2012), "The 'Healthy Immigrant' Effect": Does It Exist in Europe Today?", *Italian Journal of Public Health*, Vol. 9/3, Italian Society of Medical Statistics and Clinical Epidemiology, Milan, pp. e7532-1-7.

Downs, A. (1960), "Why the Government Budget Is too Small in a Democracy", *World Politics*, Vol. 12/4, pp. 541-563.

European Community Economic Policy Commission (2000), "Progress Report to the ECOFIN Council on the Impact of Ageing Populations on Public Pension Systems", *www.consilium.europa.eu/uedocs/cmsUpload/Progress%20Report%20on%20the%20impact%20of%20ageing%20population.pdf*.

Gale, W.G. and P.R. Orszag (2003), "Economic Effects of Sustained Budget Deficits", *National Tax Journal*, Vol. 56, No. 3, National Tax Association, Washington, DC, *www.brookings.edu/views/papers/gale/20030717.pdf*.

GAO – United States Government Accountability Office (1999), "Medicare: Outpatient Rehabilitation Therapy Caps Are Important Controls but should Be Adjusted for Patient Need", HEHS 00-15R, Washington, DC, *www.gao.gov/products/GAO/HEHS-00-15R*.

Glaser, W.A. (1991), "Health Insurance in Practice: International Variations in Financing, Benefits and Problems", Jossey-Bass, San Francisco.

Gruber, J. and D. Wise (2002), "An International Perspective on Policies for an Ageing Society", in S.H. Altman and D.I. Shactman (eds.), *Policies for an Ageing Society*, The Johns Hopkins University Press, Baltimore, pp. 34-62.

Henke, K.L. (2011), "Improving Value for Money from a Health Economics Perspective", presented at the First Annual Meeting of Senior Budget Officials (SBO) Network on Health Expenditure; OECD Conference Centre, Paris, 21-22 November 2011, *www.oecd.org/gov/budgeting/49094979.pdf*.

Henke, K.D. and K. Martin (2008), "Health as a Driving Economic Force", *Diskussionspapier 2008/2*, Technische Universität Berlin, *www.wm.tu-berlin.de/fileadmin/f8/wiwidok/diskussionspapiere_wiwidok/dp02-2008.pdf*.

Herd, R. (1989), "The Impact of Increased Government Saving on the Economy", *OECD Department of Economics and Statistics Working Paper*, No. 68. *www.kingsfund.org.uk/projects/general-election-2010/key-election-questions/performance-targets*.

Joumard, I. et al. (2010), "Healthcare Systems: Efficiency and Institutions", *OECD Economics Department Working Papers*, No. 769, *http://search.oecd.org/officialdocuments/displaydocumentpdf/?doclanguage=en&cote=eco/wkp%282010%2925*.

Kaiser Family Foundation (2007), "Snapshots: How Changes in Medical Technology Affect Healthcare Costs", *http://kff.org/health-costs/issue-brief/snapshots-how-changes-in-medical-technology-affect/*.

Karlsson, M. and F. Klohn (2011), "Some Notes on How to Catch a Red Herring: Ageing, Time-to-Death and Care Costs for Older People in Sweden", *Working Paper* No. 2011/6, University of Oslo Health Economics Research Program, *www.med.uio.no/helsam/forskning/nettverk/hero/publikasjoner/skriftserie/2011/2011+6.pdf*.

Labonte, M. (2012), "The Sustainability of the Federal Budget Deficit: Market Confidence and Economic Effects", Report No. R40770, United States Congress, Congressional Research Service, *www.fas.org/sgp/crs/misc/R40770.pdf*.

Medicare Actuaries (1998), "Memorandum: Physician Volume and Intensity Response", *www.cms.gov/Research-Statistics-Data-and-Systems/Research/ActuarialStudies/downloads/PhysicianResponse.pdf*.

Meyers, R.T. (1996), *Strategic Budgeting*, University of Michigan Press, Ann Arbor.

Moran, M. (2000), "Understanding the Welfare State: The Case of Health Care", *British Journal of Politics and International Relations*, Vol. 2/2, John Wiley and Sons, pp. 136-160.

Moreno-Serra, R. (forthcoming), "The Impact of Cost-containment Policies on Health Expenditure: Evidence from Recent OECD Experiences", *OECD Journal on Budgeting* No. 2013/3, OECD Publishing, Paris.

Morgan, D. and R. Astolfi (2013), "Health Spending Growth at Zero: Which Countries, Which Sectors Are Most Affected?" in *OECD Health Working Papers*, No. 60, OECD, Paris, *http://dx.doi.org/10.1787/5k4dd1st95xv-en*.

Nelson, R.M. et al. (2010), "Greece's Debt Crisis: Overview, Policy Responses, and Implications", Report No. R-41167, United States Congress, Congressional Research Service, p. 5, *http://fpc.state.gov/documents/organization/142363.pdf*.

Nolte, E. and M. McKee (2011), "Variations in Amenable Mortality – Trends in 16 High-Income Nations", *Health Policy*, Vol. 103, No. 1, Elsevier, Amsterdam, pp. 47-52.

Nordhaus, W.D. (2006), "Baumol's Diseases: A Macroeconomic Perspective", *NBER Working Paper* No. 12218, National Bureau of Economic Research, *www.nber.org/papers/w12218.pdf?new_window=1*.

OECD (2014a), *Society at a Glance 2014: OECD Social Indicators*, OECD, Paris, *http://dx.doi.org/10.1787/soc_glance-2014-en*.

OECD (2014b), *OECD Economic Outlook* No. 76, Chapter 5, p. 2, December, *www.oecd.org/eco/outlook/34081006.pdf*.

OECD (2013a), "Public Expenditure on Health as a Percentage of Total Expenditure on Health", *OECD Health Statistics Database*, OECD, Paris, *http://dx.doi.org/10.1787/hlthxp-pub-table-2013-2-en*.

OECD (2013b), "Total Expenditure on Health, as a Percentage of Gross Domestic Product", *OECD Health Statistics*, OECD, Paris, *http://dx.doi.org/10.1787/hlthxp-total-table-2013-2-en*.

OECD (2013c), *Education at a Glance 2013: OECD Indicators*, OECD, Paris, *http://dx.doi.org/10.1787/eag-2013-en*.

OECD (2013d), *OECD Factbook: Economic, Environmental and Social Statistics*, p. 249, OECD, Paris, *http://dx.doi.org/10.1787/factbook-2013-en*.

OECD (2013e), "Health Policies and Data", OECD, Paris, *www.oecd.org/newsroom/health-spending-continues-to-stagnate-says-oecd.htm*, accessed 27 June, 2013.

OECD (2012), "Labour Losing to Capital: What Explains the Declining Labour Share?" in *OECD Employment Outlook 2012*, OECD, Paris, *http://dx.doi.org/10.1787/empl_outlook-2012-en*.

OECD (2006), "Projecting Health and Long-Term Care Expenditures: What Are the Main Drivers?" in *OECD Economics Department Working Paper*, No. 477, p. 11, OECD, Paris, *www.oecd.org/tax/public-finance/36085940.pdf*.

OECD (2004), *OECD Economic Outlook*, No. 76, p. 2, OECD, Paris, *http://dx.doi.org/10.1787/eco_outlook-v2004-2-en*.

OECD (1998), "Work Force Ageing: Consequences and Policy Responses", *OECD Working Paper* No. AWP4.1, OECD, Paris, *www.oecd.org/els/public-pensions/2429096.pdf*.

Office of the Assistant Secretary for Planning and Evaluation (ASPE), United States Department of Health and Human Services (2008), "The Effect of Healthcare Cost Growth on the US Economy", Final Report for Task Order, No. HP-06-12, *aspe.hhs.gov/health/reports/o8/healthcarecost/report.pdf*.

Patashnik, E. (2000), *Putting Trust in the US Budget: Federal Trust Funds and the Politics of Commitment*, Cambridge University Press, Cambridge, United Kingdom.

Pearson, M. (2009), "Written Statement to Senate Special Committee on Ageing", *www.oecd.org/unitedstates/43800977.pdf*.

Plumer, B. (2013), "Coal Pollution in China is Cutting Life Expectancy by 5.5 Years", *Washington Post Wonkblog*, July 8, 2013, *www.washingtonpost.com/blogs/wonkblog/wp/2013/07/08/chinas-coal-pollution-is-much-deadlier-than-anyone-realized/*.

Propper, C. et al. (2007), "Did 'Targets and Terror' Reduce Waiting Times in England for Hospital Care?", *Centre for Market and Public Organisation Working Paper*, No. 07/179, *www.bris.ac.uk/cmpo/publications/papers/2007/wp179.pdf*.

Rechel, B. et al. (2009), "How Can Health Systems Respond to Population Ageing?", *European Observatory on Health Systems and Policies Policy Brief*, No. 10, *www.euro.who.int/__data/assets/pdf_file/0004/64966/E92560.pdf*.

Reinhardt, U.E. (1996), "Spending More through 'Cost Control': Our Obsessive Quest to Gut the Hospital", *Health Affairs*, Vol. 15, No. 2, pp. 145-154.

Remler, D.K. and J. Greene (2009), "Cost-Sharing: A Blunt Instrument", *American Journal of Public Health*, Vol. 30, pp. 293-311.

Rice, T.E. (2002), *The Economics of Health Reconsidered*, second ed., Health Administration Press, Chicago.

Rothgang, H. et al. (2010), *The State and Health Care: Comparing OECD Countries*, Palgrave MacMillan, New York.

Schick, A. (2013), "The Metamorphoses of Performance Budgeting", *OECD Journal on Budgeting*, Vol. 13/2, OECD Publishing, Paris, *www.keepeek.com/Digital-Asset-Management/oecd/governance/the-metamorphoses-of-performance-budgeting_budget-13-5jz2jw9szgs8#page1*.

Schick, A. (2009), "Budgeting for Fiscal Space", *OECD Journal on Budgeting*, Vol. 9/2, OECD Publishing, Paris, *http://dx.doi.org/10.1787/budget-9-5ksb4ssm56q2*.

Stock, S., M. Redaelli and K. Wilhelm Lauterbach (2006), "The Influence of the Labour Market on German Healthcare Reforms", *Health Affairs*, Vol. 25, No. 4, July/August 2006, pp. 1146-1148.

Technical Review Panel on the Medicare Trustees Reports (2000), "Review of the Medicare Trustees' Financial Projections", *www.cms.gov/Research-Statistics-Data-and-Systems/Statistics-Trends-and Reports/ReportsTrustFunds/downloads/TechnicalPanelReport2000.pdf*.

United States Government, White House Office of Homeland Security (2002), "National Strategy for Homeland Security", p. 65, *http://permanent.access.gpo.gov/lps20641/nat_strat_hls.pdf*.

Vladeck, B. (1999), "Managed Care's 15 Minutes of Fame", *Journal of Health Politics, Policy and Law*, Vol. 24/5, pp. 1207-1211.

Wallace, A. (2012), "The Case for Calm over Rising Health Costs", *New York Times*, Oct. 6, 2012, *www.nytimes.com/2012/10/07/business/cost-disease-offers-a-case-for-healthcare-calm.html?_r=0*.

Warrell, D.A., T.M. Cox and J.D. Firth (eds.) (2010), "Cost of Health Care in Western Countries", *Oxford Textbook of Medicine*, fifth edition, Vol. 1, pp. 112-116, Oxford University Press, Oxford.

Warren, N. (2008), "A Review of Studies on the Distributional Impact of Consumption Taxes in OECD Countries", *OECD Social, Employment and Migration Working Papers*, No. 64, *http://dx.doi.org/10.1787/241103736767*.

White, J. (2012), "Playing the Wrong PART: The Programme Assessment Rating Tool and the Functions of the President's Budget", *Public Administration Review*, Vol. 72/1, pp. 112-120.

White, J. (2009), "Gap and Parallel Insurance in Healthcare Systems with Mandatory Contributions to a Single Funding Pool for Core Medical and Hospital Benefits for All Citizens in any given Geographic Area", *Journal of Health Politics, Policy and Law*, Vol. 34:4, pp. 543-583.

White, J. (2004), "(How) is Ageing a Health Policy Problem?", *Yale Journal of Health Policy, Law and Ethics*, Vol. 4/1.

White, J. (2003), *False Alarm: Why the Greatest Threat to Social Security and Medicare is the Campaign to "Save" Them*, The Johns Hopkins University Press, Baltimore, pp. 79-80.

White, J. (1999), "Targets and Systems of Healthcare Cost Control", *Journal of Health Politics, Policy and Law*, Vol. 24:4.

White, J. (1998a), "Entitlement Budgeting vs. Bureau Budgeting", *Public Administration Review*, Vol. 58, No. 6, November/December 1998, American Society for Public Administration, John Wiley and Sons.

White, J. (1998b), "Healthcare Reform: What is the Problem?", in T.R. Marmor and P.R. De Jong (eds.), *Ageing, Social Security and Affordability*, Ashgate, Aldershot, United Kingdom, and Brookfield, United States.

White, J. (1998c), "Making 'Common Sense' of Federal Budgeting", *Public Administration Review*, Vol. 58/2, March/April.

Wilensky, H.L. (2002), *Rich Democracies: Political Economy, Public Policy and Performance*, University of California Press, Berkeley.

Wilson, J.Q. (1989), *Bureaucracy: What Government Agencies Do and Why They Do It*, Basic Books, New York.

Fiscal Sustainability of Health Systems
Bridging Health and Finance Perspectives

Chapter 3

Budgeting practices for health in OECD countries

by
Camila Vammalle, Ankit Kumar, Claudia Hulbert and Gijs van der Vlugt*

This chapter presents the results of an OECD survey of budget officials on budgeting practices for health, which aims at shedding light on the different institutional frameworks, and the instruments available to control health care expenditure in OECD countries. Health represents an important share of public spending, and one that has consistently increased faster than other areas of spending, and faster than GDP. However, controlling public health expenditure growth is particularly difficult for budget officials. A number of factors and institutions are necessary to allow governments to control health expenditure and ensure their fiscal sustainability: long-term forecasts, medium-term projections, timely information on expenditure, adequate revenues, expenditure management tools, monitoring and evaluation procedures, political agreement on targets and co-ordination mechanisms.

* Camila Vammalle and Ankit Kumar are with the OECD, Claudia Hulbert is a consultant and Gijs van der Vlugt is with the Ministry of Finance in the Netherlands.

3.1. Introduction

Health represents an important share of public spending, and one that has consistently increased faster than other areas of spending and faster than GDP. However, as the previous chapter shows, controlling public health expenditure growth is particularly difficult for budget officials. There are two main reasons for this. First, health care is perceived by citizens as a very high priority, with government policies in this area highly scrutinised. Second, there are a great number of stakeholders that intervene between the beneficiary of health care (the citizen/patient) and public resources that finance it. These include: purchasers (such as Ministries of Health, social security institutions, social insurance funds or sub-national governments), a wide range of providers of services (clinicians with different specialities, operating within hospitals and other health facilities), and providers of medicines, tests and equipment (such as pharmaceutical companies and laboratories).

A number of specific factors and institutions are therefore necessary for governments to be able to control health care expenditure growth and ensure its fiscal sustainability (Figure 3.1).

First, governments need accurate information about health care spending and funding sources to "diagnose" its fiscal sustainability. This includes:

- long-term forecasts of the likely evolution of health care spending, given demographic and economic factors, to anticipate trends and drive policy reforms;
- medium-term (three-year to five-year) spending requirements governments can use to draft their budgets;
- timely information about actual spending to enable governments to take early corrective measures if spending targets are likely to be broken;
- evaluation of the evolution of possible revenue sources (taxes and/or contributions) to link spending requirements and projections to available resources.

Second, political and institutional factors that shape the context must be taken into account. While these can be influenced in the medium to long term, they can be taken as given in the short term. Lack of these political and institutional factors could be "risk factors" for the fiscal sustainability of health systems. These factors include:

- political agreement on the need to control health expenditure growth and on specific spending targets;
- effective co-ordination mechanisms among all the different stakeholders, which respond to different incentives;
- the degree of decentralisation of health services (in terms of functions and revenues);
- the boundaries between public and private spending on health, i.e. the definition of the health benefits basket.

Finally, there are a number of policy levers and tools ("treatments") that governments can put in place to ensure greater sustainability of health spending without compromising important achievements in access and quality of health care. These will be further discussed in Chapters 5 and 6. They can be grouped into four categories: supply-side, demand-side, public management and co-ordination, and revenues:

- *Supply-side policy levers include*: developing provider payment methods that ensure the right incentives; provider competition; generic substitution; and joint purchasing.
- *Demand-side tools include*: gatekeeping and preferred drug lists. Cost sharing may help to control costs but risk have negative effects on health.
- *Public management and co-ordination policies include*: direct controls on pharmaceutical prices/profits, health technology assessment and monitoring and evaluation.
- *Financing policies*: increased revenues or changing revenue sources for health care.

Figure 3.1. **Fiscal sustainability framework**

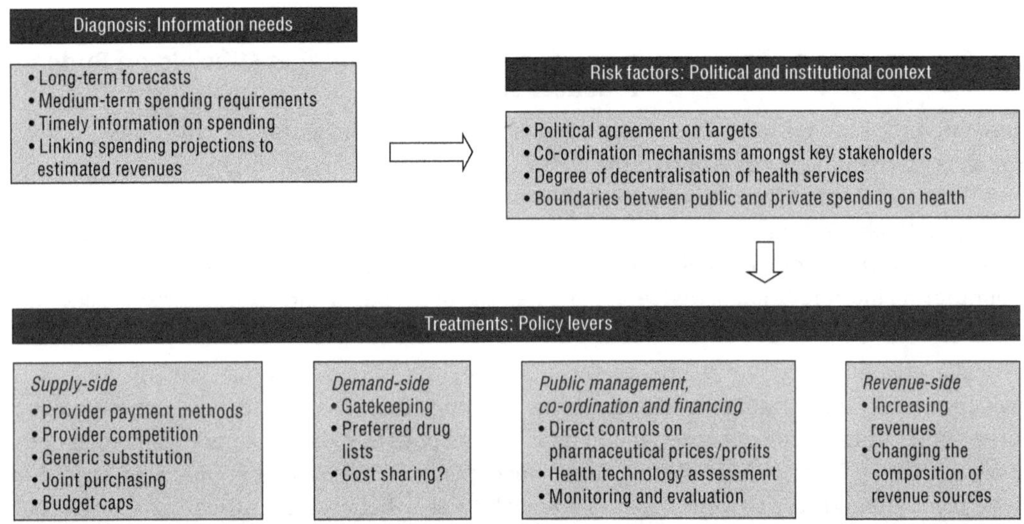

OECD countries have developed different institutional frameworks to address the above requisites. To shed light on these institutional frameworks, and the instruments available to control health care expenditure, the OECD surveyed budget officials on budgeting practices in the health sector. This survey was answered by 27 countries[1] and six sub-national governments (Canadian provinces). The results were discussed at a workshop of budget officials held in January 2014 and at the OECD SBO-Health Joint Network on Fiscal Sustainability of Health Systems in April 2014.

This chapter summarises the key results from the survey. It is organised into four sections which cover respectively: the role of health in the budget process, policies used by budget agencies to influence health spending, decision-making by budget agencies and the challenges of budgeting for health in decentralised contexts.

The majority of results obtained from the survey are descriptive; but a few challenge popular perceptions about the relationship between health and finance. The survey finds that:

- Budget agencies do not perceive co-operation with Ministries of Health to be poor, despite the common view of other commentators that this is a major problem.
- Budget Ministries' main role consists of setting overall fiscal objectives, not exercising detailed control over spending and leaving allocation decisions to Health Ministries.

- While Health Ministries (and academic health policy circles) increasingly emphasise economic assessments of health and labour market impacts of health policies, in many countries, these have little or no influence on budget agencies. This is due to a combination of insufficient capacity in Ministries of Finance to process them and a focus and presentation of these evaluations which may not be optimal to facilitate their use.
- Although long-term projections for health expenditure complement short-term budget policy decisions and help to shape medium-term to long-term policies, the usefulness of such spending projections may be limited by the uncertainty surrounding their estimates, and because budget agencies are principally concerned with the immediate fiscal years.

Box 3.1. **Caveats and challenges of the OECD Survey of Budget Officials on Budgeting Practices for Health**

Implemented for the first time, the survey used to derive these insights is a novel but blunt tool. The survey sought to combine information in the OECD's Budgeting Survey (on budgeting at large) and those from the Health Systems Characteristics Survey. Comments were sought from the WHO, the European Observatory on Health Systems and Policies and selected country officials before this was put to countries. At the workshop of budget officials held in Paris in January 2014, countries noted that there was considerable scope for differing interpretation of budgeting and health vocabularies and efforts have subsequently been made to improve the accuracy of responses provided.

A particular area of difficulty remains decentralised health care systems (particularly, Austria, Canada and Sweden) which found it difficult to answer the questions from the central government point of view or pointed out that their influence extended to only a small portion of health spending. Canada presented the survey to the provinces, and six provinces provided answers. Differences in practices, procedures and challenges faced among these provinces are as large as those seen between countries. The specific challenges of decentralised countries for health care sustainability are further discussed in Chapter 4. Furthermore, a number of questions that sought to gauge performance through self-reporting had potentially inconsistent results, such as budget agencies noting that health has been a difficult area to achieve savings and then reporting positively in terms of their self-perceived success in containing spending.

The survey nonetheless confirmed the popular perception that health is considered by budget officials to be one of the most difficult areas to achieving savings. Some preliminary operational and policy implications include:

- Health Ministries should work with Budget Ministries to make their economic evaluations of health and labour market benefits better understood and more influential in prioritising policies.
- Further efforts to return efficiency gains to budget could help avoid the use of tools that indiscriminately reduce broad categories of health spending.
- Some countries have scope to improve timeliness of spending data to help them track spending, take corrective measures and avoid the need for unplanned savings to meet end-of-year targets.
- Finance Ministries share Health Ministries' concerns about spending in hospital and pharmaceutical sectors, and are concerned about the fiscal sustainability of sub-national governments.

3.2. Approaches in budgeting for health care

There is considerable diversity in how much health spending is included in the government budget; in social insurance countries this can complicate achieving a fiscal position for the public sector

The budgeting process for health tends to be modelled around the key institutions responsible for financing health in a particular country. Three typologies stand out from the results of this survey:

1. Centralised national health systems, where the bulk of health care expenditure is in the central government's budget and determined along with the rest of government spending.
2. Social insurance systems, which have a separate budget for health, with specific revenues assigned to it unlike other government spending. The central government budget often provides subsidies towards the cost of insurance and support for public health programmes.
3. Decentralised health systems, where most health care expenditure is controlled by sub-national governments and is therefore included in a combination of central government and sub-national governments' budgets.

In all OECD countries, some or all health spending is included in the government budget. Most budget-funded countries predictably identified that they include health care in the government budget. Even in the 18 countries (out of 27), with independent social security or insurance funds, or where health is a sub-national responsibility, some expenditures were noted to be part of the central government budget (Table 3.1).

Table 3.1. **Is health care expenditure part of central government budget?**

Partly	Fully
Austria (1)	Hungary
Canada (2)	Iceland
Chile (3)	New Zealand
Czech Rep. (4)	United Kingdom
Denmark (5)	
Estonia (6)	
Finland	
France (7)	
Germany (8)	
Italy (9)	
Japan (10)	
Korea (11)	
Netherlands	
Norway (12)	
Poland (13)	
Portugal	
Slovak Republic (14)	
Slovenia	
South Africa	
Sweden (15)	
Switzerland	
Turkey (16)	

Notes

1. In Austria, a small part (2010: 4.2%) of overall public health expenditure is in the central government´s (Ministry of Health) budget. The public health care system is mainly financed by the Social Security System (65.2%) and via the automatic transfer system to state and local governments (30.7%).

2. In Canada, the federal government provides transfers to sub-national governments for health. The Canada Health Transfer provides funding to all provinces and territories for health care, and supports the principles of the Canada Health Act which are: universality; comprehensiveness; portability; accessibility; and, public administration. Equalisation, for those provinces that receive it, and Territorial Formula Financing provide unconditional funding for receiving provinces and the territories to fund their priorities, including heath care. Outside of federal transfers, the rest of provincial and territorial health care is financed through provincial and territorial revenues. The federal government also provides direct health care spending in areas of federal responsibility, consisting of First Nations' and veterans' health care, health promotion, disease prevention, and health-related research.

3. In Chile, central government budget encompasses 97.7% of public expenditure on health (including the compulsory contribution to health of 7% of wages). Only the expenditure carried out by municipalities, which represent 2.3% of total public health expenditure, are not included in the central government budget.

4. The Czech Republic operates a public health insurance system. Each citizen pays public health insurance contributions as a percentage of their income, and these are not considered as state revenue for budget purposes. The government funds contributions for lower-income citizens. This represents about 23% of total revenues of the public health insurance.

5. In Denmark, government funding of regions (health) and municipalities (partly health) is part of the central government budget.

6. In Estonia, Social tax revenue for health insurance which transferred to Estonian Health Insurance Fund is a component of central government budget.

7. Only a small share of total health spending appears in the central government budget. Most health expenditure are within the Social Security institution, and are included in a separate social security budget law, which is voted annually by the Parliament, together with the "national target for health insurance spending" (*Objectif national des dépenses d'assurance maladie*, ONDAM).

8. In Germany, the federal budget contains a large federal grant to the statutory health insurance (SHI).

9. In Italy, only the share of health expenditure financed by VAT revenue is included in the central government budget.

10. In Japan, almost all health expenditures (such as the National Health Insurance and the elderly medical insurance system) are shared between central and local governments. Therefore, only part of this expenditure appears in the central government budget.

11. In Korea, the National Health Insurance Corporation collects the premiums. However, the central government funds 20% of contributions.

12. In Norway, municipalities are responsible for primary health care and care for the elderly, and the counties are responsible for dental care. These expenditures do not appear in the central government budget.

13. In Poland, most of health care expenditure is carried out by the National Health Fund and financed by health care premiums, and are not included in the central government budget. The role of the budget is limited. It provides funds for health programmes of special importance concerning overall health policy targets (such as development of transplantology, or counteraction of modern civilisation diseases), health insurance premiums for specific groups of the population (the unemployed receiving social security benefits, persons receiving social pensions, farmers, war veterans and others), and investments in public health care institutions, highly specialised services, as well as general expenditures concerning formulation, administration, co-ordination and monitoring of overall health policies, plans, programmes and budgets, preparation and enforcement of legislation, etc. executed by the Ministry of Health.

14. In the Slovak Republic, the budget includes expenditures of the Ministry of Health and of the Office for Health Care Surveillance.

15. In Sweden, most of health expenditure is carried out by sub-national government and thus does not appear in the central government budget. However, the central government budget includes expenditures for OTC pharmaceuticals, general government grants to the county councils, and some earmarked special grants and expenditures on government agencies in the health sector.

16. In Turkey, the majority of health expenditures is in the Social Security Institution budget and does not appear in the central government budget.

Source: OECD Survey of Budget Officials on Budgeting Practices for Health, 2013, Question 1.

Many social insurance countries provide subsidies on insurance contributions for low-income or specific groups such as veterans (Estonia, France, Germany, Korea, Poland and Switzerland) direct from their budget. In decentralised countries, the central government often provides transfers for health to sub-national governments, which appear as health care spending in the government budget (Austria, Canada, Denmark, Norway and Sweden). The central government also usually finances prevention or special interest programmes, medical research or investments (Canada, France and Poland) and the allocation of funds to cover general expenditures for formulation, co-ordination and monitoring of overall health policies, plans, programmes and budgets, and for the enforcement of legislation by the Ministry of Health (Austria, Poland, France and the Slovak Republic). These results suggest that the government's budgetary process is an important tool in determining overall spending and achieving policy objectives.

Challenges arise for budget agencies where social security spending is either not subject to legislative review or occurs on a different timeline to the government budget. In most countries (10 out of 18) which have separate health/social security budgets, the latter does not require separate legislative approval, and more than half do not present information about health/social security budgeting in the general budget documentation. These indicators are symptomatic of what is often a broader disconnect between budgets for health spending and for the government at large.

Where social security budgets occur at a different timeline to the rest of the government budget, it can complicate the task of budget officials. The evolution of revenues from or spending in social health insurance results in a need to modify spending in other parts of government to ensure that these both fit within the overall fiscal target for the public sector. In some cases, deficits in social insurance can require additional funding from government budgets and crowd out other budgetary priorities (e.g. spending in another area or fiscal consolidation). This has been an area where certain countries, such as France, have undertaken considerable efforts to align the process for the social security budget with that of the government budget so they are determined simultaneously and the government can decide the extent to which fiscal objectives are met through health or other areas.

Finance Ministries do not tend to prescribe the allocation of funds within health

Budget agencies noted that, more so than in other areas of government spending, they generally leave the allocation of spending and its scrutiny to a combination of Ministries of Health and social insurance agencies. Since the 1990s, the prevailing trend across OECD countries has been a shift towards "top-down" budgeting practices where the executive determines aggregate public finance targets (spending and revenue levels) given medium-term fiscal objectives and prevailing economic conditions. Sectoral ceilings are then set (and approved by the executive), reflecting existing commitments, political priorities and key new policy initiatives. The detailed allocation decisions are then usually delegated to the individual line ministries. Top-down budgeting marks a shift in budgetary roles from a more controlling budget agency and provides line ministries with relatively greater responsibility for resource allocation and for supervising spending.

This shift towards a more supervisory role is evident in the extent to which budget agencies do not allocate budgets on the basis of achieving specific health objectives nor towards sub-categories within health spending. About half of the countries (14 out of 27) allocate funds to specific health objectives (preventing cancer, palliative care, Alzheimer, etc.) (Table 3.A1.3). Roughly the same proportion (13 out of 27) specify sub-categories of health care spending (such as hospital in-patient service, primary care, pharmaceuticals), of which five countries only use them for informative (non-binding) purposes (Table 3.A1.3). In countries which specify sub-categories of health care spending in the budget, the number of such categories varies from seven in Australia and France, to above 200 in Iceland, with Hungary and Netherlands being more typical in specifying

18 and 50 respectively. Even in these countries, there is a considerable disparity on the extent to which different sub-categories are actually used to determine the budget at large; they are often focused on funding a supplementary function.

Most countries produce long-term projections, but these are rarely used for decision making

Almost all OECD countries now produce long-term projections of health spending and these are generally publicly available. Among the 26 countries which answered this question, only the Czech Republic, Hungary, Poland and the Slovak Republic do not. In the majority of cases (16 out of 26 countries), these cover 31 to 50 years. Denmark has the longest horizon, as its technical projections run until 2100. These projections are usually publicly available (except in five countries). Long-term projections cover public health expenditure in all the countries surveyed, and most of them (20) provide projections by categories of health spending (e.g. hospitals, primary care, pharmaceuticals) (Figure 3.2 and Table 3.A1.4). Expenditure projections by age group are also quite frequent (ten countries). Fewer countries provide total health expenditure (public, private and by social insurance institutions) and private health expenditure projections (eight and four countries respectively). The responsibility for carrying out long-term projections lies usually in the Ministry of Health (15 of 27 countries); but in almost half of the countries (12 of 27), the Ministry of Finance also carries out these projections, with some countries having both ministries doing so (eight of 27). Independent institutions are also frequent sources of long-term projections (five of 27), as well as other institutions (such as health insurance funds) (seven of 24).

Figure 3.2. **Coverage of long-term health expenditure projections**

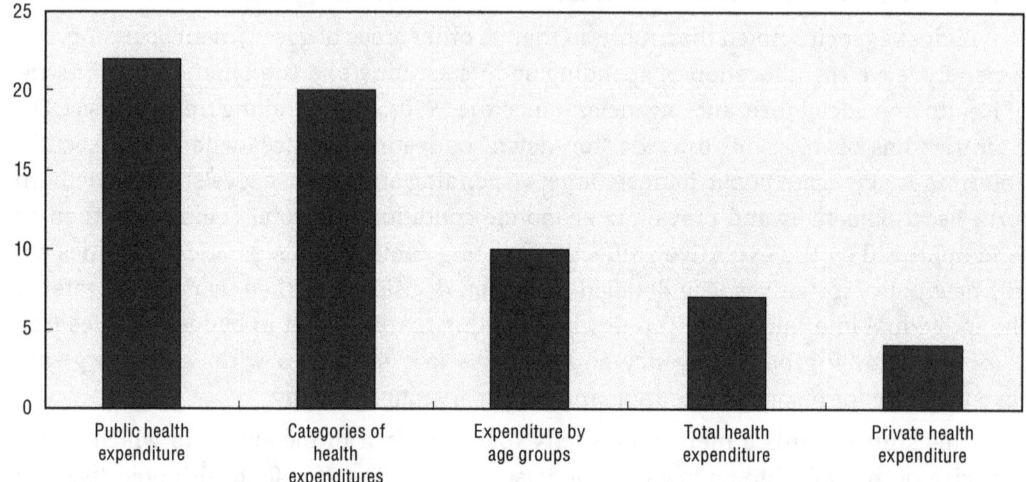

Note: For Finland, private health expenditure projections only concern those expenditures covered by health insurance and public-funded compensation.

Source: OECD Survey of budget officials on budgeting practices for health, 2013, Question 11, OECD, Paris.

StatLink http://dx.doi.org/10.1787/888933218666

While considerable effort is invested in long-term projections, these are more often used to influence public debate for difficult reforms than to guide decision making in the current year. The majority of countries responded that the key function of long-term projections is to identify challenges future governments will face and provide information to and raise the awareness of the public. In Australia these projections were used to justify recent health financing reforms, as they showed that under the existing framework, health care expenditure would soon exceed states' revenue-raising capacity. In the European Union, the ageing working group forecasts long-term sustainability of public spending, including health care. In European Union countries, the results of forecasts feed into the assessment by the Commission and Council of governments' financial sustainability. The relationship between forecasts and policy is probably most explicit in the United States, where legislation on health is evaluated on its supposed effects several decades into the future. Congress has an obligation to ensure the financial solvency of the trust fund from which Medicare's hospital insurance is funded, or payments are reduced to levels such that it can be financed entirely through tax revenues and premiums. However, in practice, law makers have overridden these planned reductions every year since 2003.

The utility of long-term projections is limited by the considerable uncertainty surrounding their estimates, and because budget agencies are ultimately held accountable for the immediate years. Budget agencies noted that the denominator in these forecasts – generally GDP or government spending – is difficult to predict meaningfully, reducing the utility of projections for them. With discussions about health often involving arguments that new policies require considerable lags to take effect (e.g. electronic health, prevention policies), it was noted that longer-term fiscal evaluations may justify some policies which would not seem interesting if only the short-term was considered, but there was scepticism about whether these would lead to actual savings.

3.3. Expenditure control tools

With most countries seeking to target a budget trajectory as well a fiscal position in a certain year, it has become important for budget agencies to have a multi-year vision of health spending.

Most countries have targets or ceilings for spending over several years, though ultimately it is economic and not health-specific factors that determine their level

As they are obliged to publish estimates for public spending for several years, most OECD countries publish health expenditure estimates for the coming three to five years. While the majority of countries provide three-year estimates, it ranges from zero (in Portugal) to five (in Netherlands and Korea) (Figure 3.3).

Most OECD countries use some kind of budget ceiling over several years for central government's expenditure on health. In 80% of surveyed countries, budget agencies developed a desired level of spending for health, and this target was reached in about two-thirds of cases. Even in countries that specify targets and not ceilings, these have become more and more binding over time. This survey only enquired about ceilings that apply to central government expenditure which is included in the budget, not those that may apply to expenditure by social security institutions, private insurers or sub-national governments (Box 3.2). Ceilings may be overall ceilings on expenditure by the Ministry of Health (36%), constrain specific categories of health services (e.g. hospitals, primary care) (35%) or be set for particular programmes (16%) (Table 3.A1.5). The popularity of ceilings reflects the perception by Budget Ministries that Health Ministries are best placed to determine where potential efficiency gains lie in their portfolio.

Figure 3.3. **Years of estimates for health spending in the budget**

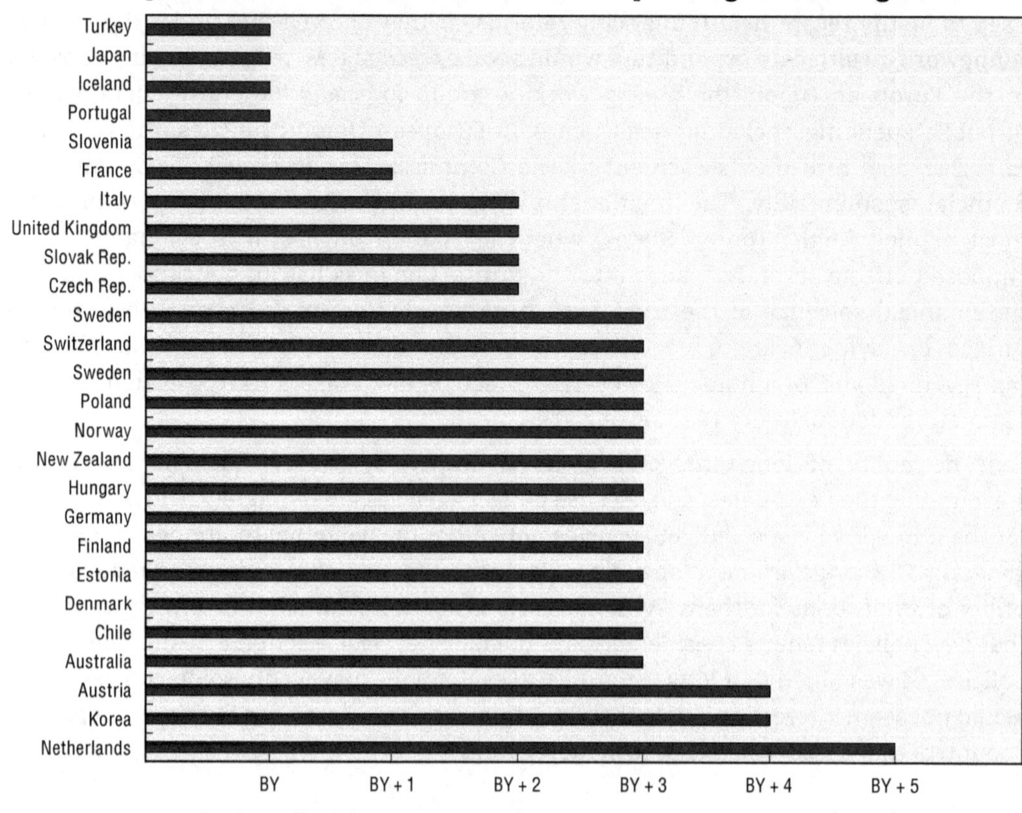

Source: OECD Survey of Budget Officials on Budgeting Practices for Health, 2013, Question 7.

StatLink http://dx.doi.org/10.1787/888933218675

Box 3.2. **Ceilings on health expenditure by sub-national governments or social security institutions**

Austria: There are ceilings on health expenditure by the social security system and states, but these are approved by other laws (agreement between the states and the federal level and a law on health reform).

Denmark: Since 2014, all government spending is subject to real expenditure ceilings. This implies a separate four-year budget ceiling for regional governments' expenditure on health (which represent more than 75% of total public health spending), as well as a specific expenditure ceiling for municipalities, which includes health. This system sets a flat spending level for four budget years, which is the basis for subsequent annual negotiations between the central government and local authorities on the spending level for the forthcoming year. Any upward change in the ceilings for sub-national governments must be compensated by the same reduction in the budget ceiling for central government expenditure. A violation of these fixed expenditure ceilings would entail economic sanctions.

Poland: The expenditure ceiling for the National Health Fund is set for the budget year and consists of an overall ceiling and ceilings by categories of health services. Procedures for amending these ceilings are stipulated in law. Financial plans of the National Health Fund cover three subsequent years (BY+3), but they are only estimates and not ceilings.

Source: OECD Survey of Budget Officials on Budgeting Practices for Health, 2013, Question 45.

Ceilings for health expenditure tend to reflect executive priorities about the budget and not factors specific to health. These are most frequently set by the central budget authority (43% of countries), by the Parliament (24%), by executive branches of government and their agencies (e.g. the Prime Minister, President and their offices), and by independent bodies (5%) (Table 3.A1.6). The objectives for the fiscal position and the outlook for GDP growth were identified as the key priorities for setting ceilings in most countries (Figure 3.4). The results show that economic factors dominate over considerations of health policy in the perspective of Finance Ministries and governments, as is to be expected.

Figure 3.4. **Factors influencing ceilings for health**

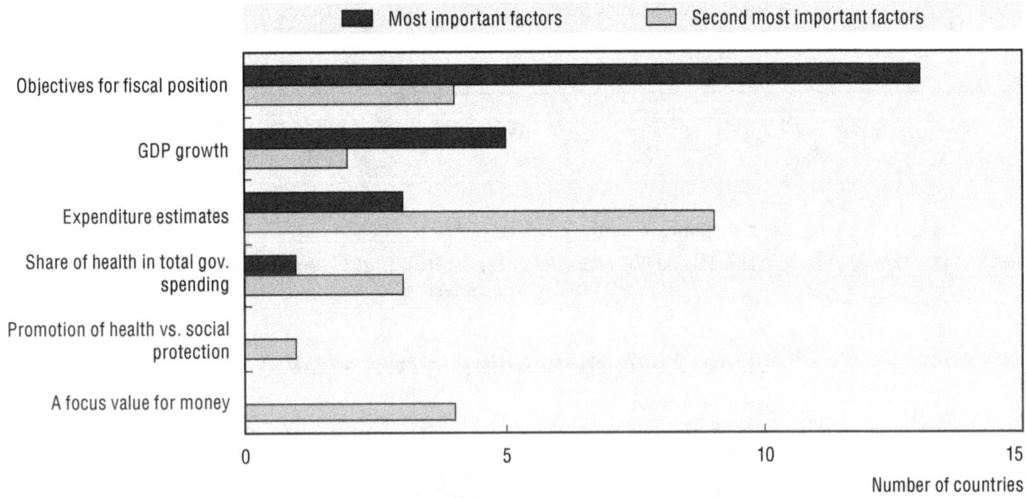

Source: OECD Survey of Budget Officials on Budgeting Practices for Health, 2013, Question 47.

StatLink http://dx.doi.org/10.1787/888933218689

Despite ceilings, budget overruns in health remains common and often leads to unplanned savings demands at the end of the year

A crude measure of the success of both ceilings and the accuracy of central government budget estimates is the extent of budget overruns and underspending. Many countries have frequent budget overruns (i.e. actual health care expenditure exceeding budgeted expenditure) though the average varies greatly between countries. More importantly, the dispersion around the average was very large and there was no systematic correlation with countries that identified themselves as having ceilings or targets. In the last seven years, most countries have experienced both budget overruns and underspending (Figure 3.5). The few countries with consistently low average variations were predominately budget-funded (Australia, New Zealand and the United Kingdom), which may reflect that their control over health system management provides them with greater budgetary control. France was an exception to this rule, perhaps reflecting recent policy efforts to impose spending targets on social security spending.

In response to persistent budget overruns, a majority of countries have developed early warning mechanisms to follow the path of health expenditure through the year and identify when targets may be broken (Figure 3.6, Table 3.A1.8 and Box 3.1).

Figure 3.5. **Size of budget overruns and underspending in percentage of budgeted spending, 2006-12**

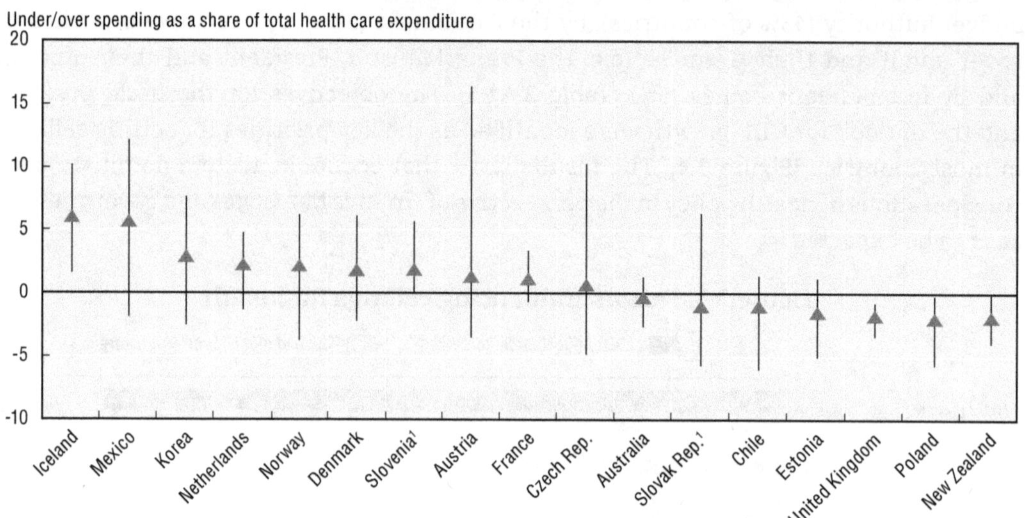

1. Slovenia and the Slovak Republic data are for the past five years.

Source: OECD Survey of Budget Officials on Budgeting Practices for Health, 2013, Question 48.

StatLink http://dx.doi.org/10.1787/888933218691

Figure 3.6. **Early-warning systems (EWS)**

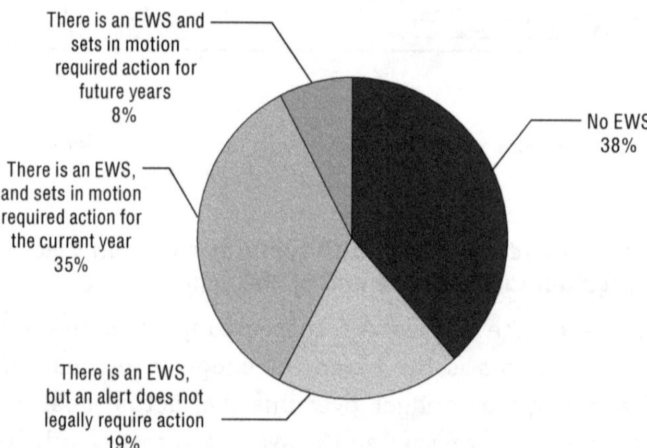

Source: OECD Survey of Budget Officials on Budgeting Practices for Health, 2013, Question 49.

StatLink http://dx.doi.org/10.1787/888933218701

A prerequisite for an early warning mechanism – and to monitor and control budgets in general – is to have timely information. This is a challenge for many countries, particularly those with a social-health-insurance-based system. In most countries, the central budget authority receives information from one to six months after the spending occurs (Figure 3.8). In others, it may take up to two years for some spending information to reach budget authorities (such as spending by hospitals and psychiatric institutions in Netherlands). In most cases, the delay is explained by data-collection issues or reporting from health care institutions/insurers (Netherlands) or sub-national governments (Switzerland). Budget agencies noted that delays in information made it harder for them to work with Health Ministries to take corrective measures through the year and in some cases prompt additional savings within a short time frame to meet end-of-year fiscal objectives.

Box 3.3. **Early warning mechanism in France**

The national objective for health care expenditure (ONDAM) was introduced in France in 1996. During the first decades, the ONDAM targets were consistently overrun, leading to large social security deficits (see Figure 3.7). In 2004, the administration decided to introduce stricter monitoring of health care spending through the creation of an Alert Committee. The committee's responsibilities, progressively enlarged over time, are to alert the Parliament, the government and the National Health Insurance Fund about increases in health care expenditure that could exceed the ONDAM targets.

The government annually sets the level of accepted deficits for national objectives (0.5% since 1 January 2013). The Alert Committee must follow a defined schedule throughout the year. First, it must assess health care spending in the previous year to re-evaluate the basis for the national objective and assess whether planned policies are in line with them. Secondly, it must state whether objectives for the current year are likely to be met or to remain within authorised overruns. If this is not the case, the committee must notify the three institutions, which have to propose correcting measures within a month. The committee must then provide an evaluation of the possible impact of these recovery measures. Finally, the committee must publish an evaluation of the current year's prospects for meeting the national objectives, and the determinants for the following year's target. It can raise concerns if it estimates that growth-rate projections and proposed savings are not realistic.

Figure 3.7. **Voted ONDAM vs. achieved health expenditures**

Percentage growth

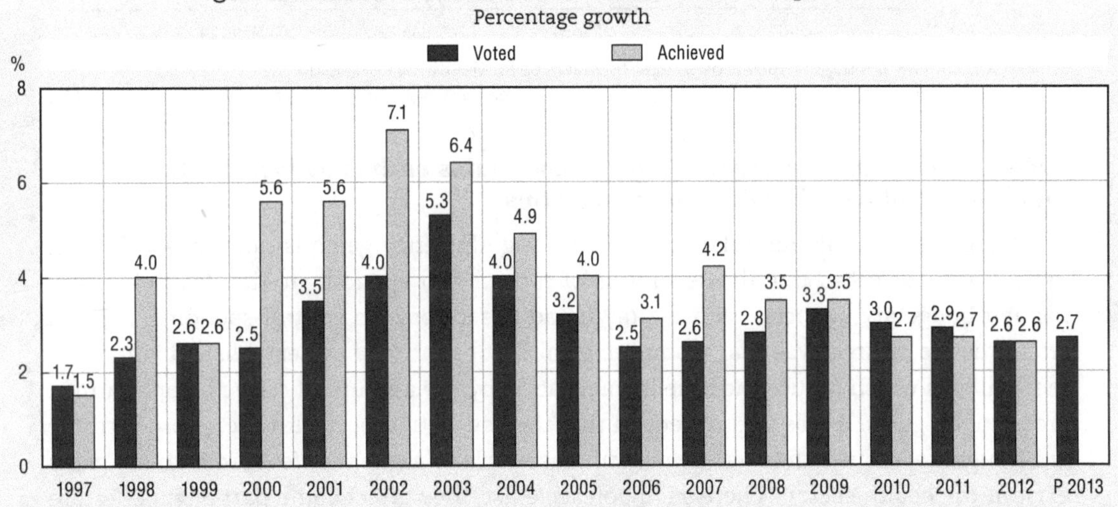

Source: Projet de Loi de Financement de la Sécurité Sociale, Social Security Accounts, Social Security Directorate, Paris.

StatLink http://dx.doi.org/10.1787/888933218716

The introduction of the Alert Committee led to a significant decrease in the growth rate of health care expenditure in France over the last decade (from 7% in 2002 to 3% in 2010). National objectives have been met since 2010. However, future target forecasts should allow for a 2.5% growth in health care spending (instead of 3%), hence introducing further savings to be made in the health care sector.

Source: see Chapter 8 on French case study.

Figure 3.8. **Delay in reporting health expenditure to central budget authority (CBA)**

In months, maximum value

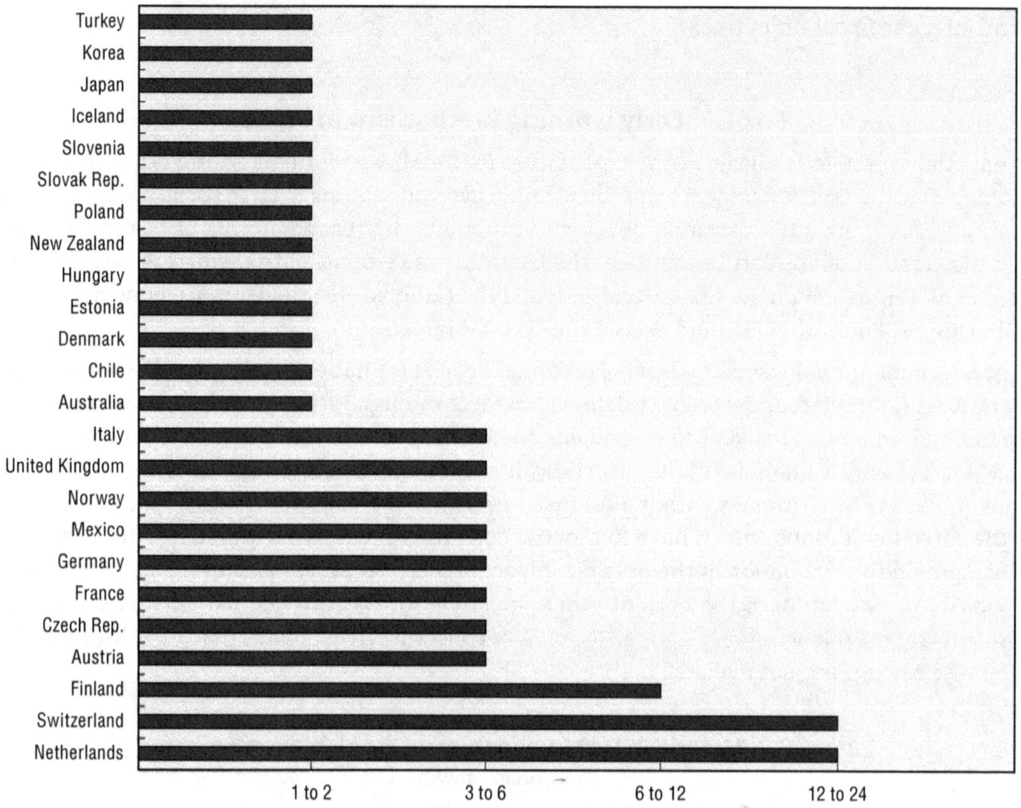

Source: OECD Survey of Budget Officials on Budgeting Practices for Health, 2013, Question 22.

StatLink http://dx.doi.org/10.1787/888933218726

Budget agencies are seeking to bring efficiency gains back to budget, but feel they have blunt tools by which to try to do this

Budgetary officials remarked that harvesting efficiency gains is notoriously difficult in health. It was noted that the devolution of control over spending to the Health Ministry has left budgetary agencies with mainly broad-based tools to control spending. A novel alternative to ceilings was that around one-third of countries have established automatic mechanisms which reduce the baseline allocation by the amount of expected or assumed productivity gains. It was acknowledged that the estimation of health sector productivity is a fraught task, but that it was equally unreasonable to argue that few productivity gains exist in the health sector. Where such policies exist, they affect some part of expenditure only (e.g. hospital budgets) (Table 3.A1.9). In some countries, the growth rate of health care expenditure is capped (Austria). In Canada, the growth of the federal block transfer for health (the Canada Health Transfer) provided to provinces and territories is fixed. However, there are not targets for the total health care expenditures of the country: most expenditure decisions are made at the provincial/territorial level, and their governments have the option, but not the obligation, to set caps on their expenditures. In other countries, objectives or budgets are set in terms of productivity gains to be reached (Denmark and the United Kingdom); New Zealand and Israel do not compensate fully for health price inflation. The main category of spending affected by automatic cuts is pharmaceuticals.

Spending reviews have been used in about half of surveyed countries to pinpoint savings in particular areas. In Australia, Denmark and Netherlands, these often do not target overall health care expenditure, but some sub-category of spending. Reviews are implemented yearly in only a few countries (Chile, Netherlands and Turkey). A few countries have conducted yearly reviews only since the beginning of the global financial crisis (France). In the United Kingdom, reviews are systematic but cover a three-year period. Canada conducted Strategic Reviews over the 2007-11 period, targeting different ministries each year. In this context, the Department of Health was reviewed in 2011. Most countries conduct regular reviews, according to governments' priorities (Australia, Hungary, Italy and Poland). Mexico and New Zealand conducted a single evaluation review in 2009.

Some countries also use incentive-based mechanisms to reach efficiency gains. In Denmark, for example, 2% of hospital budgets is provided in the form of a crude "pay for performance" arrangement that is only granted if the hospital provides 2% more activity with the same budget. In Israel, the formula by which the central government transfers funds to the health funds has a component to compensate for price inflation. But in practice, price inflation is not fully compensated, which is a way of pushing health funds to seek productivity gains. Finally, about half of the countries surveyed have performance agreements for the Ministry of Health, with the executive usually in charge of setting performance indicators.

3.4. Decision making and assessment

Perhaps the area that causes the most consternation for Health Ministries is the gatekeeping role of budget agencies in assessing new policy proposals. Budget agencies noted that their assessment predominately focused on fiscal considerations and the robustness of the policy's design.

Health care is usually an open-ended entitlement, possibly making spending control more difficult

There is enormous variation in the extent to which health care spending is considered as an entitlement or a discretionary programme. Mandatory health spending was defined as an open-ended entitlement (i.e. demand driven) which requires the Legislature to modify a law in order to change the level of spending. While on average, about half of health spending is mandatory, there are wide variations (Figure 3.9). While it is possible that countries with higher mandatory spending may simply engage Parliaments more frequently, in practice budget agencies noted this made changes more difficult to achieve.

Central budget authorities mainly focus on macro-fiscal aspects of health care spending

The survey found that central budget authorities see themselves as being mainly occupied with macrofiscal supervision of health care and are less involved in designing or implementing policy in health. The most commonly identified responsibilities for budget agencies were assessing health policy proposals, estimating future health spending, proposing desirable amounts of health care expenditure and/or advising on spending priorities (Figure 3.10). In most countries, central budget authorities are not involved in the development or implementation of health policies (Table 3.A1.10).

Figure 3.9. **Share of discretionary vs. mandatory health spending, average 2006-12**

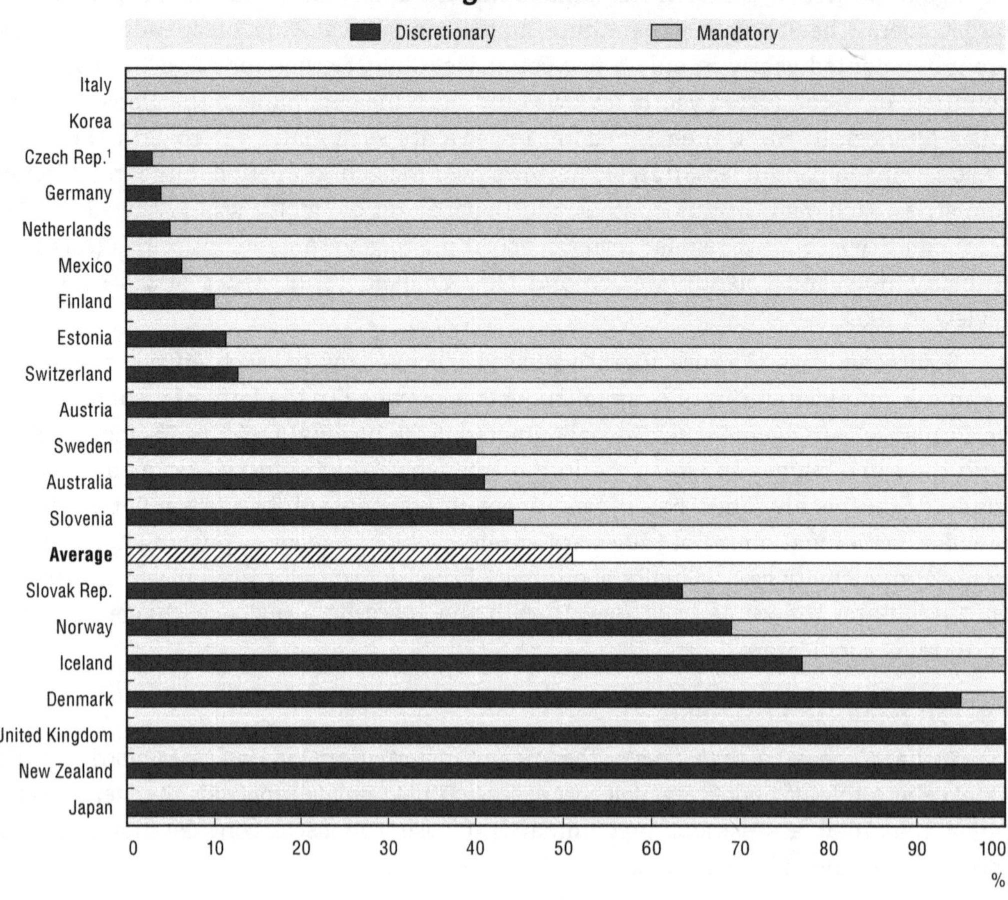

1. In the Czech Republic, the 3% of health expenditure included in the government budget are discretionary. The remaining 97% can be considered as mandatory.

Source: OECD Survey of Budget Officials on Budgeting Practices for Health, 2013, Question 5.

StatLink http://dx.doi.org/10.1787/888933218731

Central budget authorities tend to perceive that they have little influence on health policy issues such as listing new drugs or medical services, while they perceive themselves to have considerable influence on spending on health programmes and payments to doctors or pharmaceutical prices (Figure 3.11). In most countries, the central budget authority also plays a crucial role along with the Ministry of Health in estimating financial changes from a modification to existing health programmes (Table 3.A1.11).

The survey shows that the two highest priority areas for cost control for budget agencies are hospital expenditure and pharmaceutical costs (Figure 3.12 and Table 3.A1.12). This suggests a degree of consensus with the policy ambitions of their colleagues in health.

Economic evaluations provided by Health Ministries are often not influential for budget agencies, which acknowledge they struggle with having capacity to assess such issues

While in most countries budget authorities receive economic evaluations of the expected health benefits from new policy proposals suggested by the Ministry of Health, these are not reported to be a major factor in the prioritisation of policies. Around 70% of budget agencies noted that they received economic evaluations from Health Ministries for all or some policies (Table 3.A1.14). However, they also noted that these assessments count "to a lesser extent" in their assessment of policy proposals (Table 3.A1.15). This suggests a lack of connection between the economic evaluations being conducted within Health Ministries (and academic health policy circles) and their perceived utility to budget agencies. Similarly, 68% of budget agencies responded that equity considerations are either the responsibility of the Health Ministry or something they are not actively engaged with (Table 3.A1.16).

Figure 3.10. **Main healthcare-related functions undertaken by the central budget authority**

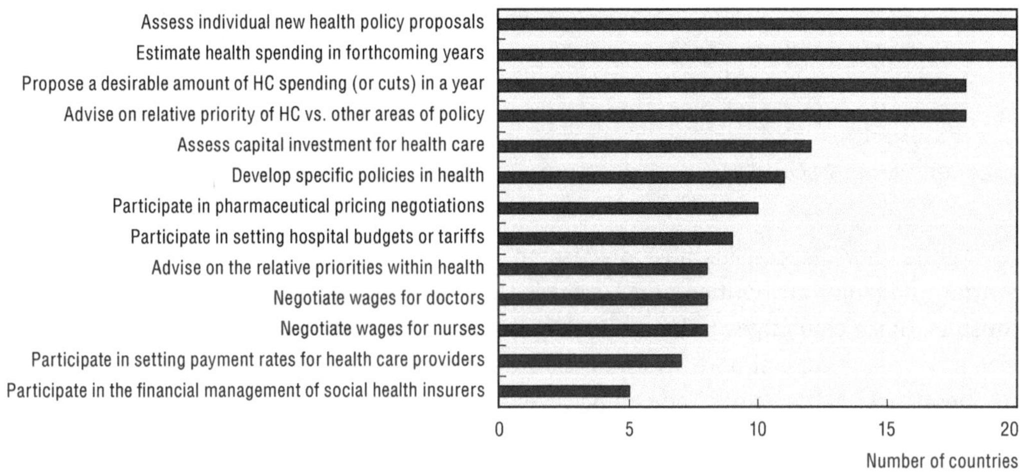

Source: OECD Survey of Budget Officials on Budgeting Practices for Health, 2013, Question 24.

StatLink http://dx.doi.org/10.1787/888933218743

Figure 3.11. **Influence of the central budget authority (CBA) over healthcare-related policies**

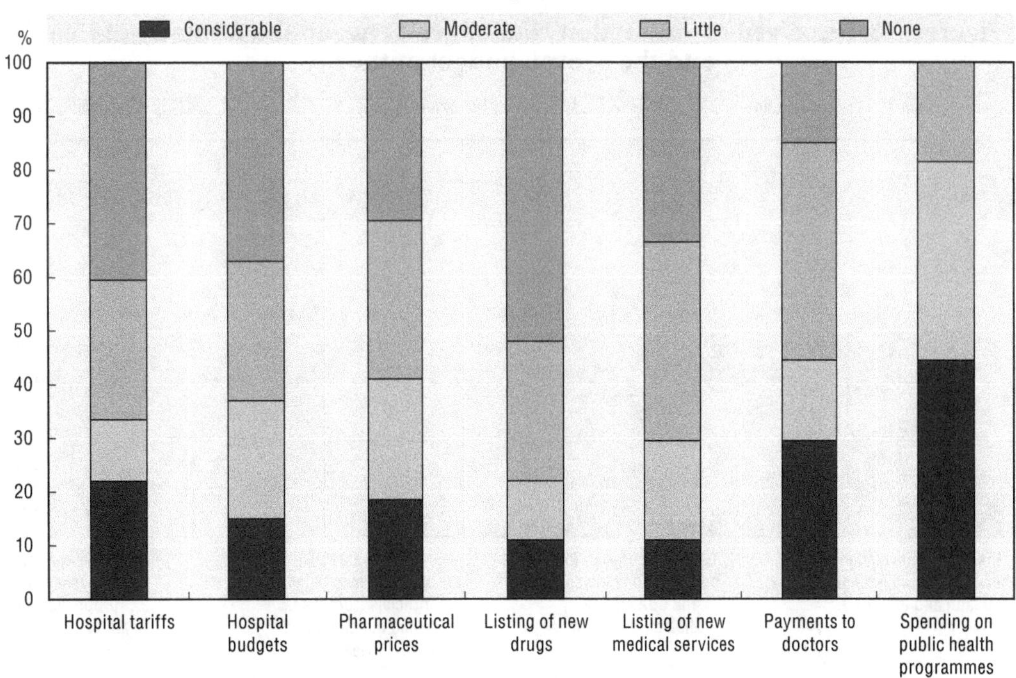

Source: OECD Survey of Budget Officials on Budgeting Practices for Health, 2013, Question 34.

StatLink http://dx.doi.org/10.1787/888933218758

Figure 3.12. **Top priority areas for health expenditure control for budget officials**

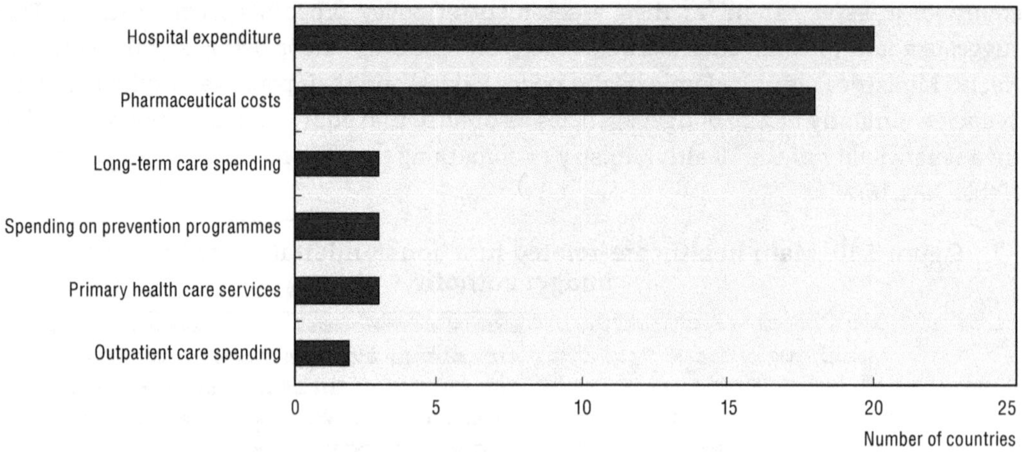

Source: OECD Survey of Budget Officials on Budgeting Practices for Health, 2013, Question 37.

StatLink http://dx.doi.org/10.1787/888933218768

While there is considerable discussion about challenges in co-operation between central budgetary authorities and Ministries of Health, most budget authorities did not consider these challenges to be major (Figure 3.13 and Table 3.A1.17). Many countries in fact have many formal and informal institutions through which these two bodies can co-operate, with the survey revealing several successful examples of co-operation: the taskforce "towards sustainable health care spending" between the Dutch Ministries of Health and Finance; France highlighted that its social spending team is jointly supervised by Ministries of Budget and Health; and Australia established *ad hoc* committees with officials from both in developing specific reforms. Only the Czech Republic, Portugal and Poland reported that they do not have any formal or informal co-ordination mechanism between both ministries (Table 3.A1.18).

Figure 3.13. **Perceived co-ordination challenges between the Ministry of Health and the central budget authority**

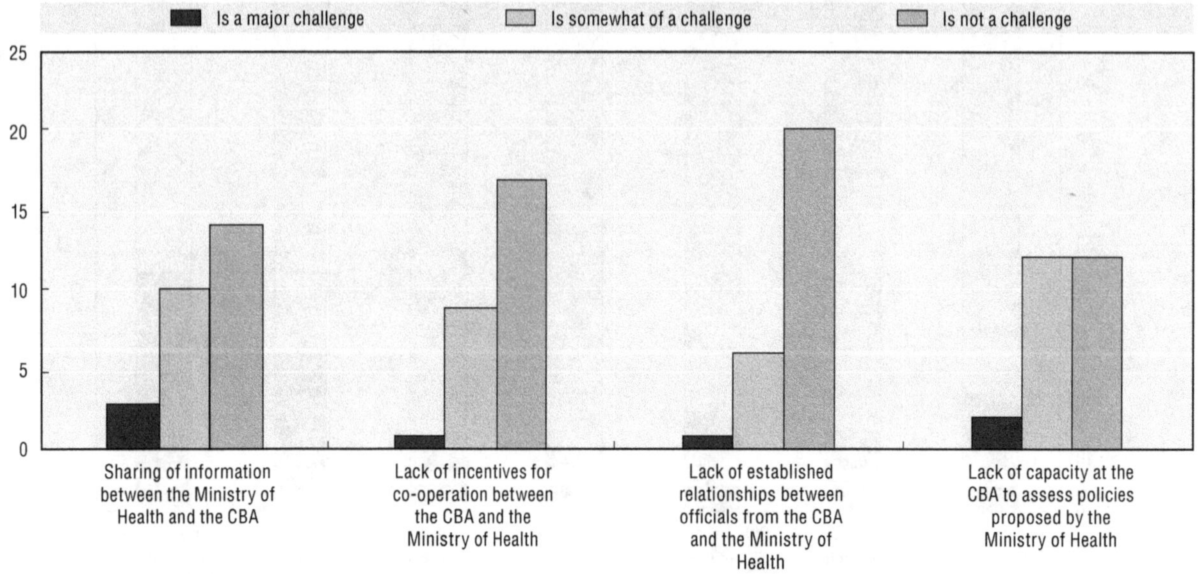

Source: OECD Survey of Budget Officials on Budgeting Practices for Health h, 2013, Question 26.

StatLink http://dx.doi.org/10.1787/888933218777

However, just over half of budget agencies noted that they have a lack of capacity for assessing policies. The number of central budget authority staff working on health varies widely across countries, from 35 in Mexico to less than one fulltime in Austria and Slovenia. This number reflects a range of factors specific to the structure of the health system and the institutional culture of the country. France, Mexico and the Netherlands have high results, which reflect the fact that those working on health also have responsibilities covering other social policy areas. The loss of sector-specific knowledge in central budget authorities that is a consequence of a "top-down" budgeting approach may have come at the cost of limiting resources to assess proposals emerging from Health Ministries.

3.5. Decentralisation of health financing and expenditure

Decentralised governments (or entities) are often dependent on transfers from central governments and social security bodies to meet their obligations to the population on health care. In many OECD countries, the share of sub-national government budgets allocated to health care has increased from 2000 to 2011. Rising health care costs are reported to be generating pressure on sub-national government budgets. This is complicated by their (generally) lesser revenue-raising capabilities and the effect of internal migration, particularly of retiring populations. These trends were sometimes noted to potentially threaten sub-national governments' finances in the medium to long term. This section gives a summary of the main issues related to fiscal decentralisation of health. More detailed analysis is presented in Chapter 4.

Sub-national government budget decisions can have a substantial influence on health spending

The survey sought to collect new data on how sub-national governments financed health care spending, as current sources only provide data on financing of sub-national government at large. As expected, this showed that sub-national governments (and entities, in the case of the United Kingdom) rely both on transfers from central authorities and on their own sources of revenues to finance health care expenditure (Figure 3.14). At both ends of the spectrum, sub-national governments in Netherlands rely exclusively on transfers, while in Switzerland, more than 90% of spending is funded by own revenues. The survey also helped identify the extent to which sub-national governments (SNG) receive transfers from social security bodies to finance health care (in Austria, Finland, the Slovak Republic and Slovenia).

Most transfers from central authorities are general purpose (not earmarked to health), suggesting that the budgetary decisions by sub-national governments have a significant influence in determining how much is spent on health in many countries. These represent the largest share of transfers in Australia, Austria and Norway (Figure 3.15). Block grants earmarked for health are mainly used in Denmark, Finland and Canada. Grants may also be attached to specific health objectives (Mexico, the Netherlands and the Slovak Republic). The highest degree of control from central governments over spending decisions is financing through grants earmarked for specific health programmes (Korea, Mexico) or reimbursement on the basis of services delivered (Denmark, Mexico and Norway).

Figure 3.14. **Sources of revenues financing SNG health expenditure**

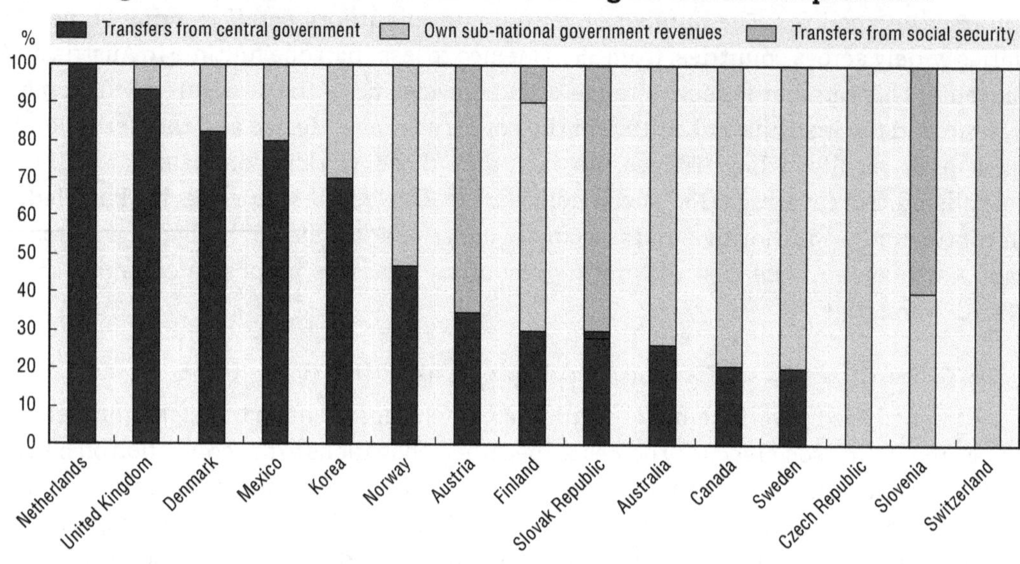

Source: OECD Survey of Budget Officials on Budgeting Practices for Health, 2013, Question 14.

StatLink http://dx.doi.org/10.1787/888933218784

Figure 3.15. **Composition of transfers from central authorities as a share of total SNG health care spending**

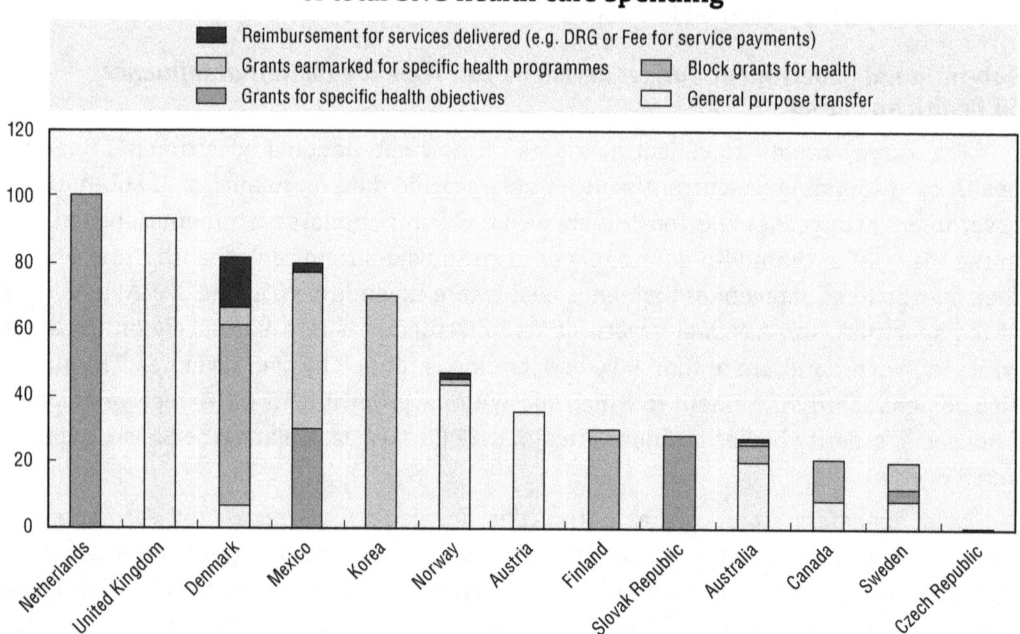

Source: OECD Survey of Budget Officials on Budgeting Practices for Health, 2013, Question 15.

StatLink http://dx.doi.org/10.1787/888933218798

Sub-national governments have relative stability in their funding and are often responsible for ensuring spending targets are adhered to

Few countries reported that there are major variations in funds provided to sub-national governments from year to year (Table 3.A1.19). Generally, central authorities may only modify resources on a multiyear basis, or have a limited capacity to vary resources from year to year (Denmark, Finland, Italy, Switzerland, etc.). In Austria, funds collected by the central government are automatically transferred to the state governments according to multiannual regulations. In contrast, central governments may significantly modify resources allocated to sub-national government spending from one year to another in the Czech Republic, France and Norway. When the parameters under which funds are allocated (e.g. a formula or share of revenues) change, half of the countries surveyed reported that this occurred unilaterally by central government or social security agencies (Figure 3.16). In Australia, Chile, Denmark and Slovenia, negotiations to change the formula are necessary (Table 3.A1.20).

Figure 3.16. **What is the procedure for central government (CG) or social security (SS) to vary total resources transferred?**

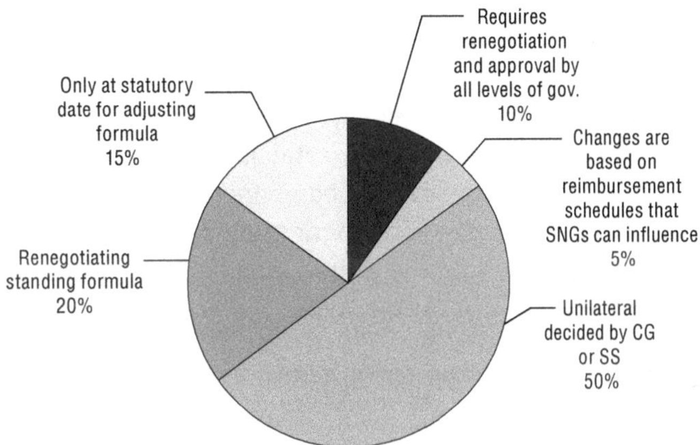

Source: OECD Survey of Budget Officials on Budgeting Practices for Health, 2013, Question 17.

StatLink http://dx.doi.org/10.1787/888933218801

A majority of countries reported that central governments are not the lender of last resort should sub-national governments fail to meet their obligations for financing health care. Central governments are ultimately responsible for funding health care expenditures in Chile, Denmark, France, Hungary, Italy, Japan, Korea and Netherlands. Central governments are not ultimately responsible for financing in countries where sub-national governments play the largest role in financing health care (Australia, Austria, Canada,[2] Finland, Mexico, Sweden and Switzerland) (Table 3.A1.21). The credibility of institutional arrangements to stop the central government from stepping in if a sub-national government cannot finance health services is questionable. Budget agencies pointed out that the lack of a legal obligation to step in may reduce moral hazard by lower levels of government, particularly where they hold responsibility for hospital capital planning. Nonetheless, most countries have mechanisms in place to provide financing of last resort for sub-national governments at large (if not specifically for their financial obligations related to health).

Central governments commonly set spending targets for health to be met by sub-national governments. Twelve out of 20 countries reported spending targets that were either a subset of a more general framework of expenditure ceilings for sub-national governments (e.g. Denmark), or temporary ceilings within the framework of recent consolidation plans, such as Austria where the federal and sub-national governments agreed to limit health care spending to nominal GDP growth and, from 2016 onwards, to not exceed 3.6% growth (OECD, 2013). In some cases, sub-national governments themselves introduce targets to limit health expenditures, such as in Canada's province of Ontario, which has capped growth in health care spending to 2.1% a year over 2013-16. In half of the countries that responded, the Ministry of Health was responsible for controlling sub-national health care expenditure (Finland, France, Hungary, Japan, Korea, Netherlands and Slovak Republic). The central budget authority is responsible for supervising sub-national government health expenditure in 36% of cases (the Czech Republic, Denmark, France, Italy and Sweden). The Social Security Agency is responsible for such control only in Slovenia (Table 3.A1.22).

While spending targets for sub-national government are common, specific performance targets and measures of outputs and outcomes are less so. When central governments monitor the performance of sub-national governments this more often tends to be through specific performance targets rather than measures of outputs and outcomes or analyses. Half of the countries surveyed reported using performance targets. In comparison, 35% of countries required sub-national governments to have output or outcome measures and only 10% required value-for-money analyses. In a large majority of countries surveyed, the Ministry of Health is primarily responsible for establishing this policy framework for sub-national governments. Other policy-setting bodies include the central budget authority (Italy), the executive (Australia) or the Parliament (the Czech Republic, Germany, Hungary and Switzerland). Only in Canada and the United Kingdom are sub-national governments responsible for setting their own policy objectives.

Taking responsibility for the governance of health systems is a challenge in decentralised contexts

There was a divergence of views on whether controlling public health expenditure was different in centralised or decentralised systems, suggesting that institutional factors broader than just health mattered more. Sweden reported that they found it easier to control costs when health is financed and provided by sub-national governments. Others noted that this complicates affairs: citizens tend to complain directly to the Ministry of Health of the central government when there is a problem and local governments do not bear the full political cost of unpopular decisions. Similarly, an increase in the number of stakeholders (particularly elected stakeholders), can soften budget constraints. The occurrence of a "blame game" between levels of government for the provision of health care services is a frequent feature of countries where sub-national governments play an important role in health provision.

A number of countries noted that determining the appropriate size of sub-national government to effectively manage health care services has been a challenge in recent years. In Sweden, for example, there are 21 county councils, but studies show that six would be more efficient (Blomqvist and Bergman, 2007). Reducing the number of sub-national governments is politically difficult – and sometimes constitutionally or historically impossible, in particular in federal countries where states pre-existed the federation (Austria, for instance). Denmark conducted a successful reform of municipal mergers in 2007, reducing the total number of municipalities from 300 to 100 and the number of regions from 14 to 5. One of the main drivers of this reform was precisely to reach a more adequate size for health care service provision (OECD, 2012). Finland has also been implementing a gradual reform of its health care system since 2007. In March 2014, it reached a political agreement to transfer health and welfare services from municipalities to five regions.

3.6. Conclusion

This chapter shows the variety of budgeting practices and procedures for health expenditure across OECD countries. These practices and procedures depend on institutional factors such as the origin of public health systems, the role of autonomous social security institutions or the degree of decentralisation. These institutional considerations, in particular relative to budgeting, shed some light on the capacity of governments to control health care expenditure growth.

Since the 1990s, there has been a gradual shift towards top-down budgeting in OECD countries, leading to a reallocation of responsibilities between the central budget authority and the Ministry of Health. Central budget authorities are mainly responsible for macro-fiscal tasks in the health sector and are content to leave policy development and implementation to Health Ministries.

There are challenges in reconciling these two perspectives, most notably whether efficiency gains in health are being returned to taxpayers. To aid the certainty of their fiscal estimates, most OECD countries use some kind of budget ceiling to limit the growth of health care expenditure, and a large majority of countries use a medium-term expenditure framework. These are often complemented by specific mechanisms to control the evolution of health care spending. Early warning systems have been introduced in most countries and usually help to reduce the growth in health care spending. Other mechanisms used to enhance spending efficiency include automatic cuts or spending reviews. Most of these tools remain quite blunt – and are often the source of disagreements between ministries on whether savings sought are appropriate. Co-ordination between the central budget authority and the Ministry of Health in better harvesting efficiency gains might help this difficult process become a more rational one.

Notes

1. Australia, Austria, Canada, Chile, the Czech Republic, Denmark, Estonia, Finland, France, Germany, Hungary, Iceland, Italy, Japan, Korea, Mexico, the Netherlands, New Zealand, Norway, Poland, Portugal, the Slovak Republic, Slovenia, Sweden, Switzerland, Turkey, the United Kingdom.
2. Except for certain population groups, such as veterans and First Nations, for which the federal government is responsible for the funding of health care.

References

ASISP – Analytical Support on the Socio-Economic Impact of Social Protection Reforms (Europe) (2012), *Annual Report 2012, Pensions, Health Care and Long-Time Care, Norway*, European Commission.

ASISP (2011), *Annual Report 2011, Pensions, Health Care and Long-Time Care, Greece*, European Commission.

Blomqvist, P. and P. Bergman (2007), "Does Regionalisation of Nordic Health Care Systems Make Them Less Democratic? An Empirical Test of the Swedish Case", Uppsala University Working Paper No. 4, Sweden.

Dexia (2012), *Les finances publiques territoriales dans l'Union européenne*, Paris.

OECD (2013a), *OECD Economic Surveys: Austria 2013*, OECD, Paris, *http://dx.doi.org/10.1787/eco_surveys-aut-2013-en*.

OECD (2013b), *Budgeting Practices and Procedures in OECD Countries*, OECD Publishing, Paris, *http://dx.doi.org/10.1787/9789264059696-en*.

OECD (2012), *Reforming Fiscal Federalism and Local Government: Beyond the Zero-Sum Game*, OECD Fiscal Federalism Studies, OECD, Paris, *http://dx.doi.org/10.1787/9789264119970-en*.

ANNEX 3.A1

Survey answers by country

Table 3.A1.1. **Perception of difficulty in reducing health care expenditure**

	Yes – Health is one of the top two policy areas from which it is hardest to achieve savings	Yes – in general, it is harder to achieve savings in health than in most areas	Same – Health is as hard as any other area of government spending	No – It is easier to achieve savings in health than in other areas of government spending	No – Health is one of the easiest policy areas from which to achieve savings
Australia			X		
Austria		X			
Canada			X		
Chile	X				
Czech Republic		X			
Denmark			X		
Estonia		X			
Finland		X			
France			X		
Germany		X			
Hungary		X			
Iceland	X				
Italy			X		
Japan		X			
Korea	X				
Mexico	X				
Netherlands		X			
New Zealand			X		
Norway		X			
Poland		X			
Slovak Republic			X		
Slovenia	X				
Sweden			X		
Switzerland		X			
Turkey		X			
United Kingdom		X			
Total	**5**	**13**	**8**	**0**	**0**

Source: OECD Survey of Budget Officials on Budgeting Practices for Health, 2013, Question 42.

Table 3.A1.2. **Success of the central budget authority (CBA) in keeping health care spending within desired parameters in the last four years**

More successful than in other areas of policy	As successful as in other areas of policy	Less successful than in other areas of policy
Italy	Australia	Iceland
Mexico	Austria	Chile
Poland	Czech Republic	Finland
Turkey	Denmark	Korea
United Kingdom	Estonia	Netherlands
	France	Slovenia
	Germany	
	Japan	
	Hungary	
	New Zealand	
	Norway	
	Slovak Republic	
	Sweden	
	Switzerland	

Source: OECD Survey of Budget Officials on Budgeting Practices for Health, 2013, Question 29.

Table 3.A1.3. **Types of budget allocation**[1]

	Budget allocated to specific health objective?		Budget allocated by sub-categories of health care services?			
					If Yes	
	NO	YES	NO	YES	These categories are used for informative (non-binding) purposes	These categories form the basis of appropriation
Australia		X		X	X	
Austria	X		X			
Canada	X		X			
Chile			X			
Czech Republic		X	X			
Denmark		X	X			
Estonia		X	X			
Finland		X	X			
France		X		X		X
Germany	X		X			
Hungary		X		X		X
Iceland	X			X		X
Italy		X		X	X	
Japan		X		X		X
Korea		X		X	X	
Mexico		X		X		X
Netherlands		X		X		X
New Zealand		X		X		X
Norway	X			X		X
Poland	X		X			
Portugal		X		X	X	
Slovak Republic	X		X			
Slovenia	X		X			
Sweden	X		X			
Switzerland	X		X			
Turkey	X			X	X	
United Kingdom	X		X			
Total (27 answers)	**12**	**14**	**14**	**13**	**5**	**8**

1. These answers only refer to the health expenditure which is included in the (central/federal) government budget.

Source: OECD Survey of Budget Officials on Budgeting Practices for Health, 2013, Question 6.

Table 3.A1.4. **Categories included in projections**

	Total health expenditure	Public health expenditure	Private health expenditure	Expenditure by age groups	Categories of health expenditures (e.g. primary care, hospital, long-term care)
Australia		X			X
Austria		X		X	X
Canada	X	X	X	X	X
Chile		X			X
Denmark		X		X	X
Estonia	X	X	X	X	X
Finland	X	X	X	X	X
France		X			X
Germany		X			
Hungary		X			X
Iceland					X
Italy	X	X		X	X
Japan		X			X
Korea	X	X		X	X
Mexico		X			X
Netherlands	X	X	X	X	X
New Zealand		X			X
Norway					X
Poland		X			X
Slovenia		X			X
Switzerland	X	X		X	X
Sweden	X	X		X	
Turkey		X			
United Kingdom		X			
Total	**8**	**23**	**4**	**10**	**20**

Source: OECD Survey of Budget Officials on Budgeting Practices for Health, 2013, Question 11.

Table 3.A1.5. **Existence of specific ceilings for health expenditures**[1]

No	Yes, it sets expenditure ceilings for overall expenditure by the Ministry of Health (or Social Affairs)	Yes, it sets expenditure ceilings by programme	Yes, it sets expenditure ceilings by category of health services (e.g. hospitals, primary care, etc.)
Australia[2]	Chile	Korea	Austria
Finland	Czech Rep.	Norway	Denmark
Japan	Estonia	Poland	France
Sweden	Germany[3]	Portugal	Hungary
Switzerland	Hungary		Italy
	Iceland		Mexico
	Mexico		Netherlands
	Netherlands		New Zealand
	Slovak Rep.		Poland
	Slovenia		Slovak Rep.
	Turkey		United Kingdom

1. These answers only refer to the health expenditure which is included in the (central/federal) government budget.

2. The majority of Australian government health expenditure is based on entitlement (e.g. Medicare benefits), and does not have an expenditure ceiling. However, non-entitlement expenditure (e.g. prevention activities) is capped.

3. In Germany, ceilings do not include expenditure of Statutory Health Insurance.

Source: OECD Survey of Budget Officials on Budgeting Practices for Health, 2013, Question 45.

Table 3.A1.6. Entity primarily responsible for setting the health expenditure ceiling(s)[1]

	Ministry of Health	Central budget authority (e.g. Ministry of Finance)	Executive Branch: Prime ministers or president's office or cabinet	Executive agency	Legislative Branch; Parliament	Independent Body	Not applicable
Australia							X[2]
Austria	X						
Canada							X
Chile		X					
Czech Republic		X	X		X		
Denmark		X			X		
Estonia		X			X		
Germany					X		
Korea		X					
Netherlands		X				X	
New Zealand					X		
Poland	X	X		X			
Portugal			X				
Slovak Republic		X					
Slovenia				X			
United Kingdom		X					
Total	**2**	**9**	**2**	**2**	**5**	**1**	**2**

1. These answers only refer to the health expenditure which is included in the (central/federal) government budget.

2. The majority of Australian government health expenditure is not subject to ceilings. However, for the specific items which are subject to ceilings, the Ministry of Health is primarily responsible for setting these.

Source: OECD Survey of Budget Officials on Budgeting Practices for Health, 2013, Question 47a.

Table 3.A1.7. Most important factors when establishing ceilings or targets for health[1]

	Estimated GDP growth			General government objectives for the fiscal position			Share of health spending in total public spending			Expenditure estimates and projections			Value for money analysis of specific health policies			The balance of public versus private spending on health by households			The balance of health promotion versus social protection in health spending		
	1	2	3	1	2	3	1	2	3	1	2	3	1	2	3	1	2	3	1	2	3
Australia				X								X		X							
Austria		X		X								X									
Chile				X					X		X										
Czech Republic	X				X							X									
Denmark			X	X				X			X			X				X			X
Estonia		X				X				X											
Finland		X		X														X			
France				X							X				X						
Germany				X					X		X										
Hungary	X			X			X				X			X				X		X	
Iceland		X		X								X									
Italy				X					X		X										
Japan	X									X						X					
Korea	X				X							X									
Mexico	X			X				X		X					X			X			X
Netherlands					X				X	X											
New Zealand				X					X		X										

Table 3.A1.7. **Most important factors when establishing ceilings or targets for health**[1] *(cont.)*

	Estimated GDP growth			General government objectives for the fiscal position			Share of health spending in total public spending			Expenditure estimates and projections			Value for money analysis of specific health policies			The balance of public versus private spending on health by households			The balance of health promotion versus social protection in health spending		
	1	2	3	1	2	3	1	2	3	1	2	3	1	2	3	1	2	3	1	2	3
Norway					X					X											X
Poland			X		X					X											
Slovak Republic				X					X		X										
Slovenia	X			X				X			X			X				X			X
Switzerland		X		X																	
Turkey			X	X							X										
United Kingdom				X							X				X						
Total	**6**	**5**	**3**	**17**	**5**	**1**	**1**	**3**	**6**	**6**	**11**	**5**	**0**	**4**	**3**	**1**	**0**	**5**	**0**	**1**	**4**

Note: 1 for the most important factor, 2 for the second most important and 3 for the third.

1. These answers only refer to the health expenditure which is included in the (central/federal) government budget.

Source: OECD Survey of budget officials on budgeting practices for health, 2013, Question 47.

Table 3.A1.8. **Existence of an early warning system to alert that health expenditures may exceed targets or legally binding levels**

No, there is not such a system	Yes, there is a system that detects overruns, but an alert *does not legally require* action	Yes, there is a system that detects overruns and sets in motion *required action for the current year*	Yes, there is a system that detects overruns and sets in motion *required action for future years*
Czech Republic	Chile	Iceland	Austria
Estonia	Norway	Australia	Denmark
Finland	Slovak Republic	Denmark	
Germany	Turkey	France	
Japan	United Kingdom	Hungary	
Korea		Italy	
Netherlands		Mexico	
Poland		New Zealand	
Sweden		Slovenia	
Switzerland			

Source: OECD Survey of Budget Officials on Budgeting Practices for Health, 2013, Question 49.

Table 3.A1.9. **Use of automatic reductions in health expenditure**

No	Only a part of health spending is subject to automatic reductions	Yes, all health spending is subject to an automatic reduction every year
Australia	Denmark	
Canada	France	
Chile	Italy	
Czech Republic	New Zealand	
Estonia	Slovenia	
Finland	Switzerland	
Germany	Turkey	
Hungary		
Iceland		
Japan		
Korea		

Table 3.A1.9. Use of automatic reductions in health expenditure (cont.)

No	Only a part of health spending is subject to automatic reductions	Yes, all health spending is subject to an automatic reduction every year
Mexico		
Netherlands		
Norway		
Poland		
Slovak Republic		
Sweden		
United Kingdom		

Source: OECD Survey of Budget Officials on Budgeting Practices for Health, 2013, Question 38.

Table 3.A1.10. Functions undertaken by the CBA

	Advise on the relative priorities across sectors	Estimate future health spending	Propose a desirable amount of health care spending	Advise on the relative priorities within health	Assess individual new health policy proposals	Develop specific policies in health	Participate in pharmaceutical pricing negotiations	Participate in setting hospital budgets or tariffs	Participate in setting payment rates for health care providers	Negotiate wages for doctors	Negotiate wages for nurses	Assess capital investment for health care	Participate in the financial management of health insurers
Australia	X	X			X	X		X					
Austria	X		X		X		X						
Canada	X				X								
Chile	X	X	X		X			X		X	X	X	
Czech Republic		X	X		X							X	X
Denmark	X	X	X	X	X	X				X	X	X	
Estonia		X											
Finland		X			X		X		X				
France	X	X	X	X	X	X	X	X	X			X	X
Germany		X			X								
Hungary		X	X				X	X					
Iceland	X	X			X		X	X	X	X	X	X	
Italy		X	X			X	X	X		X	X	X	
Japan	X	X		X									
Korea	X	X	X		X								
Mexico	X		X		X			X		X	X	X	X
Netherlands	X	X	X	X	X	X							
New Zealand	X	X	X	X	X							X	
Norway	X		X	X	X	X		X	X			X	
Poland		X	X		X				X				
Portugal			X										
Slovak Republic	X	X	X	X	X	X							
Slovenia									X	X	X	X	X
Switzerland	X	X			X	X	X						
Sweden	X		X		X	X	X						
Turkey	X	X	X			X	X	X	X	X	X	X	X
United Kingdom	X	X	X	X	X	X	X			X	X	X	
Total	**18**	**20**	**18**	**8**	**20**	**11**	**10**	**9**	**7**	**8**	**8**	**12**	**5**

Source: OECD Survey of Budget Officials on Budgeting Practices for Health, 2013, Question 24.

Table 3.A1.11. **Extent to which the CBA can influence health care policies**

	Policies																											
	Hospital tariffs				Hospital budgets				Pharmaceut-ical prices				Listing of new drugs				Listing of new medical services				Payments to doctors				Spending on public health programmes			
	C	M	L	N	C	M	L	N	C	M	L	N	C	M	L	N	C	M	L	N	C	M	L	N	C	M	L	N
Australia					X						X				X				X				X			X		
Austria				X				X			X					X			X				X			X		
Canada				X				X				X				X				X				X			X	
Chile	X					X						X				X		X			X				X			
Czech Republic			X				X				X				X				X				X				X	
Denmark			X		X					X					X				X		X				X			
Estonia			X				X				X				X				X				X				X	
Finland				X			X			X			X					X					X		X			
France	X				X						X					X		X					X		X			
Germany			X				X				X				X				X				X			X		
Hungary	X					X			X				X				X					X			X			
Iceland		X				X					X				X				X			X				X		
Italy	X							X		X						X	X				X				X			
Japan	X							X	X							X				X	X				X			
Korea				X				X				X				X				X				X		X		
Mexico		X				X						X				X				X	X					X		
Netherlands				X			X					X			X				X				X				X	
New Zealand				X			X					X				X				X			X			X		
Norway		X				X				X				X					X			X				X		
Poland				X				X			X					X			X				X			X		
Portugal			X		X					X				X				X				X			X			
Slovak Republic				X				X				X				X				X				X		X		
Slovenia				X			X					X				X				X	X						X	
Switzerland				X				X	X				X				X						X		X			
Sweden	X							X	X							X				X				X	X			
Turkey			X			X			X					X				X			X				X			
United Kingdom			X					X		X						X				X	X				X			

C: considerable; L: little; M: moderate; N: none.

Source: OECD Survey of Budget Officials on Budgeting Practices for Health, 2013, Question 34.

Table 3.A1.12. **Areas which have been key priorities for expenditure control in health in recent years**

	Hospital expenditure	Outpatient care spending	Primary health care services	Long-term care spending	Spending on prevention programmes	Pharmaceutical costs	Other
Australia			X			X	X
Austria	X			X			
Chile	X						X
Czech Republic	X					X	
Denmark	X					X	
Estonia							X
Finland			X	X			
France	X					X	
Germany	X					X	
Hungary	X					X	
Iceland	X					X	

Table 3.A1.12. **Areas which have been key priorities for expenditure control in health in recent years** *(cont.)*

	Hospital expenditure	Outpatient care spending	Primary health care services	Long-term care spending	Spending on prevention programmes	Pharmaceutical costs	Other
Italy	X					X	
Japan	X	X	X	X	X	X	X
Korea	X	X				X	
Mexico		X			X		
Netherlands	X			X			
New Zealand	X					X	
Norway	X					X	
Poland	X					X	
Portugal	X					X	
Slovak Republic					X		
Slovenia	X					X	
Sweden			X			X	
Switzerland	X					X	
Turkey	X				X	X	
United Kingdom	X						X
Total	**20**	**3**	**4**	**4**	**4**	**18**	**5**

Source: OECD Survey of Budget Officials on Budgeting Practices for Health, 2013, Question 37.

Table 3.A1.13. **Existence of a "desirable" level of spending for health care set by the CBA**

No	Yes, and the "desired" level of spending has been reached	Yes, but the "desired" level of spending was not reached
Japan	Austria	Chile
Australia	Czech Republic	Korea
Germany	Denmark	Netherlands
Korea	Estonia	Slovenia
Slovenia	Finland	Switzerland
	France	
	Hungary	
	Italy	
	Mexico	
	New Zealand	
	Norway	
	Poland	
	Sweden	
	Slovak Republic	
	Turkey	
	United Kingdom	

Source: OECD Survey of Budget Officials on Budgeting Practices for Health, 2013, Questions 30 and 31.

Table 3.A1.14. Countries in which the CBA receives economic evaluations of expected health benefits from new policy proposals suggested by the Health Ministry

Yes, accompanying all new health policy proposals	For some health policies	Rarely	Other	Only for pharmaceuticals or listing new medical services
Austria	Australia	Chile	Korea	
Hungary	Canada	Czech Republic		
Japan	Denmark	Estonia		
Poland	Finland	Germany		
Slovak Republic	France	Iceland		
Slovenia	Italy	Mexico		
	Netherlands	Sweden		
	New Zealand			
	Norway			
	Switzerland			
	Turkey			
	United Kingdom			

Source: OECD Survey of Budget Officials on Budgeting Practices for Health, 2013, Question 32.

Table 3.A1.15. Assessment of health policy proposals (on the basis of economic assessments of their expected benefits) by the CBA

To a large extent: Policy proposals are prioritised or supported on the basis of their expected life-years saved ahead of all other factors	*To some extent:* Policy proposals are prioritised or supported on the basis of expected life-years saved along with other factors	*To a lesser extent:* It is the job of the Health Ministry to indicate priorities and the CBA is principally concerned with their fiscal implications	Other
Australia	Finland	Austria	Japan
	Mexico	Canada	Switzerland
	New Zealand	Chile	
	Norway	Czech Republic	
	United Kingdom	Denmark	
		Estonia	
		France	
		Germany	
		Hungary	
		Iceland	
		Italy	
		Korea	
		Netherlands	
		Poland	
		Slovak Republic	
		Slovenia	
		Sweden	
		Turkey	

Source: OECD Survey of Budget Officials on Budgeting Practices for Health, 2013, Question 33.

Table 3.A1.16. **Assessment of the impact of health policies on equity by the CBA**

To a large extent, health policies are often assessed for their impact on equity	To some extent, equity is an important consideration but not a primary concern	Assessing the impact on equity of health policies is usually the responsibility of the Health Ministry	Budget policy makers are not actively engaged with equity issues in health
New Zealand	Australia	Austria	Chile
	Finland	Canada	Czech Republic
	Germany	Denmark	Estonia
	Iceland	France	Netherlands
	Italy	Hungary	Slovak Republic
	Korea	Japan	Slovenia
	Mexico	Poland	Switzerland
	Norway	Portugal	
		Sweden	

Source: OECD Survey of Budget Officials on Budgeting Practices for Health, 2013, Question 35.

Table 3.A1.17. **Major challenges encountered in the co-operation between the CBA and the Ministry of Health**

	Is a major challenge	Is somewhat of a challenge	Is not a challenge
Sharing of information between the Ministry of Health and the CBA	Chile, Korea, New Zealand	Australia, Estonia, France, Germany, Iceland, Mexico, Netherlands, Portugal, Slovenia, Switzerland	Austria, Canada, Czech Republic, Denmark, Finland, Hungary, Italy, Japan, Norway, Poland, Slovak Republic, Sweden, Turkey, United Kingdom
Lack of incentives for co-operation between the CBA and the Ministry of Health	Korea	Chile, Denmark, Estonia, France, Germany, Iceland, New Zealand, Norway, Slovenia	Australia, Austria, Canada, Czech Republic, Finland, Hungary, Italy, Japan, Mexico, Netherlands, Poland, Portugal, Slovak Republic, Sweden, Switzerland, Turkey, United Kingdom
Lack of established relationships between officials from the CBA and the Ministry of Health	Korea	Chile, Estonia, Germany, Iceland, New Zealand, Slovak Republic	Australia, Austria, Canada, Czech Republic, Denmark, Finland, France, Hungary, Italy, Japan, Korea, Mexico, Netherlands, Norway, Poland, Portugal, Slovak Republic, Sweden, Switzerland, Turkey, United Kingdom
Lack of capacity at the CBA to assess policies proposed by the Ministry of Health	Korea, Portugal	Austria, Denmark, Estonia, Finland, Germany, Mexico, New Zealand, Norway, Poland, Slovenia, Sweden, United Kingdom	Australia, Canada, Chile, Czech Rep., France, Hungary, Iceland, Italy, Japan, Netherlands, Slovak Rep., Switzerland, Turkey

Source: OECD Survey of Budget Officials on Budgeting Practices for Health, 2013, Question 26.

Table 3.A1.18. **Existence of a formal co-ordination body between the CBA and Ministry of Health, and other institutions for co-ordination**

Yes	Regular informal consultation and meetings	Ad hoc bodies created for specific needs (discussing a reform, etc.)	Consultation for budget preparation only	None
Italy	Australia	Austria	Germany	Czech Republic
Finland	Canada		Hungary	Portugal
Mexico	Chile		Iceland	Poland
Norway	Denmark		Japan	Slovenia
Turkey	Estonia		Korea	
	France		New Zealand	

Table 3.A1.18. Existence of a formal co-ordination body between the CBA and Ministry of Health, and other institutions for co-ordination *(cont.)*

Yes	Regular informal consultation and meetings	Ad hoc bodies created for specific needs (discussing a reform, etc.)	Consultation for budget preparation only	None
	Netherlands		Slovak Republic	
	Sweden		Switzerland	
			United Kingdom	

Source: OECD Survey of Budget Officials on Budgeting Practices for Health, 2013, Question 25.

Table 3.A1.19. Ability of the central government (or social security) to vary total resources transferred to sub-national governments for health from one year to the next

To a large extent – central government can significantly vary total resources from one year to the next	To a moderate extent – central government can make changes within a specified margins	To a small extent – central government has little capacity to vary total resources from year to year	Resources are varied on a multi-year basis (every 3-5 years) and not generally year to year
Czech Republic	Australia	Denmark	Austria
France	Chile	Finland	Canada
Norway	Korea	Mexico	Italy
	Slovak Republic	Netherlands	United Kingdom
	Sweden	Slovenia	
		Switzerland	

Source: OECD Survey of Budget Officials on Budgeting Practices for Health, 2013, Question 16.

Table 3.A1.20. Procedure for central government (or social security) to vary total resources transferred to sub-national governments from one year to the next

	Unilateral changes can be decided at the central (or social security) level	Changes require re-negotiating a formula for the distribution of funds	Changes cannot be made until the next statutory date for the revision of the formula	Changes require negotiation and approval by all levels of government concerned but are not based on a formula	Changes are based on reimbursement schedules that sub-national governments can influence	Other
Australia	X	X		X		
Austria			X			
Canada			X			
Chile	X	X				
Czech Republic	X					
Denmark	X	X				X
Finland					X	
France	X					
Hungary	X					
Korea	X					
Mexico			X			
Netherlands				X		
Norway	X					
Slovak Republic	X					
Slovenia		X				
Switzerland						X
Sweden	X					
Turkey	X					
United Kingdom	X					
Total	**12**	**4**	**3**	**2**	**1**	**2**

Source: OECD Survey of Budget Officials on Budgeting Practices for Health, 2013, Question 17.

Table 3.A1.21. **Influence of the central government (CG) on overall health spending by sub-national governments**

	CG has ultimate responsibility for health care financing		CG sets targets for health spending by sub-national governments		CG establishes performance targets for sub-national governments		CG prescribes outputs or outcome measures for sub-national governments on health		CG requires sub-national governments to carry out value-for-money analysis	
	YES	NO	YES	NO	YES	NO	YES	NO	YES	NO
Australia		X	X		X		X			X
Austria		X	X		X			X		X
Canada		X		X		X		X		X
Chile	X			X	X		X			X
Czech Republic		X		X		X		X		X
Denmark	X		X		X		X			X
Finland		X	X			X		X		X
France	X		X		X		X		X	
Hungary	X			X		X	X			X
Italy	X		X		X		X			X
Japan	X		X			X		X		X
Korea	X		X		X		X		X	
Mexico		X	X		X			X		X
Netherlands	X		X		X			X		X
Norway		X		X	X			X		X
Slovak Republic		X	X			X		X		X
Slovenia		X	X			X		X		X
Switzerland		X		X		X		X		X
Sweden		X		X		X		X		X
United Kingdom		X		X		X		X		X
Total	**8**	**12**	**12**	**8**	**10**	**10**	**7**	**13**	**2**	**18**

Source: OECD Survey of Budget Officials on Budgeting Practices for Health, 2013, Question 19.

Table 3.A1.22. **Institution primarily responsible for controlling health spending by sub-national governments**

	Ministry of Health	Central budget authority (CBA)	Ministry of Interior or of Local Administrations	Social Security Agency	Other
Australia					X
Austria					X
Canada					X
Chile					X
Czech Republic		X			X
Denmark		X			
Finland	X				
France	X	X			
Hungary	X				X
Italy		X			
Japan	X				
Korea	X				
Mexico					X
Netherlands	X				
Norway					X
Slovak Republic	X				
Slovenia				X	
Switzerland					X
Sweden		X			
Turkey			X		
United Kingdom					X
Total	**7**	**5**	**1**	**1**	**10**

Source: OECD Survey of Budget Officials on Budgeting Practices for Health, 2013, Question 20.

Fiscal Sustainability of Health Systems
Bridging Health and Finance Perspectives

Chapter 4

Decentralisation of health financing and expenditure

by
Claudia Hulbert and Camila Vammalle*

In a majority of OECD countries, sub-national governments (SNGs) play some role in health-care spending. The allocation of health care expenditure between central, state and local levels has significant repercussions over the design, financing and sustainability of health care systems. This chapter gives an overview of health care decentralisation in OECD countries, and analyses the main differences in spending allocations between levels of government, as well as revenue distribution (taxes, transfers, etc.). It also focuses on recent reforms in OECD countries devolving further responsibilities for health expenditure to sub-national governments.

* Claudia Hulbert is a consultant and Camila Vammalle is with the OECD.

The statistical data for Israel are supplied by and under the responsibility of the relevant Israeli authorities. The use of such data by the OECD is without prejudice to the status of the Golan Heights, East Jerusalem and Israeli settlements in the West Bank under the terms of international law.

4.1. Introduction

In a majority of OECD countries, sub-national governments (SNGs) play some role in health care spending. The allocation of health care expenditure between central, state and local levels has significant repercussions over the design and financing of health care systems.

While such allocations may result from historical developments (for instance, federal countries typically assign a higher share of health care spending to SNGs), a trend towards greater decentralisation of health expenditure is under way in a number of OECD countries, often to alleviate fiscal pressure on central governments. Reforms to increase the size of territories to obtain greater efficiency in health expenditure have also been introduced recently in a number of countries.

The issue of the allocation of health expenditure between levels of governments and the organisation of tax and transfer systems financing sub-national health care services is therefore crucial in the light of recent reforms. While there is no consensus on an "ideal" system, international differences in health expenditure decentralisation, revenue distribution and related problems faced by governments can yield insightful comparisons.

This chapter gives an overview of health care decentralisation in OECD countries, and analyses the main differences in spending allocations between levels of government, as well as revenue distribution (taxes, transfers, etc.). It also focuses on recent reforms in OECD countries devolving further responsibilities for health expenditure to sub-national governments.

4.2. Role of sub-national governments in health care provision and financing

Sub-national governments are the main actors in health care spending in some decentralised countries (in particular in federal, quasi-federal and North European countries) (Figure 4.1).

A trend towards greater decentralisation of health care spending is under way in a significant number of OECD countries (Box 4.1), often to alleviate pressure faced by central governments' budgets. This additional devolution of responsibilities to sub-national governments is not always accompanied by an equivalent transfer of financial resources.

Increased decentralisation of health care expenditure and increasing health care costs have generated pressure on sub-national government budgets over the last decade. In many OECD countries, the share of sub-national government budget allocated to health care has increased significantly over 2000-11 (Figure 4.2). Such a trend may threaten sub-national governments' finances in the medium-to-long term, and generate difficulties in public service provision.

Figure 4.1. **Division of public health care spending between levels of government, 2012**

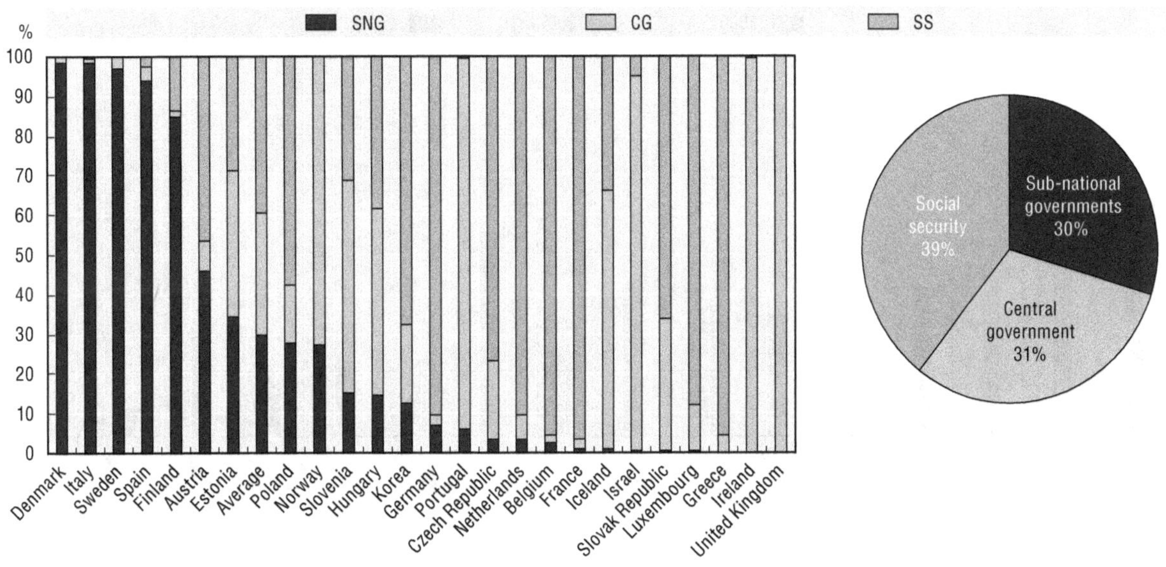

Note: Data for Austria and Korea are for 2011 instead of 2012. CG: Central government; SNG: Sub-national government.

Source: OECD National Accounts Statistics, http://dx.doi.org/10.1787/na-data-en.

StatLink http://dx.doi.org/10.1787/888933218812

Box 4.1. **Recent reforms towards greater decentralisation in health care spending in OECD countries**

Belgium passed a reform in 2012 granting to regions and communities more spending responsibilities for health care (hospital infrastructures, mental health services and preventive medicine). In parallel, the fiscal autonomy of sub-national governments is expected to be reinforced as transfers by the federal government are expected to be replaced by new autonomous revenues (the equalisation system will be maintained).

In the **Czech Republic**, central authorities, insurance companies and local health authorities are currently planning a reform in order to optimise the distribution of central, local and private funding, with the aim of generating savings in the health care sector.

In **Greece**, in parallel to the Kallikratis reform (2011), a health care reform transferred some responsibilities to local governments relative to elderly care, health care and health prevention. Health and social care committees were introduced at the municipal and regional level. They are responsible for monitoring health care needs, making proposals for increasing efficiency and improving planning capacity. These committees were also given authority over spending control (over accountability and performance evaluations) (ASISP, 2011).

In **Finland**, significant reform of health care spending is under consideration (see Box 4.4).

In **the Netherlands**, central authorities decided to transfer some responsibilities to municipalities regarding health care and social expenditures. These transfers of responsibilities are not compensated by an equivalent transfer of revenues to local authorities. Sub-national governments will therefore have to reach efficiency gains from 5 to 30% (Dexia, 2012).

In **Norway**, municipalities were granted additional responsibilities for health care from January 2012. This reform was to rearrange the allocation of responsibilities between the central government and municipalities, and between primary and specialised health care services (ASISP, 2012).

Figure 4.2. **SNG health care expenditure as a share of total SNG expenditure, 2000-12**

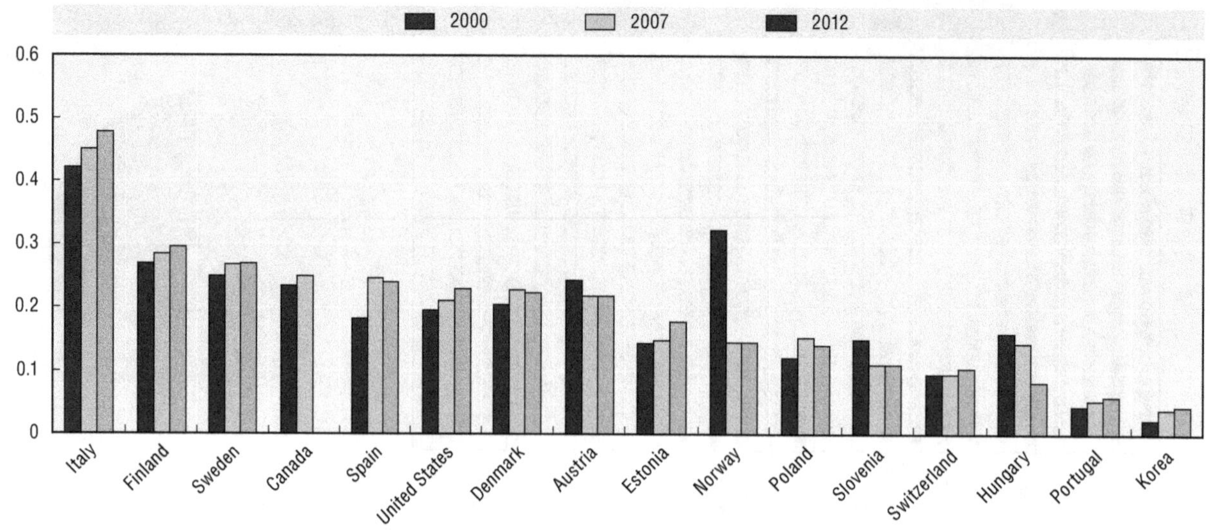

SNG: Sub-national government.

Note: Data for Poland: 2002 instead of 2000. Switzerland: 2005 instead of 2000. Austria, Korea and the United States: 2011 instead of 2012. Canada: 2009 instead of 2012.

Source: OECD National Accounts Statistics, http://dx.doi.org/10.1787/na-data-en.

StatLink http://dx.doi.org/10.1787/888933218821

In addition to the widespread challenge of ageing populations, sub-national governments face an additional challenge compared to central governments. Indeed, they may be subject to faster changes in population, especially in countries with a high mobility of population. Some countries may also experience internal migrations of population, whereby people may not wish to retire in the same region as they have been working. These changes of population imply changes both in needs and in the financial capacity to pay for the services. For instance, in Japan the rapidly-ageing population is seen as a major challenge to the sustainability of municipal health care spending. Municipalities in Japan are responsible for the National Health Insurance, one of the major health insurance schemes in the nation. As aged citizens may be concentrated in specific areas (in particular rural), and as the shrinking population creates a significant pressure on tax bases, financing health expenditure is a major challenge for some municipalities. Japan decided to increase its VAT rate in 2013. All revenues generated by this rate increase will fund expenditures on health care, long-term care, child care and pensions, of which around half will be used for enhancing the current social security system and the remainder for reducing the deficit financing of current social security expenditures. As Japanese provinces and municipalities are major actors in these areas and will benefit from these additional revenues, sub-national spending should increase significantly.

4.3. Overview of sub-national revenues for funding health care expenditures

Composition of sub-national government revenues for health

In most OECD countries, sub-national governments rely both on transfers from central authorities and on own revenues to finance health care expenditure (Figure 4.3). However, the share of these two main sources of revenue varies widely between countries. At both ends of the spectrum, sub-national governments in the Netherlands rely exclusively on transfers, while in Switzerland, more than 90% of spending is funded by own revenues. In a few OECD countries, sub-national governments also receive transfers from social security bodies to finance health care spending (Austria, Finland, Slovak Republic and Slovenia).

Figure 4.3. **Sources of revenues financing SNG health expenditure**

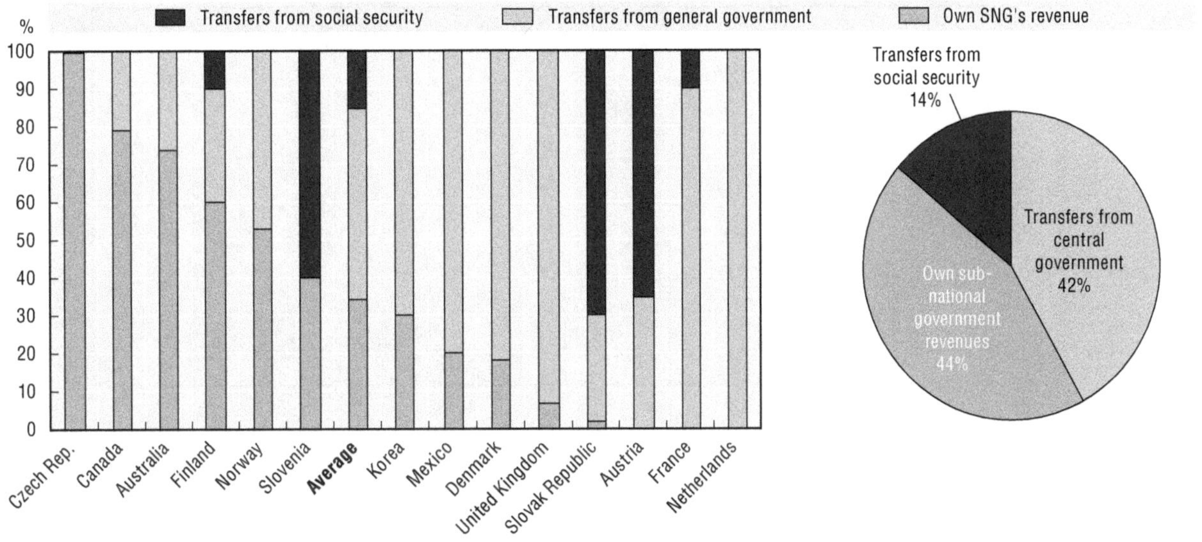

SNG: Sub-national government.

Note: In Switzerland (not shown), more than 90% of sub-national spending is funded by own revenues.

Source: OECD Survey of Budget Officials on Budgeting Practices for Health, 2013, Question 14.

StatLink http://dx.doi.org/10.1787/888933218832

Most transfers from central authorities are general-purpose, i.e. non earmarked (Figure 4.4). In such systems, sub-national governments have a high degree of autonomy over the use of funds to finance their health care expenditure. In parallel, Korea, Mexico and Sweden rely to a large extent on transfers earmarked for specific health programmes, hence limiting sub-national government spending autonomy and/or focusing resources on governments' priorities.

General purpose transfers give sub-national governments the most room for manoeuvre on how to spend the money (they represent the largest share of transfers in Australia, Austria, Notway and the United Kingdom) (Figure 4.4). These are contained quite frequently in the composition of sub-national government resources allocated to health. Block grants for health also provide spending autonomy, as their only conditionality is to be spent within the health sector respecting the general policy framework, leaving sub-national governments free to determine specifically how. These are mainly used in Canada, Denmark and Finland. In Canada, for example, provinces and territories are free to decide how to spend the amounts received from the Canadian Health Transfer, as long as they respect the conditions specified in the Canada Health Act (universality, portability, accessibility, public administration and comprehensiveness, and the prohibition of extra-billing and user charges). Grants may also be attached to specific health objectives (Mexico, Netherlands and the Slovak Republic). The highest degree of control from central governments over spending decisions is financing through grants earmarked for specific health programmes (Korea and Mexico).

Figure 4.4. **Composition of transfers from central authorities as a share of total SNG health care spending**

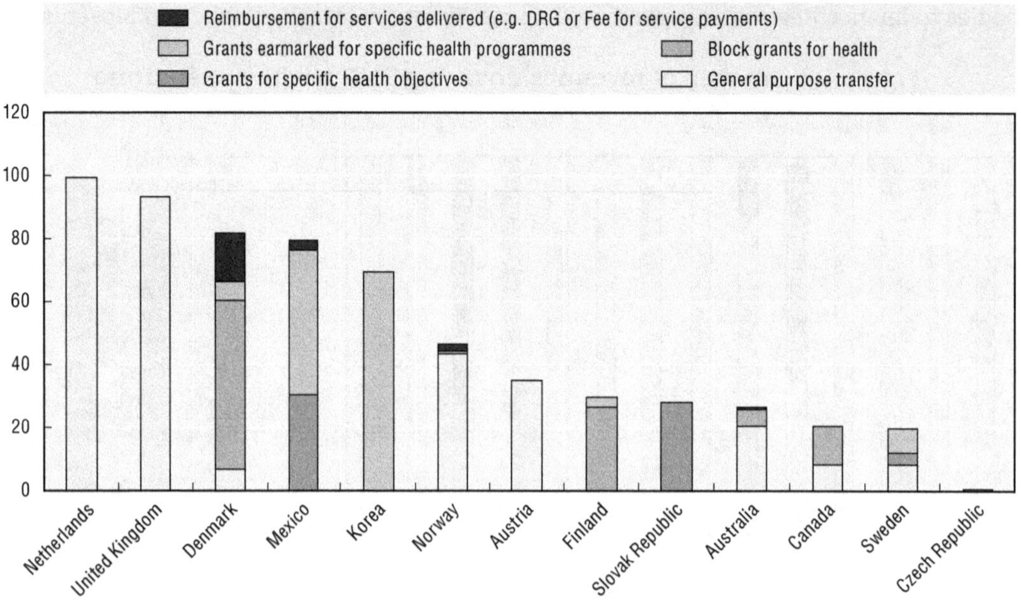

SNG: Sub-national government.

Source: OECD Survey of Budget Officials on Budgeting Practices for Health, 2013, Question 15.

StatLink http://dx.doi.org/10.1787/888933218848

Stability and predictability of sub-national government revenues for health

The ability of central authorities to modify sub-national health care resources from one year to another is critical for the stability of health care policies and of sub-national government finances. In countries where sub-national governments play a major role in health care expenditure, the degree of central government discretion over such funding is typically limited – central authorities may only modify resources on a multi-year basis, or have a limited capacity to vary resources from year to year (Denmark, Finland, Italy, Switzerland, etc.) (Figure 4.5). In Austria, funds collected by the central government are automatically transferred to the state governments according to multi-annual regulations governing the financing of state and local governments (including financing for hospitals). The funds collected by the autonomous social security system are distributed by the system and cannot be checked or influenced by the government. In contrast, central governments in some countries may significantly modify resources allocated to sub-national government spending from one year to another. In the Czech Republic, this concerns only 0.2% of SNG health expenditure and corresponds to subsidies from the central government, excluding EU financial support. In addition, sub-national governments only play a minor role in health care spending.

In most cases, variations in resources transferred to sub-national governments are decided unilaterally by central authorities or social security bodies (Figure 4.6). In Australia, Chile, Denmark and Slovenia, negotiations to change the formula are necessary to modify sub-national government revenues for health care. In most federal countries, such a modification is not possible without reaching an agreement between levels of governments and/or waiting for the next statutory date to modify the existing formula.

Figure 4.5. **To what extent can the central government or social security authority vary total resources transferred to SNGs for health from one year to the next?**

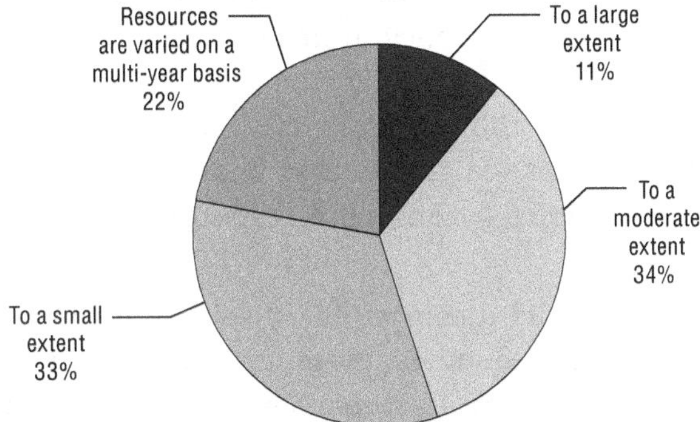

Source: OECD Survey of Budget Officials on Budgeting Practices for Health, 2013, Question 16.

StatLink http://dx.doi.org/10.1787/888933218852

Figure 4.6. **What is the procedure for the central government or social security authority to vary total resources transferred?**

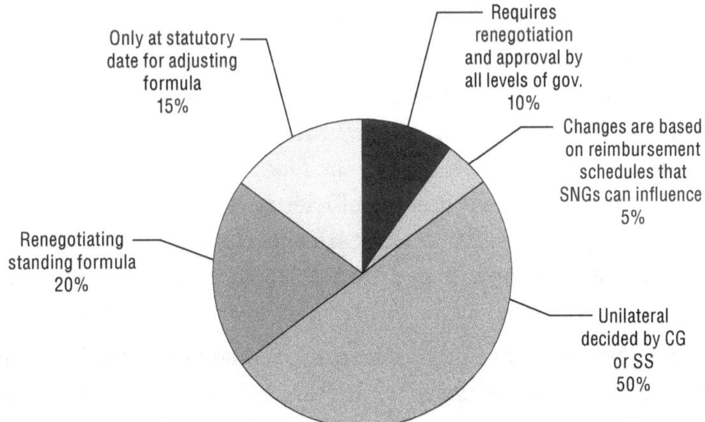

Source: OECD Survey of Budget Officials on Budgeting Practices for Health, 2013, Question 17.

StatLink http://dx.doi.org/10.1787/888933218863

Responsibility of last resort for financing health expenditure

In 40% of surveyed countries, central governments are ultimately responsible for funding health care expenditures (Chile, Denmark, France, Hungary, Italy, Japan, Korea and Netherlands). Usually, in countries where sub-national governments play the largest role in financing health care, central governments are not explicitly ultimately responsible for financing health (Australia, Austria, Canada, Finland, Mexico, Sweden and Switzerland). As health is such a visible, high-priority expenditure for citizens, it is questionable whether the central government would not step in when a sub-national government cannot finance the health services for which it is responsible. But the fact that there is no legal obligation to do so probably reduces moral hazard. The "blame game" between levels of government for problems in the provision of health care services is a frequent occurrence in countries where sub-national governments play an important role in health provision.

4.4. Policy setting and control over sub-national health care expenditures

In a large majority of surveyed countries, the Ministry of Health is primarily responsible for establishing the policy framework for sub-national governments (Question 18). Other policy-setting bodies include the central budget authority (Italy), the executive (Australia) and the Parliament (Czech Republic, Germany, Hungary and Switzerland). Only in Canada (provinces) and the United Kingdom (devolved administrations) are sub-national governments responsible for setting their own health policy framework.

This control of central authorities over policy setting in the health sector is hence widespread throughout OECD countries. A number of countries consider that the responsibility of the Ministry of Finance is to manage overall public expenditure. Ultimately, most central governments will be held responsible for health-related services, as well as for the financial sustainability of sub-national authorities if they are threatened by increasing health expenditures.

Central governments often set spending targets for health to be met by sub-national governments to ensure compliance with national objectives and monitor aggregate public spending (Table 4.1). These targets may be part of a more general framework of expenditure ceilings for sub-national governments (for example, in the case of Denmark). Other countries have introduced temporary ceilings to limit health care spending within the framework of recent consolidation plans. In Austria, the 2012 health care reform was undertaken to enhance co-ordination among the federal government, provinces and social security bodies in order to achieve greater efficiency in spending. The federal and sub-national governments agreed to limit health care expenditure: until 2016, spending should not exceed the nominal GDP growth and from 2016 onwards it should not exceed 3.6% (OECD, 2013).

In some cases, sub-national governments themselves introduce targets to limit health expenditures. This is the case, for instance, in Canada where the province of Ontario announced that it would cap growth in health care spending at 2.1% a year over 2013-15, and the province's 2013-14 budget forecast an increase of 2.0% for 2012-13 to 2015-16.

The use of performance targets for sub-national governments seems to be widespread among OECD countries, with over half of the surveyed countries using such targets (Table 4.1). In comparison, requiring sub-national governments to carry out output or outcome measures or value-for-money analyses is not as common (even in countries where sub-national governments are major players in health care provision and financing) (Figure 4.7). In some countries, central governments may take drastic actions regarding non-efficient health care services. For instance, in Poland in 2013 municipalities were forced to privatise hospitals that were losing money. This decision came as part of a large-scale trend towards privatisation of the Polish health care system.

Table 4.1. **Central governments set targets for health spending by SNGs**

Yes	No
Australia	Canada
Austria	Chile
Denmark	Czech Republic

Table 4.1. **Central governments set targets for health spending by SNGs** *(cont.)*

Yes	No
Finland	Hungary
France	Norway
Italy	Switzerland
Japan	Sweden
Korea	United Kingdom
Mexico	
Netherlands	
Slovak Republic	
Slovenia	

SNGs: Sub-national governments.

Source: OECD Survey of Budget Officials on Budgeting Practices for Health, 2013, Question 19.

Figure 4.7. **Central government monitoring of sub-national government performance for health expenditure**

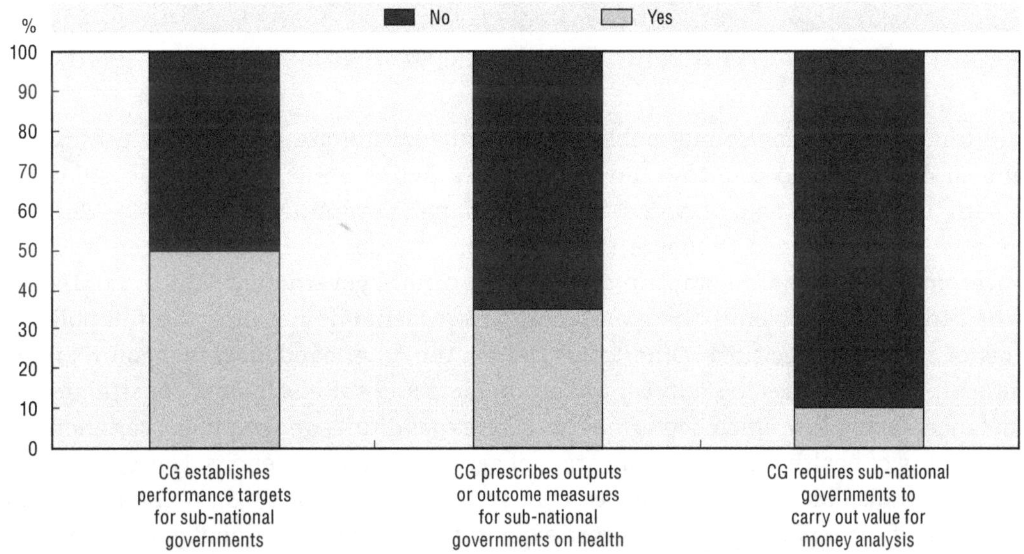

Source: OECD Survey of Budget Officials on Budgeting Practices for Health, 2013, Question 19.

StatLink http://dx.doi.org/10.1787/888933218877

It is often the Ministry of Health which is responsible for controlling sub-national health care expenditure (Figure 4.8) (Finland, France, Hungary, Japan, Korea, Netherlands and Slovak Republic). The central budget authority is responsible for supervising sub-national government health expenditure in 36% of the cases (Czech Republic, Denmark, France, Italy and Sweden). The social security agency is responsible for such control only in Slovenia.

Figure 4.8. **Institutions in charge of controlling SNG health care spending**

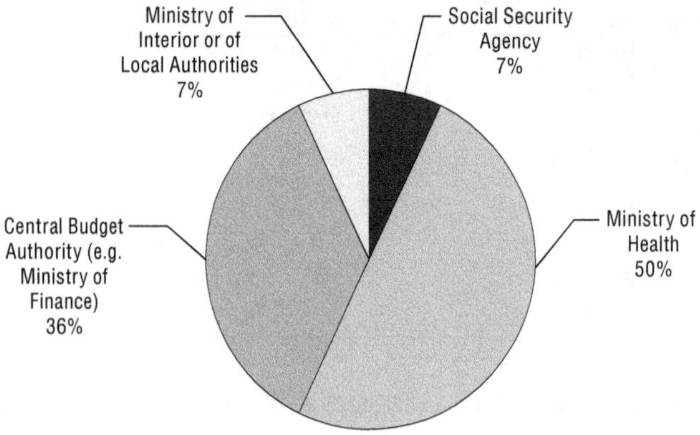

SNG: Sub-national government.

Source: OECD Survey of Budget Officials on Budgeting Practices for Health, 2013, Question 20.

StatLink http://dx.doi.org/10.1787/888933218885

4.5. Specific challenges in controlling health expenditure in decentralised settings

Challenges in controlling public health expenditure are different in centralised and in decentralised countries. Some countries find it easier to control costs when health is financed and provided by sub-national governments (Box 4.2). Citizens in most countries tend to ignore the allocation of responsibilities between levels of government and usually complain direct to the central government Ministry of Health when there is a problem – therefore, local governments do not bear the full political cost of unpopular decisions. Other countries, on the other hand, may find control more difficult as it increases the number of stakeholders and softens budget constraints. For instance, facing low efficiency of health care expenditure, geographical variations in the quality of health services, duplication of services and high deficits, Norway decided to re-centralise its specialised health care system in 2002 (Box 4.3). A challenge may also arise if the reporting of health care expenditure from sub-national governments to central authorities is not prompt.

The size of sub-national governments is not always optimal for the provision of health services. In Sweden, for example, there are 21 county councils; but studies show that six would be more efficient (Blomqvist and Bergman, 2007). Reducing the number of sub-national governments is politically difficult – and sometimes constitutionally or historically impossible, in particular in federal countries where states/Lander pre-existed the federation (Austria, for instance). Denmark successfully merged municipalities in 2007, reducing the total number to 100 from 300 and the number of councils to 5 from 14. One of the main drivers of this reform was to reach a more adequate size for health care service provision. The reform was implemented in parallel to the Health Act of 2007. New medical technologies in Denmark increased specialisation and called for larger regions (OECD, 2012). These problems had already led to hospital reform in the region of Copenhagen, when several small municipalities merged their hospitals to provide better service. Finland has also been implementing a gradual reform of its health care system since 2007 (Box 4.4). In March 2014, it reached an initial political agreement to take health and welfare services away from municipalities and give the responsibility for them to five regions. The reform is still under negotiation at the time of writing and details are not available.

Box 4.2. **Controlling health care expenditure in decentralised frameworks: The case of Sweden**

The Swedish health care system ranks amongst the most decentralised health care systems of OECD countries, with sub-national governments responsible for 80% of public health expenditure. Sweden is also one of the OECD countries with below-average growth in health expenditure during the period 2000-09. The decentralised framework is perceived as helping to control health care expenditure growth.

The Swedish health care system is organised into three levels: national, regional (county councils) and local. The central government is responsible for the overall health care policy. County councils are responsible for funding and providing health care services to their population, while municipalities are in charge of long-term care for elderly and disabled people. The Health and Medical Services Act gives county councils and municipalities considerable freedom with regard to the organisation of their health services.

Eighty per cent of health care expenditure by sub-national governments is covered by their own revenues (income taxes, patient fees and sales taxes) Both the county councils and the municipalities levy proportional income taxes to cover services that they provide. They also generate income through user charges. The central government provides funding for prescription drug subsidies and financial support to county councils and municipalities through grants allocated using a risk-adjusted capitation formula. It may also provide one-off grants to focus on specific problem areas such as geographical inequalities in access to health care.

Figure 4.9. **Health care resources for county councils, Sweden, 2011**

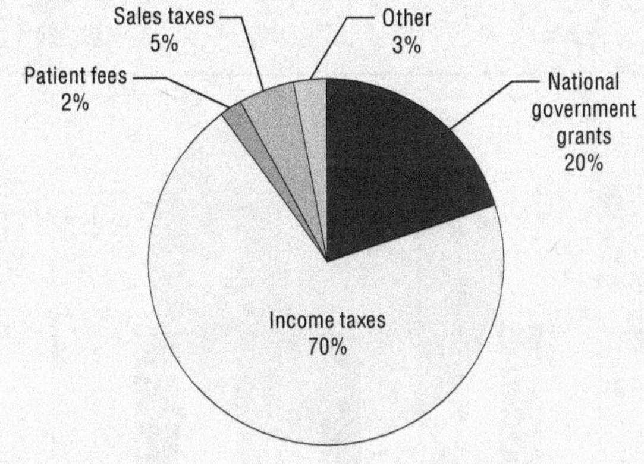

Source: OECD Survey of Budget Officials on Budgeting Practices for Health, 2013.

StatLink http://dx.doi.org/10.1787/888933218890

Since 2000, the county councils and municipalities have been required to balance their budgets (a deficit should be compensated for within three years). This implies that an increase in health care expenditure in a given year requires a similar decrease in other spending or an increase in the tax burden that year. This gives great incentives to sub-national governments and citizens to control health care expenditure growth.

Source: OECD Survey of Budget Officials on Budgeting Practices for Health, 2013.

Box 4.3. **Re-centralisation of specialised health care services in Norway in 2002**

Norway was characterised by highly decentralised health care spending over 1980-2002. During that period, counties were responsible for funding specialised health care services and municipalities were responsible for primary health services. The central government retained authority regarding supervision, control and planning.

However, a number of concerns arose and led ultimately to services being returned to the central government. First, the decentralised system had led to large geographic variations across counties/ municipalities for health care services. Secondly, competition for capacity between counties produced excess capacity and duplication of services. Finally, this system introduced a soft budget constraint, large deficits and a "blame game" between counties and the central government.

To alleviate these issues, Norway decided in 2002 to re-centralise specialised health care services. The provision of services was organised into five "regional health enterprises" (RHE) and funding was set as a combination of block and earmarked grants to the RHE.

Source: Magnussen, J. (2009), "Healthcare in Norway: Re-centralisation with a Twist", AcademyHealth, Washington, DC, *www.academyhealth.org/files/2009/monday/magnussen.pdf*.

Box 4.4. **Reform of health care in Finland**

Municipalities are key actors of health care expenditure in Finland and spending in this area has increased steadily over the last decade. Growth in spending per inhabitant has been particularly strong in smaller municipalities (see Figure 4.10).

Figure 4.10. **Evolution of social and health care services in Finnish municipalities**

Net expenditures, EUR/resident, base year 2005

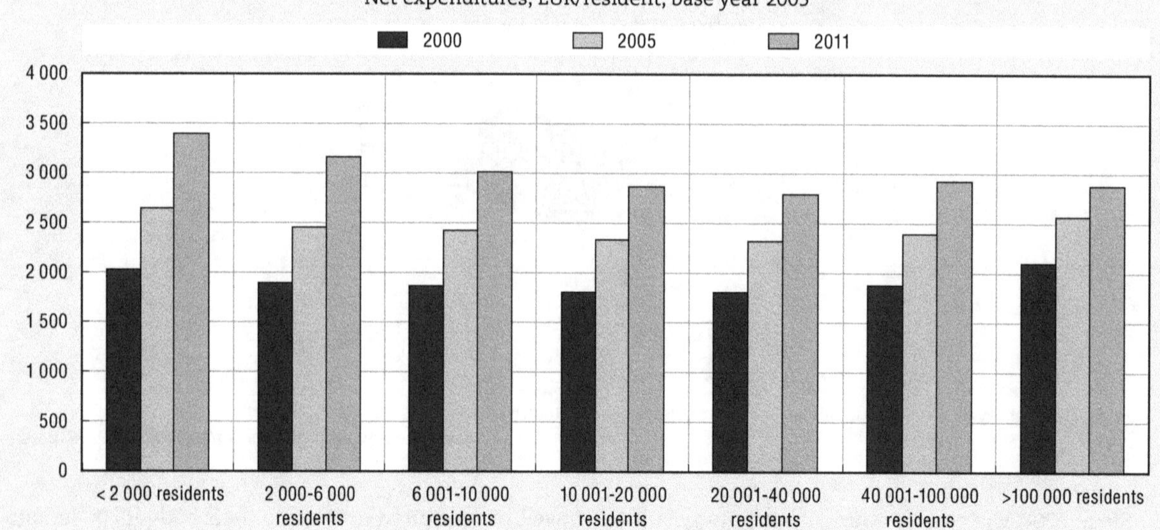

Source: OECD questionnaire (Directorate for Public Governance and Territorial Development) and OECD calculations.

StatLink http://dx.doi.org/10.1787/888933218909

In 2007, a first reform to achieve greater efficiency was carried out through municipal mergers (PARAS reform). With a similar objective, the Finnish government is currently discussing a new reform in which municipalities were being strongly encouraged to merge and to provide merger plans before July 2014, for mergers to be implemented between 2015 and 2017.

Box 4.4. **Reform of health care in Finland** *(cont.)*

In parallel, an agreement between the government and opposition parties was reached in late March 2014 on a major reform of the health care system. New regions are to be introduced on 1 January 2017 and will be run by a joint municipal authority.

The reform aims at delivering health care services on a larger scale through the creation of five "social welfare and health care regions". Services will be provided by these large regions instead of by municipalities. The concentration of health care services in larger organisations is to close efficiency gaps between specialised care units, make a more efficient use of information technologies and labour division, and introduce more efficient control at the national level, in particular regarding the strategic development of future health care policies. Some service provision will remain at the municipal level, in particular for every-day services. However these services will be organised by the five large regions.

The funding on the "social welfare and health care regions" will be provided by the municipalities, weighted according to each municipality's population. Moreover, in order to achieve fair funding, the population will be weighted by demographic structure and morbidity.

Source: Finnish Ministry of Social Affairs and Health, Helsinki.

4.6. Conclusion

Sub-national governments are responsible on average for 30% of health care expenditure in OECD countries, and this share reaches over 90% in some federal, quasi-federal and northern European countries (Denmark, Italy, Switzerland, Spain and Finland).

While some of the most efficient health care systems rely heavily on SNGs, decentralisation may introduce geographical differences in service provision, soften SNG budget constraints (as the central government may, at least implicitly, be responsible for bailouts) and induce excess capacity. Efficient, decentralised systems typically allocate precise responsibilities to each level of government in order to avoid duplication of services, and they may rely on sub-national fiscal rules to alleviate moral hazard behaviours.

The issue of the optimal size for health service provision in a decentralised context has been much discussed over recent years and was at the heart of Denmark's territorial reform in 2007. In a similar way, Finland plans to decrease the number of regions responsible for health expenditure in the years to come, and studies show that a similar reform in Sweden may significantly increase performance. However, large territorial reforms may be politically costly and more time may be needed to assess their impact on health spending efficiency.

There seems to exist no clear link between decentralisation of health expenditure and the composition of SNG revenues (i.e. distribution of sub-national revenues between taxes, transfers, etc.). However, countries in which SNGs are major actors in health expenditure typically protect sub-national governments from large variations in revenues from one year to another by making changes possible only on a multi-year basis or through the indexation of revenues to specific formulae.

References

ASISP – Analytical Support on the Socio-economic Impact of Social Protection Reforms (Europe) (2012), *Annual Report 2012, Pensions, Health Care and Long-Time Care, Norway*, European Commission.

ASISP (2011), *Annual Report 2011, Pensions, Health Care and Long-Time Care, Greece*, European Commission.

Blomqvist, P. and P. Bergman (2007), "Does Regionalisation of Nordic Health Care Systems Make Them Less Democratic? An Empirical Test of the Swedish Case", Uppsala University Working Paper No. 4, Sweden.

Dexia and CCRE – Conseil des Communes et Régions d'Europe (2012), *Les Finances publiques territoriales dans l'Union européenne*, 11th edition, July, *www.eetaa.gr/enimeroseis/17-01-13/Note_CCRE_Dexia_FR.pdf*.

Magnussen, J. (2009), *Health Care in Norway: Re-centralisation with a Twist*, *www.academyhealth.org/files/2009/monday/magnussen.pdf*.

OECD (2013), *Budgeting Practices and Procedures in OECD Countries*, OECD Publishing, Paris, *http://dx.doi.org/10.1787/9789264059696-en*.

OECD (2012), *Reforming Fiscal Federalism and Local Government: Beyond the Zero-Sum Game*, OECD Fiscal Federalism Studies, OECD Publishing, Paris, *http://dx.doi.org/10.1787/9789264119970-en*.

Fiscal Sustainability of Health Systems
Bridging Health and Finance Perspectives

Chapter 5

The impact of cost-containment policies on health expenditure

by
Rodrigo Moreno-Serra*

Many governments have enacted health cost-containment policies in recent years, and many are currently considering further reform alternatives to tackle growing health spending and promote efficiency in the health system, particularly in light of projections regarding future cost pressures in this sector. This chapter assesses the most robust empirical evidence on the public spending effects of health policy alternatives to contain excess cost growth in the system. A stylised theoretical framework for the relationships between potential cost-containment measures, economic incentives and quantities, and health expenditure is suggested. The framework provides structural guidance for reviewing the evidence on the cost-containment impacts of various reforms implemented in OECD countries in the last decades.

* Rodrigo Moreno-Serra is a Lecturer in Economics at the University of Sheffield, United Kingdom. Many thanks are due to Tiffany Ko for excellent research assistance during this project.

The statistical data for Israel are supplied by and under the responsibility of the relevant Israeli authorities. The use of such data by the OECD is without prejudice to the status of the Golan Heights, East Jerusalem and Israeli settlements in the West Bank under the terms of international law.

5.1. Introduction

Following steady health expenditure growth in many OECD countries in recent decades and projections of continued pressure on national health budgets in future years, governments have employed – and are continuously considering – a plethora of policy options for cost containment in the health system. Since financial resources and political capital are scarce goods, it is crucial to identify those policy options with higher potential to achieve cost-containment objectives once implemented. Contrary to earlier assessments,[1] empirical evidence on the effects of several cost-containment reforms introduced in the OECD area has now been accumulated and, despite being more abundant for certain policies and country settings, certainly offers valuable elements to inform health policy decisions if adequately put into context.

This chapter gathers and summarises the most robust empirical evidence on the health spending impacts of cost-containment policies implemented by OECD countries in recent decades. The evidence refers to policy efforts that have sought to tackle "excess cost growth" in the health system by changing cost-containment incentives to health care providers, consumers, or a combination of both. In some cases the policy efforts have also aimed at influencing health system administration costs.[2] Increased efficiency in the use of existing resources has also been targeted in order to help reduce cost pressures in the public health system. The available evidence on cost-containment policies, presented in more detail in the main text, is summarised in Table 5.1. At the same time, attention should be drawn to the critical importance of context, in terms of the detail of policy design and the starting point prior to the introduction of a given cost-containment policy.

Cost-containment policies aimed at the supply side: What do we know?

- *Provider payment methods.* Reforms to the way health care providers are reimbursed have been mostly effective in influencing health expenditure patterns. The introduction of physician payment methods based on capitation (e.g., United Kingdom) and cuts in service fees within fee-for-service schemes (e.g., United States) has succeeded in containing overall costs, with no evidence of cost-shifting to higher levels of care. The implementation of hospital payment mechanisms based on diagnosis-related groups has shown more mixed effects. While the cost-containment effects of provider payment reforms enacted more recently are difficult to predict in the longer run, given their potential boosting effect on demand through lower service prices, even relatively short-lived initiatives may result in permanent cost-saving changes in physician practice patterns.[3]
- *Provider competition.* Encouraging competition among hospital care providers has been linked to lower overall costs, greater efficiency and better quality of care in the United Kingdom and the United States, provided competition for patients is based on factors other than price (e.g., quality). Regulatory strategies such as enhanced patient choice and dissemination of information regarding hospital performance seems crucial in that regard. Price-based competition among hospitals has been associated with worsening

Table 5.1. Summary of the reviewed empirical evidence on cost-containment policies in OECD countries

Cost-containment policy	Category	Primary effect on	Empirical evidence of cost containment?	Main empirical evidence from	Notes
Fee-for-service reduction	Supply-side	Price	Yes	United States	Cost-containment effect partly mitigated by increase in service demand
Capitation payment	Supply-side	Price	Yes	United Kingdom	Combined with GP fundholding and gatekeeping No evidence of cost-shifting
DRG-based payment	Supply-side	Price	Mixed	Several OECD countries	May affect quality of services
Hospital competition	Supply-side	Mixed price and quantity	Yes (but note adverse effects on quality)	United Kingdom, United States	Price-based competition linked to lower care quality
Insurer competition and selective contracting	Supply-side	Mixed price and quantity	Mixed	Netherlands, United States	Successful in the United States (but note was combined with pay-for-performance) Less successful in the Netherlands (limited selective contracting and payment-for-performance)
Mandated generic substitution	Supply-side	Price	Yes	Canada, Sweden	
Joint purchasing of pharmaceuticals	Supply-side	Price	Yes	United States	Most evidence methodologically limited
Budget caps (sector and global)	Supply-side	Mixed price and quantity	Yes	Germany, United Kingdom	Most evidence methodologically limited Some evidence of cost-shifting due to sector budget
Workforce supply and wage controls	Supply-side	Mixed price and quantity	No	Canada, United States	Evidence of cost increases due to stricter entry legislation
Malpractice award limitation	Supply-side	Quantity	Yes	United States	Magnitude of cost-savings controversial
Cost-sharing extension	Demand-side	Price	Yes (but note adverse effects on access)	Several OECD countries	Extended cost-sharing linked to reduced access to necessary and quality care Consequential deleterious impacts on inequalities and health outcomes
Private insurance subsidisation	Demand-side	Mixed price and quantity	No	Australia, Spain, United Kingdom	Subsidy removal probably cost-saving
Gatekeeping role for physicians	Demand-side	Quantity	Mixed	Several OECD countries	Most evidence methodologically limited
Pharmaceutical formularies	Demand-side	Quantity	Yes	Canada, United States	Most evidence methodologically limited
Definition of publicly funded benefit package	Demand-side	Quantity	Evidence unavailable		Direct restriction to services offered within the public health system Link to use of health technology assessment (see below)
Direct price control of pharmaceuticals	Public management, coordination and financing	Price	Yes	Several OECD countries	Magnitude of cost-savings from reference pricing schemes heavily context-dependent Long-run effects on costs controversial
Decentralisation of health system functions	Public management, coordination and financing	Mixed price and quantity	Mixed	Several OECD countries	Centralised funding associated with higher sub-national expenditures Evidence of aggravation of inter-regional spending inequalities
Recentralisation of health system functions	Public management, coordination and financing	Mixed price and quantity	No	Norway	Only one country-case, with concurrent change to provider reimbursement
Reforms to the mix of health financing sources	Public management, coordination and financing	Mixed price and quantity	Yes	Several OECD countries	Evidence of cost-savings from move away from social insurance contributions towards general taxes
Use of health technology assessment	Public management, coordination and financing	Mixed price and quantity	Evidence unavailable		Cost-containment impacts likely to arise from combination with other reforms, including definition of basic benefit package

health outcomes for inpatients. And although quality controls imposed by the public sector can in principle protect consumers, there is evidence that hospitals may focus on maintaining quality for services more easily monitored by the public authority at the expense of other unmeasured activities (Propper et al., 2008). As with many other cost-containment strategies discussed in this chapter, long-term effects on health expenditures will depend on the extent by which aspects such as quality improvements increase aggregate service demand.

- *Insurer competition and selective contracting*. The cost-control potential of insurer competition hinges to a large extent on the combined role of selective contracting, particularly in inpatient care. A strong role for selective contracting – with payment-for-performance elements – seems to magnify any cost savings from the encouragement of insurer competition. This highlights the importance of developing and improving comprehensive provider performance indicator systems in addition to effective risk equalisation schemes. Although selective contracting has been used in single-payer systems as well, most evidence on its cost-containment effects comes from the experience in multiple-payer systems that have also promoted health insurer competition (Netherlands and United States). The cost-containment impacts of insurer competition reforms seem to apply in contexts beyond health systems characterised by a unique configuration such as managed care in the United States. Yet the scope for introducing such market-based reforms depends on whether there are already multiple insurers in the system and on the extent of provider competition and patient choice.
- *Pharmaceutical policies*. Mandated generic substitution has helped curb the growth in pharmaceutical expenditures (Canada and Sweden), at least in the relatively short period of time most research has been able to analyse. Joint (multi-state) purchasing has also been suggested to decrease the pharmaceutical bill to the public sector (United States). These policies have frequently been employed alongside other pharmaceutical-related reforms affecting both the supply and demand sides (see below), enhancing their cost-containment potential. It is possible that pharmaceuticals will continue putting upward pressure on health expenditures in the longer term should they enable more people to obtain treatment, and for longer periods of time, due to price reduction.
- *Budget caps*. Ceilings on global or sector expenditures have had some success in containing health costs (Germany, United Kingdom). Some cost-shifting from sectors affected by the budget caps towards uncontrolled sectors has been identified in Germany, but the additional costs in other sectors seem outweighed by the generated savings from the cap policy. Although the OECD experience with budget controls is perceived as mostly positive, particularly in single-payer countries (Docteur and Oxley, 2003), the available hard evidence is limited. Also, concerns may be raised about the possibility of other consequences for the system, for instance increased waiting lists as hospitals adjust their activity levels. Unfortunately, there is a paucity of empirical evidence on these aspects.
- *Workforce legislation*. Reforms restricting the supply of health professionals – mainly through stricter professional entry barriers – and wage controls have proved ineffective in containing overall health expenditures (Canada and United States). In fact, empirical research has shown that tighter entry or licensure legislation may be cost-increasing for the health system as a whole due to reduced provider competition and resulting increases in the overall wage bill for "protected" professionals. It would be important for health policy design if empirical evidence was also generated about changes in the mix and quality of care resulting from workforce legislation reforms.

- *Malpractice legislation*. Limits imposed on malpractice damage awards paid by physicians have helped contain health spending growth in the United States by curbing higher volumes of care due to defensive medicine behaviour. The magnitude of these gains is controversial, however. The evidence is also unclear about the effects of such reforms on quality of care, as presumably decreased risk of litigation may encourage lenient behaviour by some providers and possibly worse patient outcomes.

Cost-containment policies aimed at the demand side: What do we know?

- *Cost-sharing*. Reforms expanding the role of cost-sharing in health financing have generally succeeded in lowering overall public spending on health in the short run. Yet expanded cost-sharing seems to lead to deleterious effects on patients' health outcomes and to inequalities by imposing barriers to access to needed and quality care, especially by more vulnerable populations. Since the demand for most medical services is relatively price-inelastic (Cutler and Zeckhauser, 2000), only by imposing substantial increases in cost-sharing can governments expect to significantly limit the demand for health services and associated costs, probably at the expense of damaging consequences on care access and health outcomes. Exemption policies, complementary private insurance and ceilings on spending targeted at vulnerable populations can help mitigate such negative consequences if carefully implemented, as attempted in France and Sweden (Docteur and Oxley, 2003).
- *Private insurance tax policies*. Subsidies to encourage the take-up of complementary private health insurance have failed to relieve public budgetary pressures (Australia, Spain and United Kingdom). In fact, studies have recommended the elimination of existing tax incentives for enrolment into private health insurance in light of potentially substantial savings for the public sector, even when increased use of publicly funded care is factored in. Any cost savings for the public sector from the removal of these subsidies may be exacerbated if private insurers reduce their premiums and succeed in keeping part of their enrolees, thereby mitigating increased use of publicly funded health care.
- *Physician gatekeeping*. The implementation of gatekeeping arrangements in OECD countries has contained health expenditure growth, at least according to cross-country evidence. The combination of gatekeeping with supply-side reforms, such as capitated payment and budget-holding for GPs applied in the United Kingdom, seems a promising strategy to curb overall health spending. However, the evidence on the system-wide cost impacts of gatekeeping implementation in individual countries is still methodologically limited.
- *Pharmaceutical formularies (preferred drug lists)*. Formularies seem to have decreased spending on pharmaceuticals and resulted in overall cost savings in the system (Canada, United States). As above, the available research on the topic is still limited. Arguably, the benefits in terms of cost control and quality of care are potentially higher if formularies tilt consumption patterns towards drugs with high cost-effectiveness and exclude those with low cost-effectiveness, highlighting the catalyst role of health technology assessment within broad cost-containment strategies.

Cost containment through public management, co-ordination and financing reforms: What do we know?

- *Direct control of pharmaceutical prices and profits*. The joint introduction of direct price controls and other regulations (such as mandated generic substitution) in pharmaceutical markets across the OECD has proved an effective policy lever to contain health expenditures. Strict price regulation has lowered drug prices in several countries (e.g., Canada, France, Germany, Japan and the United States). Differences related to some pharmaceutical market institutional features have been instrumental in exacerbating the cost-containment effect of reference pricing reforms in some contexts compared to others. For instance, mandated generic substitution was key for cost containment through reference pricing in Germany, while price controls on generics magnified cost savings from reference pricing in New Zealand compared to Germany and the Netherlands. But although direct price control policies have also been found more capable of decreasing the overall pharmaceutical bill to the public sector than cost-sharing (Sweden; Andersson et al., 2006), their long-term cost-control effects remain controversial. More research is also needed on other potential impacts of price and profit control policies, for example the extent to which revenue reductions can negatively affect innovation in the pharmaceutical industry.

- *Decentralisation and re-centralisation of health system functions.* Transfer of functions such as planning and service delivery to sub-national levels of government, with mostly centralised funding, seems to have translated into cost savings at the system level in some contexts (Italy, where the reforms took place in the context of health budget cuts) but not others (Spain). The prevalence of soft budgeting post-decentralisation has been singled out as a major caveat for effective cost containment in the health system, particularly at sub-national government levels. The scarce evidence on re-centralisation policies (Norway) also suggests a lack of cost-containment impacts in the health sector, again owing in part to the persistence of soft budgets after the reform. Sub-national inequalities in health spending seem to be aggravated after decentralisation reforms (Italy, Spain and Switzerland). In these contexts, governments must ensure the implementation of adequate co-ordination and fiscal equalisation arrangements in order to prevent spill-over effects such as residents seeking health care in a different locality due to low quality of care in their area.
- *Sources of health system financing.* Reforms aimed at increasing reliance on social insurance contributions *vis-à-vis* general taxation have led to higher total and government health expenditures in OECD countries, according to a body of empirical evidence. Due to the broad nature of health financing reforms, the corresponding hard evidence comes almost exclusively from aggregate, cross-country studies, which makes it difficult to investigate the specific channels responsible for higher health expenditures in systems moving towards social insurance financing. Some evidence has been found of higher administrative costs and provider wage bills due to higher reliance on social insurance funding. More generally, the available research suggests that movements towards social-insurance-based financing often involve costly institutional reforms (e.g., creation of a social insurance agency and the co-ordination and regulation of multiple payers) which are not usually offset by cost savings or efficiency improvements elsewhere in the health system.
- *Health technology assessment.* Reforms to enhance the role and quality of health technology assessment (HTA) activities may promote efficiency in health system funding allocation and may free up resources, thus reducing pressures on the public budget. Although no systematic evidence is available on the direct cost-containment impacts of HTA, it seems more sensible to expect HTA to have cost-containment and efficiency impacts mainly through its judicious use in defining the package of interventions publicly funded in the

health system, assisting also with decisions about public funding of new, more expensive (but potentially more clinically effective) technologies. The overall effect on health costs of adopting new technology will depend not only on prices, but also on its effects on health care demand.[4]

This chapter is structured as follows. Section 5.2 provides some background on the rationale for, and the nature of, cost-containment reforms introduced in the health system in recent years by OECD countries. It also lays out the objectives and scope for the review of the available empirical research assessing cost-containment impacts. Section 5.3 presents a stylised theoretical framework for the relationships between potential cost-containment measures, economic incentives and quantities, and health expenditure. The framework provides structural guidance for Section 5.4, which reviews the empirical evidence on the cost-containment impacts of various reforms by OECD countries in the last decades. Section 5.5 presents some concluding remarks.

5.2. Background and chapter objectives

Most OECD countries finance their health systems predominantly from public sources such as general tax revenues and social health insurance contributions (Figure 5.1). Following a steady increase in health expenditures among member countries over the 1960s and 1970s, such growth in spending slowed down over the 1980s and part of the 1990s. Yet from the early 2000s onwards countries have experienced a revival in health expenditure growth at rates that many countries find worrying for public finances given current levels of overall economic activity. Health expenditures among OECD countries represented on average 9.0% of GDP in 2012, reaching between 11-12% in countries such as Canada, France, Germany, the Netherlands and Switzerland, and 17% in the United States (Figure 5.2).

Figure 5.1. **Public expenditure on health as a share of total health expenditure, OECD countries 2012 or nearest year**

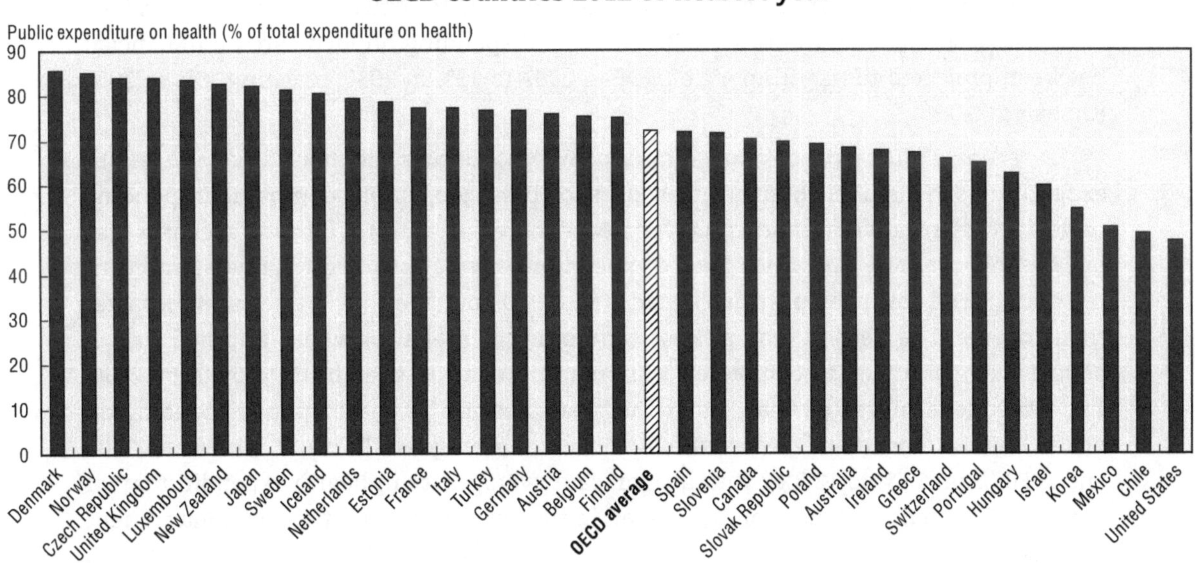

Note: Data for Australia, Netherlands, Portugal and New Zealand are from 2011. For the Netherlands, current health expenditure data are reported.

Source: *OECD Health Statistics, http://dx.doi.org/10.1787/health-data-en.*

StatLink http://dx.doi.org/10.1787/888933218918

Figure 5.2. **Total expenditure on health as a share of GDP, OECD countries 2012 or nearest year**

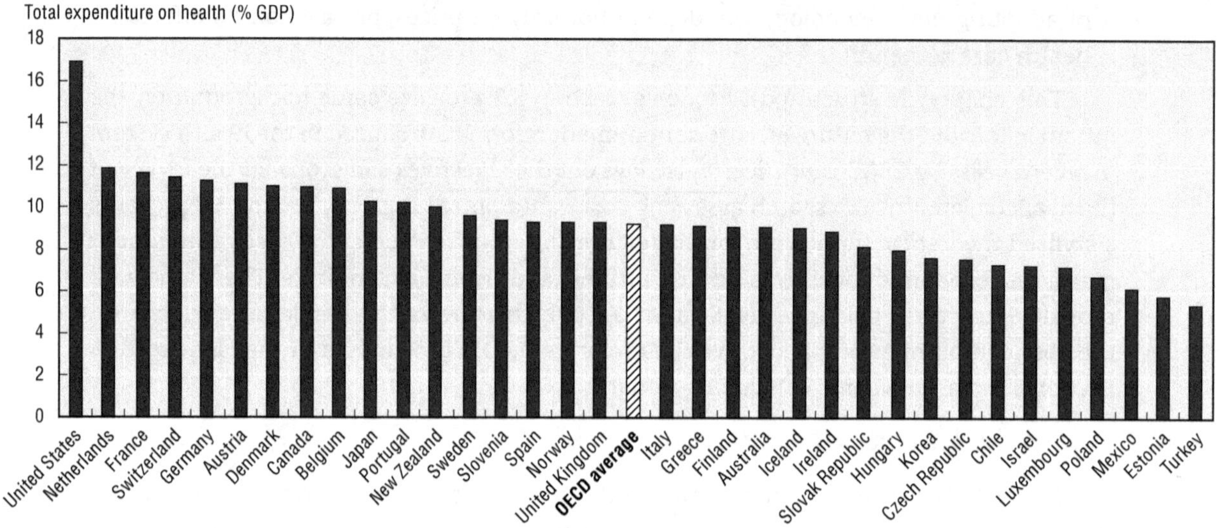

Note: Data for Australia, Portugal and New Zealand are from 2011. For the Netherlands, current health expenditure data are reported.

Source: *OECD Health Statistics, http://dx.doi.org/10.1787/health-data-en.*

StatLink http://dx.doi.org/10.1787/888933218926

Many governments have enacted health cost-containment policies in recent years, and many are currently considering further reform alternatives to tackle growing health spending and promote efficiency in the health system, particularly in light of projections regarding future cost pressures in this sector. For example, a report commissioned by the British government to examine trends in health expenditure over the following 20 years concluded that, under reasonable scenarios of health needs, technological advance, workforce use and productivity changes, total health spending in the United Kingdom would grow from less than 8% of GDP in 2002 to between 10.6% and 12.5% by 2022 (Wanless, 2002). In the United States, federal spending on Medicare and Medicaid has been projected to rise from 4% of GDP in 2007 to 12% in 2050, reaching 19% in 2082 (Orszag, 2007).[5]

A recent OECD report developed a framework to discuss the main drivers of health expenditures in member countries, as well as to obtain projections of growth in spending under two alternative scenarios (Oliveira Martins et al., 2006). The first scenario was one of "cost-pressure", in which health expenditures were assumed to grow in line with historical trends over the past two decades in OECD countries, i.e. 1% per annum faster than income. The second was a "cost-containment" scenario, where national health policies were assumed to completely eliminate that extra expenditure growth by 2050. The projections suggested that, under the "cost-pressure" scenario, public spending on health could almost double as a share of GDP in an average OECD country between 2005 and 2050 (from 6.7% to 12.8%), with a significant average rise in health expenditures – of around 3.5 percentage points of GDP – even in the event of successful cost-containment policies.

As for the major health expenditure drivers, the retrospective decompositions and projections of the growth in public spending for OECD countries broadly confirmed the conclusions from previous (and also more recent) research. Population ageing and other demographic factors, including improvements in population health status, account for only a modest share of health spending growth. Specifically, Oliveira Martins et al. (2006) estimated the age effect to account for less than one-tenth of the increase in government health expenditure per capita between 1970 and 2002. In the United States, ageing is expected to account for less than 20% of federal spending on Medicare and Medicaid by 2050 (and about 10% by 2082; Orszag, 2007). Studies for other countries have obtained similar results (e.g., France; see Dormont et al., 2006).[6]

The OECD work on projections concluded that non-demographic aspects (which include effects from income growth, technology adoption and changes in relative prices) represent by far the most important drivers of the growth in health expenditures. The expenditure growth corresponding to non-demographic factors was estimated to reach around 4% per annum between 1970 and 2002. Income growth seems to have played a significant role for the rising shares of national income devoted to health services in that period. Yet this and other studies for OECD countries indicate that economic growth is not necessarily the key underlying factor, with health spending typically growing faster than income in what is often referred to as "excess cost growth" (Orszag, 2007; White, 2007). Instead, cost pressures associated with the institutional setting around the organisation, financing and delivery of health services – including changes in medical practice and uptake of new technologies – are frequently identified as the most important cost drivers in past and projected increases in national health expenditures, representing between one-third and two-thirds of health spending growth in the OECD as a whole and in countries such as the United States and France (Wanless, 2002; Dormont et al., 2006; Oliveira Martins et al., 2006; Chernew et al., 2012).[7]

Many of the cost-containment reforms introduced in the OECD area from the late 1980s have been primarily aimed at reversing the strong increase in excess cost growth; but a systematic analysis of their effects on health spending, based on hard empirical evidence, is surprisingly lacking. Projection work such as Oliveira Martins et al. (2006) has usually simulated "cost-containment" scenarios in which policies are successful in curbing health spending by the end of the projection period, yet such policies have rarely been modelled explicitly based on actual quantitative evidence about how effective their introduction has been in the past.

This report gathers and summarises the most robust empirical evidence on the health spending impacts of cost-containment policies implemented by OECD countries in recent decades.[8] These policies have been enacted against a background of widespread acknowledgement by policy makers that changing the incentives embedded into existing arrangements for health care organisation and delivery can be fundamental to improving efficiency in the system, thereby helping to tame upward pressures in health care costs. From a policy perspective, it is crucial to examine the available evidence on the impacts of alternative measures of cost containment in the health sector. Planning and forecasting activities require quantitative information about the potential that such reforms have to curb overall spending in the system. Assumptions based on theoretical expected effects will not necessarily correspond to actual policy effects when those are implemented in real conditions. They may render less valid the conclusions from exercises that seek to estimate growth in health spending based on a strong effect of cost-containment initiatives.

The focus of this review is to assess the evidence on the public spending effects of health policy alternatives to contain excess cost growth in the system. This is, after all, the main component driving up health system costs (apart from overall economic growth), and upon which most policy options readily available for governments are suited to act.[9] A detailed description of all cost-containment reforms implemented in the OECD area is beyond the scope of the present chapter. Other studies have presented these reforms in more depth, mainly from a taxonomical perspective (cf. e.g., Mossialos and Le Grand, 1999; Docteur and Oxley, 2003; Langenbrunner et al., 2005), and the reader is referred to them for more details of each policy reform. Yet effective policy making requires hard evidence on the impact of alternative policies under different contexts, so those more likely to succeed in a particular health system configuration can be selected. Since the quantitative impacts of any policy will likely vary across countries according to institutional and historical settings, the present review has the modest goal of assisting policy makers to make more informed decisions on health cost-containment reform paths based on particular country experiences, outlining a number of more specific recommendations for governments grounded on the available empirical research.

5.3. A stylised economic framework for cost-containment reforms

Governments have several cost-containment policy options at their disposal. These options vary greatly with regard to the specific channels through which they are expected to influence health expenditures. Policies may be expected to change mainly provider or consumer behaviour and activities, or act through a combination of both. Any changes in provider or consumer behaviour may affect the prices and/or quantities of health services provided, sometimes primarily in one sub-sector but with spill-overs to other sub-sectors.

Figure 5.3 presents a suggested stylised framework to analyse the economic mechanisms and relationships at work. The framework developed here builds on earlier typologies of cost-containment health policy reforms suggested elsewhere (Oxley and MacFarlan, 1995; Joumard et al., 2010), grouping alternatives into: supply-side, demand-side or reforms in public management, co-ordination and financing. The boundaries between these categories can be blurred and sometimes debatable. Figure 5.3 offers one possible, simplified policy categorisation based on whether the cost-containment policy is primarily meant to alter provider behaviour, consumer behaviour or a combination of both (sometimes also including public administrators) through changes in public management and broad institutional arrangements.

The components of total health expenditure (THE) are disaggregated into three sub-sectors: outpatient and inpatient expenditure ($HE_{O/I}$), pharmaceutical expenditure (HE_{PH}) and public administration expenditure (HE_{ADM}). Further structure is added to the proposed framework by the introduction of basic economic parameters, the price (P) and quantity (Q) of health services, so as to generate clearer insights about the potential direction of health spending variations induced by each reform.

Policy instruments may then – at least in theory – influence health expenditure by acting directly or primarily on service prices (black lines) or quantities (light grey lines). Policies may also affect sector and overall health expenditures by indirectly stimulating administrative units, providers and consumers to adjust prices and/or quantities (dotted lines). It is sensible to expect policy reforms to exhibit important interactions among them and with institutional aspects of the health system, thus mitigating or exacerbating their "pure" cost-containment effects, as well as causing indirect knock-on effects on other sub-sectors of the system. For the sake of exposition, these are not modelled in the framework proposed here, but rather discussed on a case-by-case basis according to the available empirical evidence reviewed below.

Figure 5.3. **A stylised economic framework for cost-containment reforms**

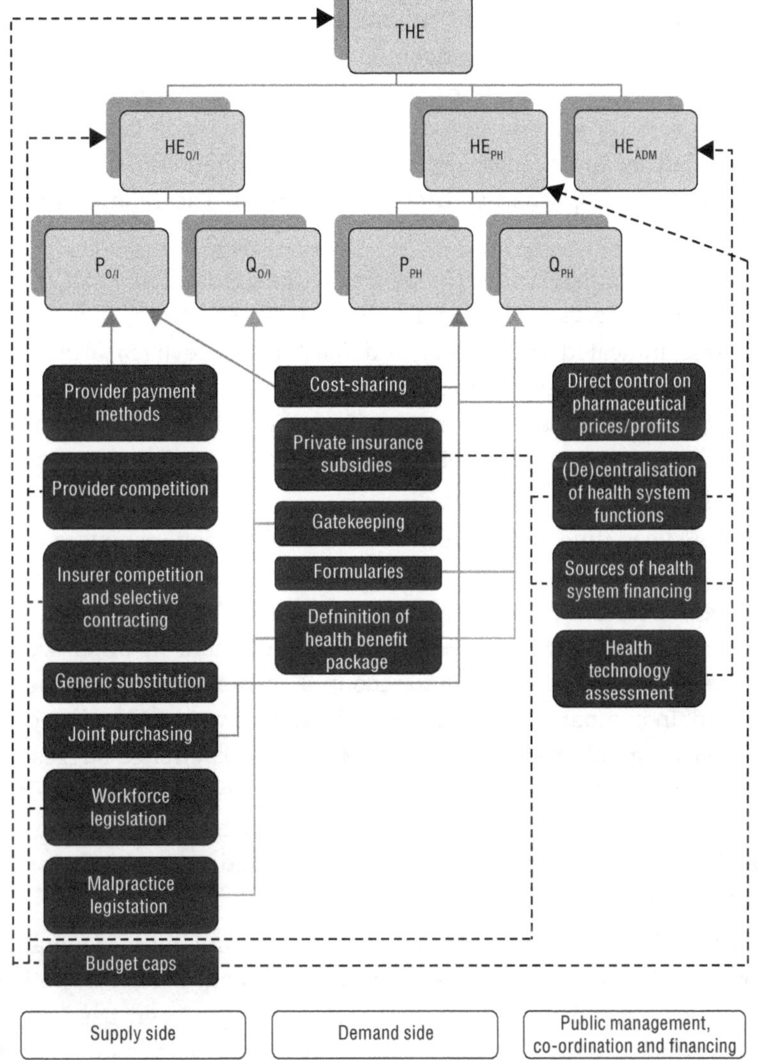

$HE_{O/I}$: outpatient and inpatient expenditure; $HE_{ADM:}$ public administration expenditure; $HE_{PH:}$ pharmaceutical expenditure; P: price; Q: quantity; THE: total health expenditure.

The policy reforms displayed in Figure 5.3 are not intended to represent the whole menu of cost-containment instruments available to policy makers. They mostly represent those interventions for which some robust empirical evidence is available on their effectiveness to control health expenditure. Despite its simplicity, the proposed framework offers a tractable and insightful structure, based on economic parameters, to think straight about the possible and observed impacts of policy reforms to address non-demographic drivers of health expenditure.

5.4. Cost-containment policy reforms in OECD countries: Reviewing the evidence

Supply-side reforms

Reforms to physician payment mechanisms

Physicians are often involved in the role of deciding how health resources are allocated, as they act as agents of their patients and are often entrusted with the authority to determine the need for and arrangement of specialist or hospital care. Effective implementation of primary-care reforms, such as the introduction or reinforcement of a gatekeeping role for general practitioners (GPs), depends largely on the financial incentives provided by the accompanying payment system for physicians. The latter operates on health costs primarily through changes in the relative price of services (Figure 5.3).

Payment methods for physicians can be crudely categorised into salary arrangements, capitation, and fee-for-service (Ellis and Miller, 2008). Economic theory and empirical studies have long indicated that salary and fee-for-service (FFS) arrangements rarely provide physicians with the incentive to contain cost (Gerdtham and Jönsson, 2000; Ellis and Miller, 2008). FFS schemes may even proliferate supplier-induced demand, although there have been attempts to control costs in such systems by directly cutting service fees or implementing FFS within a hard budget.

Nguyen (1996) used time series data to examine physician responses to fee reduction within the FFS arrangements for the United States Medicare programme. Results show that the volume of services whose fees were cut by the Omnibus Budget Reconciliation Act of 1989 increased by 3.7% for every 10% fee reduction. In other words, for every dollar cut in fees, physicians were able to recoup 37 cents through increasing volume of services provided. In comparison, procedures whose fees were not reduced did not seem to have experienced a volume increase. The Medicare experience suggests that simple fee reductions within FFS arrangements are likely to have their impacts on health cost-containment attenuated if taken in isolation, with no further provisions to curb the high-powered spending incentives possibly leading to undesired behavioural responses such as supplier-induced demand.

In contrast to FFS payments, capitation methods and more generally the use of predefined budgets for GP payment are often argued to allow funders to keep a tighter control over health expenditures. Such arrangements have been used as a strategy to transfer the responsibility over resource allocation onto physicians or GPs even though, depending on the details of implementation, they may provide GPs with little incentive to maintain or improve quality of care (Ellis and Miller, 2008).

Dusheiko et al. (2006) used the introduction of GP fundholding in the United Kingdom in 1991, and its subsequent abolition in 1999, to compare trends in hospital admission rates among fundholding and non-fundholding GP practices before and after the policy change of the late 1990s. During the existence of the GP fundholding policy, general practices could choose to be given a budget to pay for the costs of certain types of elective surgery (chargeable electives) for their patients and could retain any surplus, but they did not pay for other types of elective admissions or for emergency admissions. The removal of financial incentives associated with budget holding was found to increase chargeable elective admissions by 3.5%-5.1% among former fundholding practices, implying estimated savings in the range of GBP 46 million to GBP 67 million for the English National Health System had fundholding remained in place in 2000. Evidence from this natural experiment suggests that gatekeeping physicians are indeed likely to respond to the introduction of capitation or budget payment by cutting back service volume, through which there is potential for reduced overall spending in the health system.[10]

Reforms to hospital payment mechanisms

There is hard evidence from OECD countries also with regard to the potential impact of reforming payment methods to hospitals – the biggest spenders in a health system – as policy tools for overall cost containment. As with physician payment methods, reforms to hospital payment arrangements are expected to change the behaviour of providers by altering the relative price of health care services.

Payment mechanisms to hospitals can be broadly classified into three groups: payments based on provider characteristics (e.g., line-item budgets), payments based on service characteristics (e.g., FFS) and payments based on patient characteristics (e.g., variants of diagnosis-related groups – DRGs). In theory, under otherwise similar institutional contexts, payment arrangements based on provider or patient characteristics give hospitals stronger financial incentives to contain spending than payment methods based on the characteristics of the services, in which providers are usually remunerated according to the volume of procedures (Ellis and Miller, 2008).

A study by Kwon (2003) examined changes in hospital throughput and costs associated with the implementation of DRGs within a pilot programme in Korea, covering a selected group of diseases with voluntary provider participation. This DRG experiment was intended to pave the way for the eventual roll-out of case-based payment for all inpatient care funded by the Korean national health insurance programme, which had been paying providers by fee-for-service since its inception. Simple comparisons pre- and post-pilot showed that total medical expenses per claim case decreased by 14% after the introduction of DRG, owing in part to sizeable reductions in typical length of stay. This conclusion, although only indicative, echoes findings from studies conducted elsewhere in the OECD area (and comparative studies including OECD countries) suggesting that providers have responded to the incentives embedded in DRG-based payment towards curtailment of overprovision of services and reduced hospital expenditures (cf. e.g., Louis et al., 1999 for Italy; Gerdtham et al., 1999 for Sweden; Moreno-Serra and Wagstaff, 2010 for some recent OECD member countries).

However, the above provider response to the introduction of DRG-based payment may be linked to undesired consequences elsewhere in the health system. For example, although studies have frequently been unable to detect deleterious impacts on health care quality arising from DRG introduction or expansion reforms (Dismuke and Guimaraes, 2002; Or and Hakkinen, 2010; Moreno-Serra and Wagstaff, 2010; among others), some empirical research in the area has concluded that lack of adequate quality assurance mechanisms may be behind increased hospital readmission rates or lower-than-expected quality gains in a few contexts (Forgione et al., 2004). More generally, a European Observatory review of hospital payment mechanisms found the evidence on unit costs mixed, and in some cases increased total hospital costs (Busse et al., 2011).

Reforms to promote competition among providers

The existence of market failures mean that unregulated competition among suppliers in the health sector is unlikely to result in lower prices and improved quality of care (Arrow, 1963). In many instances, governments have fostered the development of "quasi-markets" in health care by, *inter alia*, introducing and regulating the choice of providers and insurers, and controlling the extent to which providers can compete for patients. The idea behind market-oriented reforms is that they will encourage providers and insurers to seek efficiency gains (in addition to improvements in aspects like quality of care), thereby helping to contain the growth of health expenditures. In reality, the introduction of competition reforms in OECD health systems has focused mainly on the hospital and insurer (payer) levels. Market-oriented reforms have been adopted or are under discussion in countries such as Australia, Belgium, Czech Republic, Israel, Netherlands and the United Kingdom, while in the United States markets have long been used for the delivery of health care.

The system-wide effects of different competitive regimes for providers introduced in the 1990s and 2000s in the United Kingdom offer valuable insights for policy makers, particularly concerning the aspects on which provider competition is based. Gaynor et al. (forthcoming) studied the introduction of market-oriented reforms in the English NHS in 2006, whereby GPs were required to offer patients a choice of provider for elective inpatient care, and providers started to be remunerated based on prospective fixed prices (a variant of DRGs). Examining data for all English hospitals, the authors show that the reforms encouraged providers to compete for patients through improvements in quality of care, since prices were fixed. Hospital efficiency was found to improve in that better health outcomes were achieved in hospitals more exposed to competitive pressure, with lower average length-of-stay and no general increases in hospital expenditures. One of the channels by which competitive pressure may have improved efficiency among English hospitals is through encouraging service reconfiguration (consolidation and reallocation) across hospital sites, which has been associated with elimination of excess bed capacity and sizeable cost savings for some providers (Palmer, 2011).

A word of caution regarding the set-up of provider competition comes from a previous market reform enacted in the United Kingdom in the early 1990s. Despite evidence of lower waiting times and cost reductions through lower expenditure per patient after the reform, under this previous regime prices were negotiated, hospital reimbursement was based chiefly on retrospective cost and measures of quality were very limited and not publicly available. This meant that competitive pressure ended up reducing quality of care measured by indicators not monitored (unobserved) by the regulator (Propper et al., 2008). The importance of the institutional framework for the quality-cost trade-off from enhanced provider competition is reinforced by studies of price competition in other settings, with similar results (Volpp et al., 2003).

Reforms to promote selective contracting and competition among purchasers

Insurer competition and selective contracting have also been used as policy tools for health cost containment and improved efficiency in OECD countries. In the United States since the early 1980s, this has translated into the implementation of managed care organisations which are intended to achieve cost savings relative to "traditional" private insurers (indemnity plans) by negotiating service prices from selected, competing hospitals and steering their enrolees to them, as well as shifting away from cost-based hospital reimbursement towards prospective payment mechanisms. Another example since the early 1990s is the Dutch case, where managed competition has been rolled out focusing primarily on purchaser competition and selective contracting of providers within reforms to implement a compulsory private insurance scheme.

A number of studies have concluded that purchaser competition coupled with selective contracting and payment-for-performance in the United States have delivered reductions in the growth rate of health insurance premiums by containing costs and improving system efficiency (Dranove et al., 1993; Zwanziger et al., 1994, 2000). More specifically, both for-profit and not-for-profit hospitals located in more competitive areas exhibited slower spending growth (compared to their counterparts in locations with lower pressure from other competitors) after the emergence of selective contracting (Zwanziger et al., 2000). There is also indicative evidence on spillover effects from managed care and selective contracting within the traditional Medicare system. For example, the average fee-for-service inpatient expenditure of traditional Medicare enrolees has been found to decrease by as much as 2.5% for a 10% increase in the market share of managed care organisations, with similar results for outpatient expenditure (Baker, 1999).

The available evidence for the Netherlands emphasises the substantial degree of interdependence between distinct features of "quasi-markets" in health care. In addition to encouraging price competition among health insurers, the move towards purchaser competition in the Dutch health system has been found to lower price inflation among non-price-regulated hospitals and significantly reduce generic drug prices between 2006 and 2009 (Schut and van de Ven, 2011). Nevertheless, there is no hard evidence that the pro-market reforms have played a role in reducing the growth of overall health expenditures in the Dutch health system. To some extent, this seems due to two main reasons. One is the limited practical role for selective contracting based on provider performance within current purchasing processes, since most service prices are still subject to substantial regulation and health insurers typically have most deficits on hospital expenses reimbursed retrospectively (van de Ven and Schut, 2009). This dilutes the incentive insurers have to push for lower prices from providers, and allows providers to compensate for lower prices by raising the volume of services delivered. Another possible reason is the reluctance of insurers (possibly driven by medical profession opposition) to integrate vertically with providers – one of the expected outcomes of the reform – and set up managed care organisations similar to those found in the United States and Switzerland (Schut and van de Ven, 2011).

Reforms to pharmaceutical markets

The rapid growth of expenditure on pharmaceuticals in the OECD area during most of the second half of the 20th century presented a challenge for national health budgets.[11] As a response, countries such as Canada, Germany, Spain, Sweden and the United States have enacted an array of alternative cost-containment policies targeted at all levels of the production and distribution of pharmaceuticals. Supply-side policies for cost control have focused mainly on influencing the price of individual drugs (Figure 5.4). Although pharmaceuticals still represented on average over 15.8% of total health expenditure in the OECD area in 2011 (OECD, 2013), those cost-containment policies may have played a role for the declining share of pharmaceutical spending in total health spending observed in recent years (Figure 5.4).

Figure 5.4. **Evolution of pharmaceutical expenditure as a share of total health expenditure**

Pharmaceutical expenditure (% of total health expenditure)

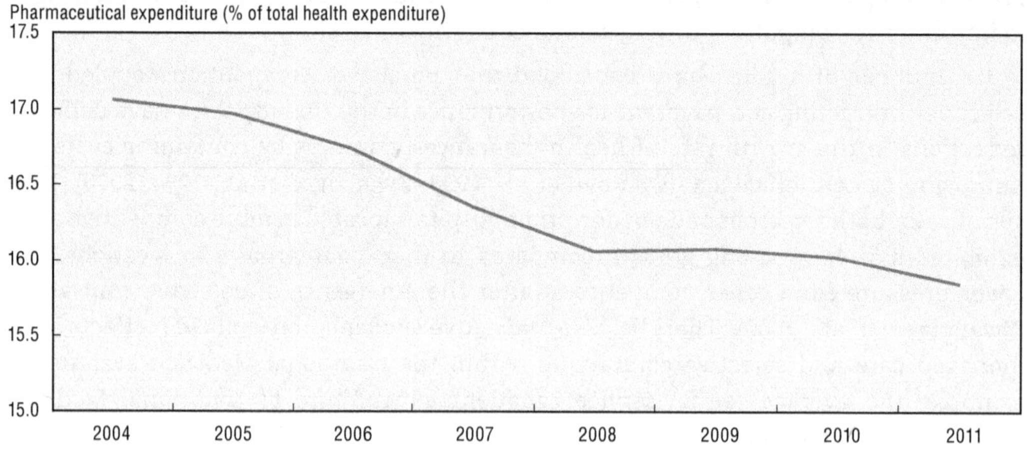

Note: Simple averages for 27 OECD countries with available data for the entire period.

Source: OECD Stat Extracts, available at: *http://stats.oecd.org*.

StatLink http://dx.doi.org/10.1787/888933218937

One example of such policies is mandated generic substitution of brand name drugs in publicly funded outpatient and inpatient care. In Canada, a reform was introduced in British Columbia in 1994 subsidising purchases of pharmaceuticals for the amount equal to the cost of generics, requiring senior citizens to pay extra for a branded drug. In spite of a gradual increase in prices charged for existing products, this trend was more than offset by increased use of generics between 1991 and 2001 (Morgan et al., 2004). A 2002 mandate for generic drug substitution in Sweden has had qualitatively similar impacts on patients' spending and on the reimbursed cost for outpatient prescription drugs under the Swedish Pharmaceutical Benefits Scheme. Increasing trends in pharmaceutical spending before mandatory generic substitution seem to have reverted after the reform, for both patient expenses and government subsidies, and at both the country and county council level (Andersson et al., 2007).

Another example of a cost-containment policy aimed at pharmaceutical providers, which is more feasible in some specific institutional settings, has been the use of joint purchasing arrangements with other states pursued by Michigan's Medicaid programme in the United States in the early 2000s. Joint purchasing and pooling for supplemental rebates were expected to generate reductions in drug manufacturers' prices and lower administrative costs for the public sector (through economies of scale). Multi-state drug purchasing arrangements were found to contribute to savings in prescription drug expenditures, yet this result should be treated with caution given the several concurrent reforms enacted at the time (Kibicho and Pinkerton, 2012).

Reforms to introduce ceilings on health expenditures

Budget caps have long been introduced by governments alongside other supply-side reforms as a way of targeting cost-containment measures, both in "older" and "recent" OECD countries (Docteur and Oxley, 2003; Schneider, 2007).[12] As displayed in Figure 5.4, ceilings on provider spending can be applied by sector (e.g., inpatient care) and/or by referring to overall (global) government health expenditure, and have sometimes been employed within broader programmes of fiscal consolidation. If implemented in isolation, one theoretical disadvantage of sector budgets compared to global budgets for effective spending control is that the former may stimulate cost-shifting and raise expenditure in sectors not subject to explicit budget ceilings (e.g., outpatient care).

Again, since the implementation of budget caps has often occurred within a broader array of cost-containment measures in health systems, hard evidence specifically about budget impacts on overall health spending is limited (Gerdtham and Jönsson, 2000). Informal assessments have concluded that the experience of most OECD countries with budget ceilings is likely positive regarding health expenditure control (Mossialos and Le Grand, 1999).[13] Moreover, country evidence on cost-shifting in the context of sector budgets indicates that additional (shifted) costs tend to be smaller than the savings obtained from imposing spending ceilings. In Germany, the imposition of a budget cap on drugs prescribed at the individual physician level (in which doctors were meant to be fined for exceeding the budget) resulted in an upsurge in the number of referrals and hospital admissions, presumably due to physicians referring their patients to other physicians or hospitals for fear of exceeding the ceiling (Schöffski and von der Schulenburg, 1997). However, the additional costs from admissions and referrals elsewhere were estimated to amount to just one-quarter of the total cost savings produced by the budget cap policy. This adds to the results of a previously mentioned analysis of the physician fundholding experience in the United Kingdom, which found no evidence of cost-shifting to other sectors (and net savings) due to the presence of capitated physician budgets (Dusheiko et al., 2006).

Reforms to workforce and malpractice legislation

The perception that the growth in overall health expenditures was to a great extent due to inflationary pressures related to the health workforce has led some governments to introduce direct or indirect controls over the total wage bill in the sector. Workforce supply and wage controls have been applied (under various alternative designs) in Denmark, France, Italy, Spain and Sweden, among others, succeeding in areas such as controlling the growth of physician numbers (Mossialos and Le Grand, 1999). Where increases in workforce cost have been attributed primarily to oversupply of professionals (especially physicians), tighter entry or licensure legislation has been enacted, apparently resulting in further inflationary pressures on the total wage bill or service prices in Canada and the United States due to reduced provider competition (Bärnighausen and Bloom, 2010). In the United States, stricter entry rules for alternative medicine providers in a given state have been linked to higher mainstream physician earnings (Anderson et al., 2000). Freezes or cuts in health sector wages have also been employed (e.g., Luxembourg and Spain during the 1990s); but there is virtually no robust quantitative evidence about whether their immediate cost saving impacts actually translate into lower growth rates of overall health costs later in time.

Financial incentives aimed at physicians and capable of influencing trends in health sector expenditures may also take forms other than distinct reimbursement arrangements, according to the specific institutional context. One such case is the enactment and operationalisation of malpractice laws that act as an incentive for health professionals to be prudent in their treatment choices. Some have argued that such laws, if not carefully implemented, may push service provision above its "optimal" level (from a social welfare perspective, for instance) by promoting defensive medicine practices, whereby physicians tend to prescribe marginally useful tests, procedures or medication for fear of litigation (Thomas et al., 2010).

The health sector spending effects of alternative designs for malpractice laws have been investigated empirically mainly in the United States, where some states have limited malpractice damage awards in the hope of reducing the health care bill associated with defensive medicine. The general message from available studies is that, although capping malpractice damages does seem to succeed in lowering costs arising from defensive medicine behaviour and contribute to slower health spending growth overall, the magnitude of such savings is controversial. Analyses of macro-level data have suggested that the existence of a cap on malpractice damages in a given state is associated with a reduction of between 3% and 4% in its annual health expenditure per capita. Yet investigations using micro-level data have estimated only modest impacts on total medical costs from reductions in medical malpractice insurance premiums (a measure of "perceived liability risk" by physicians), amounting to savings of merely 0.13% for a 10% decrease in malpractice premiums (Thomas et al., 2010; Hellinger and Encinosa, 2006).

Demand-side reforms

Reforms to expand cost-sharing

Some degree of patient cost-sharing has long been used in publicly funded health insurance schemes in most OECD "old" member countries, and countries that joined the OECD more recently have generally followed suit (e.g., Czech Republic, Hungary and Korea). Cost-sharing has taken a plethora of forms, including user payments for certain services in primary, specialist and inpatient care, as well as for prescription drugs, in the form of co-payments (fixed amount), co-insurance rates (share of costs) and/or deductibles (patient reimbursement only above a given minimum threshold cost) per prescription or service. In many instances, an enhanced role for patient cost-sharing in OECD health systems has been advocated as a policy lever to contain perceived overconsumption of specific therapies and reduce pressure on national health budgets (Schokkaert and van de Voorde, 2011).

By effectively raising the price of health care for users, it is hardly surprising that most empirical research points to lower service utilisation (particularly amongst low-income families) and reduced public health spending arising from reforms which increase reliance on cost-sharing. A prime example is the well-known Rand Health Insurance Experiment that took place in the United States in the early 1980s, where enrolees were randomly allocated to five types of health insurance plans with varying levels of co-insurance. Findings from the experiment indicated significant reductions in annual health expenditures for higher co-insurance or deductibles (though at decreasing rates), with people in the plan with no co-insurance having estimated annual expenditures 46% higher than those in the 95% co-insurance plan (Manning et al., 1987). Evidence on short-term reductions in health expenditures owing to expanded cost-sharing has since accumulated in many other OECD countries, including sub-areas such as pharmaceutical spending (cf. e.g., Rubin and Mendelson, 1996; Zweifel and Manning, 2000; Goldman and Zheng, 2007; Schokkaert and van de Voorde, 2011; Kenneally and Walshe, 2012).[14] Evidence about the longer-term effects of higher cost-sharing on the trajectory of cost growth remains scant, however. Indeed, Swartz, in a synthesis of evidence from high-income countries, finds that cost-sharing is unlikely to significantly slow health spending growth (Swartz, 2010).

Higher reliance on cost-sharing as a health policy tool has sometimes proved a politically difficult option, mainly due to the widespread public perception that increases in user charges end up translating into more difficult access to necessary and good-quality care, possibly harming people's health (Robinson, 2002). And generally the available hard evidence on cost-sharing in OECD countries does support public attitudes in this case. The Rand insurance experiment and subsequent studies in the United States have found that higher cost-sharing resulted in lower rates of initiation of needed medical care and utilisation of outpatient care, especially among low-income and high-risk populations, with adverse consequences for health status (Manning et al., 1987; Gruber, 2006; Haviland et al., 2011). Moreover, Chernew and Newhouse posits that results from the RAND study suggest cost sharing could in the longer-term actually increase costs because of delayed access to care (Chernew and Newhouse 2008). Similar patterns have been found in many other OECD countries (Rubin and Mendelson, 1996; Lundberg et al., 1998; Robinson, 2002; Jemiai et al., 2004; Kim et al., 2005).[15]

Reforms to encourage private health insurance enrolment

In light of the arguments against extended cost-sharing, some governments have turned to demand-side policies encouraging the use of private-sector health insurance to complement or supplement insurance provided within a universal health care system. These policies have usually taken the form of subsidies (tax relief on premiums) to individuals taking up insurance coverage from private companies and funds, in the hope that the value of released capacity and lower cost pressure in the public sector proves larger than the value of public subsidies towards private insurance (Mossialos and Thomson, 2002).

Yet the cost-containment promise of private insurance subsidisation does not seem to hold in practice. Analyses of the costs and benefits from such tax incentives – under various distinct designs in Australia, Ireland, Spain, the United Kingdom and elsewhere – have often concluded that they their costs to the public purse surpass the savings obtained in the public health sector, in addition to being a generally regressive tax policy (Emmerson et al., 2001; Mossialos and Thomson, 2002; López Nicolás and Vera-Hernández, 2008). In Australia, for example, there is now accumulated hard quantitative evidence that removing existing private insurance subsidies altogether would lead to substantial net reductions in government health expenditures, with one study suggesting savings in inpatient care of around AUD 1.6 billion from the elimination of subsidies, after any costs from increased public health sector use are considered (Palangkaraya et al., 2009; Cheng, 2011).[16] Therefore, the overall message from the available evidence for OECD countries is that the removal of private insurance subsidisation may actually constitute an effective tool to curb publicly funded health expenditures.

Reforms to directly contain demand through the introduction of gatekeeping and drug lists

Other policy alternatives for demand-side management of health care use and consequent reductions in expenditure have included reforms to expand the role of primary-care doctors as gatekeepers and the introduction of formularies (also known as preferred drug lists). Although formularies are meant to curb drug spending whereas gatekeeping is expected to have a more general influence on outpatient and inpatient care spending, these two sets of policies are similar in spirit. Both are intended to affect the behaviour of patients by imposing restrictions on health care demand (Figure 5.4), often according to evidence-based clinical guidelines or protocols.

Several OECD countries have introduced gatekeeping arrangements in recent decades to help control health care costs by requiring primary-care physicians to pre-authorise service use by patients, screening out unnecessary services (Docteur and Oxley, 2003). Currently in the OECD area, gatekeeping is more prevalent in, for example, Italy, the Netherlands, Norway, Spain and the United Kingdom, and somewhat more restricted in, for example, Belgium, France and Germany. The system-wide evidence on the cost-containment impacts of gatekeeping is severely limited in that many empirical studies have used claims data from only a few units (such as individual managed-care organisations in the United States), and sometimes with no cost data from an adequate comparison group of units (cf. e.g., Kralewski et al,. 2000; and research reviewed in Forrest, 2003). This makes it difficult to draw conclusions about cost effects at a more aggregate level. These studies find little association between gatekeeping and better cost containment, which is in contrast with a cross-country analysis in the OECD area (Gerdtham et al., 1998).[17]

Formularies refer to systems where some pharmaceuticals are granted a preferred status (usually based on criteria such as cost-effectiveness) so they may be dispensed without prior authorisation by a physician. There are many examples of OECD countries that have adopted formularies to deter patients from purchasing more expensive drugs where cheaper and clinically equivalent options are available, hence helping reduce public expenditure on pharmaceuticals. These include Italy, Spain, Switzerland and the United Kingdom, among others (Ess et al., 2003). Since formularies have often been introduced alongside other pharmaceutical policies (e.g., encouraging the use of generic drugs[18]), it becomes difficult to disentangle the specific cost-containment effects of formularies from those due to concurrent reforms, which tends to explain the relative scarcity of hard evidence on the topic. There is, however, some indicative empirical evidence that formularies have contributed to containing public expenditure on pharmaceuticals in Canada (Morgan et al., 2004), and resulted in lower purchase prices and overall cost savings for the public sector and managed care organisations in the United States as pharmaceutical companies avoided going off-list (Elzinga and Mills, 1997; Kibicho and Pinkerton, 2012).

Public management, co-ordination and financing reforms

Governments have also implemented policies that include health cost-containment elements through changes to public management and institutional arrangements in the health sector, at times within the context of broader macroeconomic reforms. Arguably, such policies differ conceptually from those reviewed above in that their health expenditure impacts are expected to arise from a combination of changes in incentives to providers, consumers and public administration, affecting – directly or indirectly – health care prices and quantities (Figure 5.4).

Reforms to pharmaceutical markets

Authorities in, for example, France, Italy, Japan and Spain have introduced direct price control of pharmaceuticals through unilateral reduction of the maximum selling price by drug companies, with the aims of encouraging consumption of cheaper alternatives in a given drug class and reducing the total pharmaceutical bill to the public sector. Furthermore, some OECD countries including Germany, the Netherlands, New Zealand and Sweden have determined maximum or reference reimbursement prices for all drugs with similar therapeutic effects in a particular cluster, usually based on the lowest priced product in each cluster, with the ultimate goal of stimulating price competition and cost savings. Consumers are normally required to pay the difference if manufacturers charge prices above the reference price.[19] Profit controls for the pharmaceutical industry – mark-up adjustments and maximum annual limits on profits or profit growth rates – have also been put in place by a few governments (e.g., Spain and the United Kingdom) as an indirect way of containing public expenditure on drugs. In theory, all these policy reforms may stimulate lower pharmaceutical prices; but the overall cost savings in terms of drug expenditures will depend on the extent to which such policies (and their interaction with other features of the health system) also encourage further demand for pharmaceuticals.

There is empirical evidence pointing to net cost-containment impacts of direct price control policies in OECD countries. Reviews and cross-country studies have concluded that direct price regulation does systematically lead to lower pharmaceutical prices (mainly for older and globally diffused drugs), although it is less clear that direct price controls are more effective in reducing national pharmaceutical spending than indirect price controls such as mandated generic substitution (Danzon and Chao, 2000; Danzon, 2011). By contrast, the potential cost-containment effects of reference pricing seem more heavily dependent on context. In Sweden, the implementation of a reference pricing scheme was associated with slower growth in total drug expenditures, with cost reductions in reference-priced drugs apparently extending to non-reference priced drugs as well (Andersson et al., 2006). Reference prices appeared to have pushed down brand-name drug prices shortly after introduction according to a study involving three other OECD countries, although cost reductions have been of modest magnitude in Germany and the Netherlands compared to New Zealand (Danzon and Ketcham, 2004).[20]

It is unclear whether concurrent reductions in drug expenditures driven by price controls help contain the growth of public spending on drugs in the longer run. For instance, a compulsory price reduction policy enacted in 1999 in Catalonia, Spain, was estimated to have saved 1.7% in annual pharmaceutical spending per capita in the year after its implementation, with no effects afterwards (and no effects from subsequent compulsory price reductions until 2006) (Moreno-Torres et al., 2011). A similar pattern was found for the imposition of mark-up controls in the same Spanish region, and for reference pricing in Sweden (Andersson et al., 2006). On the other hand, a study using data for a group of OECD countries concluded that the cost-reducing impacts of price controls on pharmaceuticals actually become larger over time (Sood et al., 2009). Finally, despite the best efforts of researchers, distinct price and profit control reforms have frequently been applied simultaneously as a mixed cost-containment strategy, proving a challenge to single out individual reform impacts.

Reforms to the level of centralisation of health system functions

As well as seeking to impose a priori limits on the total amount of resources going to the health sector or subsectors, many OECD countries have sought to improve efficiency in the use of existing health care resources and contain waste through decentralisation of health system functions to sub-national levels of government (including planning, management, financing and delivery of services) (Saltman et al., 2006).[21] The premise behind decentralisation is that it can accomplish cost-efficiency and control by aligning resource allocation with local preferences and cost structures. However, some national governments (e.g., Denmark, Norway, Poland and Slovak Republic) have recently taken measures to promote the re-centralisation of key functions within their health systems, partly due to perceptions that the previous decentralised system was damaging cost-containment efforts by weakening co-ordination and encouraging duplication of services (Magnussen et al., 2006). Both decentralisation and re-centralisation measures in the health system have often been part of wider public management restructuring processes involving political, economic, organisational and legal aspects.

A study for 20 OECD countries during the period 1990-2000 found that decentralised health systems have higher total health expenditures compared to more centralised systems (e.g., France and the United Kingdom) (Mosca, 2007). Nonetheless, the numerous alternative decentralisation models adopted in OECD countries makes it problematic to draw policy conclusions from comparisons between broad aggregate categories such as "decentralised" vs. "centralised" systems. Single-country studies may be more illuminating in that respect.

Some insights into cost containment can be found in analyses of the Spanish and Italian experiences with decentralisation – funding controlled by the central government while local authorities oversee the administration and execution of regional-level health policy. The 1992 health care reform in Italy sought to suppress growing health costs by delegating central funds and granting some tax-raising powers to regional authorities, accompanied by measures such as wage controls and budget cuts. This strategy was found to result in a significant spending reduction at the central level, lowering the annual rate of growth in per capita public expenditure on health from 2% (1980-91) to less than 0.5% (1992-95) (Giannoni and Hitiris, 2002).

The cost-containment effect of decentralisation observed in Italy does not seem to have taken place in Spain, which saw an increase in per capita health expenditure following the gradual process of health care decentralisation starting from the early 1980s (Costa-Font and Pons-Novell, 2007). In this case, political competition within a centralised funding system has meant that local legislators seeking public support lack the incentive to cut back on spending in regions where health care is seen as a priority. A more recent study of the Spanish process speculated that the initial increase in health spending may be due to sunk costs of decentralisation, i.e. an "experience effect" that opens the door for cost reduction in the longer run (Costa-Font and Moscone, 2008). A less encouraging policy consequence of the Spanish and Italian decentralisation reforms identified in the previous studies has been an increase in inter-regional health spending inequalities, a phenomenon also associated with decentralisation in the Swiss health system (Crivelli et al., 2006).

Contrary to the trend of decentralised health system models in Europe, Norway initiated a health sector reform in 2002 aimed at recentralising ownership or control over inpatient and outpatient specialised care, as a way of eliminating weak cost-control incentives at the sub-national levels due to soft budgets (the guarantee perceived by local governments or providers that any deficits incurred will be eventually covered by higher-level or central funding). The evidence to date on the Norwegian recentralisation reform points to a lack of general cost-containment impacts. Overall health expenditures have continued to rise in line with previous trends, likely due to the fact that soft budgets were not eliminated post-reform (the proportion of supplementary funds granted by the Parliament continued to rise according to health spending increases), coupled with the growth in activity-based financing (Magnussen et al., 2006, 2007).[22]

Reforms to alter the mix of health system financing sources

National discussions around health sector reform in the OECD area have invariably considered whether the currently employed mix of health system funding sources is in itself a potential driver of total cost (Mossialos et al., 2002). Although the crude dichotomy of Beveridge-Bismarck has lost meaning in a context where most health systems are funded by a mixture of revenue sources, it seems reasonable to enquire whether changing the mix of funding – for instance, the relative importance of general taxes *vis-à-vis* payroll-based contributions – has any potential effects on trends in total government health expenditures. While the set-up of payroll-based (social insurance) systems may promote efficiency by separating purchasing from provision and encouraging selective contracting, some predominantly tax-funded systems have also introduced such mechanisms as discussed previously, and social insurance arrangements may entail additional administrative and co-ordination costs (e.g., through the creation of sickness funds).

In the United Kingdom, an influential report concluded that there was no evidence to date that moving away from general taxation for health system funding would lower health care costs, and such a move could actually prove more costly (Wanless, 2002). Recent international evidence seems to lend empirical support to that conclusion. In an analysis of reforms to health funding systems in the OECD between 1960 and 2006, higher reliance on social health insurance (payroll-based) contributions was found to lead to an increase of between 3% and 4% in annual per capita health spending (with no apparent improvements in population health outcomes) compared to higher reliance on general taxation (Wagstaff, 2009). A similar conclusion was reached by Mosca (2007). A study including recent OECD members from Central and Eastern Europe also concluded that countries that reformed their health financing systems towards chief reliance on payroll-based contributions ended up spending more on health per capita than those countries which remained predominantly tax-funded, even after accounting for factors such as the frequent use of fee-for-service payment methods in inpatient care by social insurance countries (Wagstaff and Moreno-Serra, 2009). In the latter case, the swell of overall health expenditures from social insurance reforms seemed mainly driven by a rise in government health spending, possibly through increased wage and administration bills.

Reforms to expand the role of health technology assessment for resource allocation

Since the introduction of new technologies in the publicly funded health benefit package is not commonly cost-saving, and technological innovation is expected to become even more intense in certain areas such as diagnostic equipment (Chernew and May, 2011), some governments have sought to take a more active role in health technology assessment (HTA) in order to curb cost-explosion driven by more expensive therapies. The assessment of the costs and benefits of new technologies as a criterion for the definition of the publicly funded health benefit package is largely expected to promote value for money and reduce waste by direct restrictions on demand for specific interventions whose benefits are not worth the costs. This was a major force behind the creation of several national agencies to assess new technology in Europe in recent decades, for instance in France, Spain, Sweden and Finland (Mossialos and Le Grand, 1999). The National Institute for Clinical Excellence has long played a major role in assisting resource-allocation decisions in the United Kingdom. Notwithstanding its cost-containment potential, the creation of HTA bodies is likely to add to management and administration costs in a health system.

Quantitative evidence on the cost-containment impacts associated specifically with the introduction of or an expanded role for HTA in resource allocation is scarce. Yet it must be noted that the expected cost savings from HTA are likely to arise from its combination with other system reforms: HTA should be seen primarily as a means to an end. If the recommendations from HTA agencies are used to inform decisions about health care guidelines (for example, implementation of pharmaceutical formularies), cost-sharing schedules (for example, lower user charges for cost-effective preventive interventions that reduce the use of more expensive outpatient and inpatient care) and the broader definition of the public benefit package (for example, by providing the basis for exclusion of certain therapies with low cost-effectiveness from public funding), HTA will probably serve as a catalyst to maximise the cost-containment effects of these accompanying supply-side and demand-side reforms.

5.5. Conclusion

This chapter has sought to review the most robust empirical evidence on a fundamental policy topic: the potential to contain the growth of health system expenditures that the several options of health policy provide to national governments. There is now robust evidence on the cost-containment effects of many of the reforms implemented by OECD countries, and examining this evidence offers valuable insights for policy decisions.

As usual in the policy arena, it is clear that there is no magic bullet. The end result of cost-containment reforms is often context-dependent. Policy levers need to be carefully introduced and co-ordinated with other institutional features of the health system to ensure that cost-containment benefits in one sub-sector are not offset by poorer performance elsewhere. But if policy makers learn from the experience of past reforms, and wisely tailor interventions to their specific context, there are various alternative policies in a government's arsenal that can be combined to achieve better cost control in the health system.

Notes

1. For instance, Docteur and Oxley (2003), in their comprehensive description of health reforms in OECD countries particularly during the 1990s, concluded that most reforms had been implemented too recently for conclusions on their relative effects to be drawn. The authors acknowledged that the growth in health spending had slowed noticeably over the 1980s and 1990s; but their general assessment of the then available empirical evidence on policy reform impacts was that it constituted a very thin body of knowledge offering limited statistical support to claims that budgetary caps or other cost-containment initiatives had played an important role in reducing health care cost escalation.
2. See Section 5.2 for the definition of "excess cost growth" in health spending studies.
3. One such example is the British GP fundholding experience during the 1990s (see Section 5.4).
4. Moreover, despite not being the rule, it has been argued that some new technologies have replaced more expensive ones (for instance, some types of pharmaceuticals; Griliches and Cockburn, 1994).
5. The same study forecast an increase in total US health spending (including the private sector) from 16% of GDP in 2007 to 37% in 2050 and 49% in 2082.
6. This relatively minor role played by population ageing in projections of health spending growth is also due to the so-called "healthy ageing" assumption, which is in line with observed trends in most OECD countries (Oliveira Martins et al., 2006). Even though the extent of the older population has been increasing (and is expected to remain so in future years), elderly people today tend to enjoy better health and hence require less health care per capita than did their counterparts in the past, offsetting to some extent pressures on the demand for health services arising from the overall rise in the share of older people. Moreover, as the elderly today also live longer than in

the past, death-related costs – which constitute the major component of individuals' health care spending over the life cycle – are postponed, and their financial burden decreases in present value (see Savedoff et al., 2012 and references therein).

7. White (2007) estimates that, while rates of health spending growth due to ageing and economic growth were similar in the United States and the other OECD countries between 1970 and 2002, annual US excess cost growth was twice that of the rest of the OECD. This further highlights the crucial role of health sector institutional factors – and reforms targeted to those factors – for the effective control of national health expenditures.

8. Empirical studies on cost-containment policy impacts were included if they attempted to deal statistically with potential estimation biases arising from observable and unobservable differences across analytical units (e.g., hospitals or health systems). These studies typically used data from situations where groups of "treatment" and "comparison" units could be identified in (or were generated by) health policy reforms, often employing econometric regression models to seek causal inference instead of simple correlations. See, for example, Jones (2000).

9. This is not to say that demographic cost drivers and policies addressing them are not important for cost containment in health. Research has shown that public health interventions that affect the health status of survivors, for instance restrictions on alcohol and cigarette consumption, may be cost-saving (Kenkel and Sindelar, 2011). However, as mentioned above, the relatively small overall component of spending growth owing to demographic drivers implies that policies aimed at these factors will likely have lower aggregate cost-containment impacts. Also, cost drivers such as changes in population structure seem less readily amenable to health policy reforms.

10. Depending on the specific configuration of the health system, the introduction of capitation payment methods or budget holding may in principle encourage physicians to transfer the burden of cost through referrals to higher-level care. Although a theoretical possibility, there is no evidence from the British experience that such a phenomenon took place, or at least the net result of the GP fundholding policy seems to have been one of overall cost reduction (Dusheiko et al., 2006). Also, since fundholding was a GP choice, the cost-containment effect of the policy could in principle have been larger had it been a compulsory programme, which has implications for current discussions in the United Kingdom about a renewed fundholding role for GPs.

11. The immediate pressure on public budgets from rising pharmaceutical costs remains in practice even if part or most of such spending refers to better drugs with a beneficial impact on population health.

12. Country examples include Canada, Denmark, Finland, Poland, Slovenia and the United Kingdom among several others. Global budgets have also been developed in some countries mainly as a strategy to control volume of care where providers are paid through fee-for-service (Mossialos and Le Grand, 1999).

13. A cross-country analysis for 22 OECD countries over 20 years found the introduction of global budgets did not contain the growth of national health expenditures (Gerdtham et al., 1998). However, the authors acknowledged that their results might have been confounded by the possibility that countries with high expenditure might have been more prone (or quicker) to adopt budget caps.

14. An exception was a study of the Swedish pharmaceutical cost-sharing reforms during the 1990s, which failed to find any effect from increased co-payments in the total cost or volume of prescription drugs (Andersson et al., 2006). Nonetheless, issues pertaining to the enactment of various pharmaceutical policies during the period of analysis – including reference-based pricing and changes in the reimbursement schedule – limited the study's ability to distinguish the specific spending effects of each of these policy reforms.

15. Moreover, cost-sharing typically appears to deliver far less than expected as a supplement to pooled health sector revenues (Robinson, 2002) and has been found to be a highly regressive source of health sector financing among OECD countries (van Doorslaer et al., 1999).

16. Cheng (2011) also concluded that such public subsidies ended up disproportionately benefiting higher-income individuals in Australia, who presumably would have been able to purchase private insurance coverage without public subsidisation.

17. Although the jury is still out concerning "pure" gatekeeping impacts on health expenditures, more recent (and methodologically robust) empirical work for England has indicated some cost-containment effects from a reform coupling gatekeeping with capitated budget fundholding (Dusheiko et al., 2006; see above), as well as a beneficial impact on patient satisfaction with services provided (Dusheiko et al., 2007).

18. See the above discussion on mandated generic substitution policies.

19. In addition to the expected change in consumer behaviour and the competitive incentive theoretically provided to drug companies by reference pricing, incentives to other health sector agents have been introduced to reinforce cost savings from cheaper prescriptions. An example is allowing pharmacists to share the savings between the reference price and the manufacturer's price in the Dutch health system (Danzon and Ketcham, 2004).

20. Price competition stimulated by reference pricing seems to have been weak in Germany and the Netherlands, since manufacturers had no incentive to reduce prices below the reference price. This led those countries to implement additional measures such as mandated generic substitution. In New Zealand, reference pricing has been more successful in reducing costs of pharmaceuticals, possibly due to the requirement by the government (single purchaser) of price cuts for new generics and their subsequent application to all drugs in the cluster (Danzon and Ketcham, 2004).

21. Switzerland has fully devolved both managerial and fiscal powers to local authorities, with the public health care budget being primarily financed by cantons and municipalities (20% of funding comes from the central authority) (Crivelli et al., 2006). Other countries including Italy, Spain and Norway (until 2002) delegated managerial responsibilities to regional authorities while reserving fiscal responsibilities for the central government.

22. The damaging effect of soft budgets to cost-control in decentralised health systems has been highlighted in a recent study by Crivelli et al. (2010). The authors used data for OECD countries to find that soft budgets, in the form of large reliance on central government transfers and high borrowing autonomy, lead to higher sub-national health spending. Specifically, the authors estimated that a one percentage point increase in their measure of vertical fiscal imbalance produced a 4.5% greater increase in annual sub-national health spending per capita for countries where sub-national governments had high borrowing autonomy relative to those with less.

References

Anderson, G. et al. (2000), "Regulatory Barriers to Entry in the Healthcare Industry: The Case of Alternative Medicine", *Quarterly Review of Economics and Finance*, Vol. 40, No. 4, Bureau of Economic and Business Research, University of Illinois at Urbana-Champaign, Elsevier, pp. 485-502.

Andersson, K. et al. (2007), "Impact of a Generic Substitution Reform on Patients' and Society's Expenditure for Pharmaceuticals", *Health Policy*, Vol. 81, No. 2-3, Elsevier, Amsterdam, pp. 376-384.

Andersson, K. et al. (2006), "Do Policy Changes in the Pharmaceutical Reimbursement Schedule Affect Drug Expenditures? Interrupted Time Series Analysis of Cost, Volume and Cost per Volume Trends in Sweden 1986-2002", *Health Policy*, Vol. 79, No. 2-3, Elsevier, Amsterdam, pp. 231-243.

Arrow, K. (1963), "Uncertainty and the Welfare Economics of Medical Care", *American Economic Review*, Vol. 53, American Economic Association, Nashville, United States, pp. 941-973.

Baker, L. (1999), "Association of Managed Care Market Share and Health Expenditures for Fee-for-service Medicare Patients", *Journal of the American Medical Association*, Vol. 281, No. 5, American Medical Association, Chicago, pp. 432-437.

Bärnighausen, T. and D. Bloom (2011), "The Global Health Workforce", in S. Glied and P. Smith (eds.), *The Oxford Handbook of Health Economics*, Oxford University Press, Oxford.

Busse, R., Geissler, A., Quentin, W., Wiley, M (2011), "Diagnosis-Related Groups in Europe. *European Observatory on Health Systems and Policies.*

Cheng, C. (2011), "Measuring the Effects of Removing Subsidies for Private Insurance on Public Expenditure for Health Care", *Health, Econometrics and Data Group (HEDG) Working Paper*, University of York, York.

Chernew, M. and D. May (2011), "Healthcare Cost Growth", in S. Glied and P. Smith (eds.), *The Oxford Handbook of Health Economics*, Oxford University Press, Oxford.

Chernew, M. and J. Newhouse (2008). "What does the RAND health insurance experiment tell us about the impact of patient cost sharing on health outcomes?", *American Journal of Managed Care*, Vol. 14, No. 7, pp. 412-414.

Costa-Font, J. and F. Moscone (2008), "The Impact of Decentralization and Inter-territorial Interactions on Spanish Health Expenditure", *Empirical Economics*, Vol. 34, No. 1, Springer International Publishing, pp. 167-184.

Costa-Font, J. and J. Pons-Novell (2007), "Public Health Expenditure and Spatial Interactions in a Decentralized National Health System", *Health Economics*, Vol. 16, No. 3, John Wiley and Sons, pp. 291-306.

Crivelli, E. et al. (2010), "Sub-national Health Spending and Soft Budget Constraints in OECD Countries", *IMF Working Papers* No. 10/147, IMF, Washington.

Crivelli, L. et al. (2006), "Federalism and Regional Healthcare Expenditures: An Empirical Analysis for the Swiss Cantons", *Health Economics*, Vol. 15, No. 5, John Wiley and Sons, pp. 535-541.

Cutler, D. and R. Zeckhauser (2000), "The Anatomy of Health Insurance", in A. Culyer and J. Newhouse (eds.), *Handbook of Health Economics*, Elsevier, Amsterdam.

Danzon, P. (2011), "The Economics of the Biopharmaceutical Industry", in S. Glied and P. Smith (eds.), *The Oxford Handbook of Health Economics*, Oxford University Press, Oxford.

Danzon, P. and W. Chao (2000), "Cross-national Price Differences for Pharmaceuticals: How Large, and Why?", *Journal of Health Economics*, Vol. 19, No. 2, Elsevier, Amsterdam, pp. 159-195.

Danzon, P. and J. Ketcham (2004), "Reference Pricing of Pharmaceuticals for Medicare: Evidence from Germany, the Netherlands and New Zealand", in D. Cutler and A. Garber (eds.), *Frontiers in Health Policy Research*, Vol. 7, NBER and MIT Press, Cambridge, United States.

Dismuke, C. and P. Guimaraes (2002), "Has the Caveat of Case-mix Based Payment Influenced the Quality of Inpatient Hospital Care in Portugal?", *Applied Economics*, Vol. 34, No. 10, Taylor & Francis, pp. 1301-07.

Docteur, E. and H. Oxley (2003), "Healthcare Systems: Lessons from the Reform Experience", *OECD Economics Department Working Papers* No. 374, OECD Publishing, Paris, *http://dx.doi.org/10.1787/865047648066*.

Dormont, B. et al. (2006), "Health Expenditure Growth: Reassessing the Threat of Ageing", *Health Economics*, Vol. 15, No. 9, John Wiley and Sons, pp. 947-963.

Dranove, D. et al. (1993), "Price and Concentration in Hospital Markets: The Switch from Patient-driven to Payer-driven Competition", *Journal of Law and Economics*, Vol. 36, No. 2, The Booth School of Business of The University of Chicago and The University of Chicago Law School, Chicago, pp. 179-204.

Dusheiko, M. et al. (2007), "The Impact of Budgets for Gatekeeping Physicians on Patient Satisfaction: Evidence from Fundholding", *Journal of Health Economics*, Vol. 26, No. 4, Elsevier, Amsterdam, pp. 742-762.

Dusheiko, M. et al. (2006), "The Effect of Financial Incentives on Gatekeeping Doctors: Evidence from a Natural Experiment", *Journal of Health Economics*, Vol. 25, No. 3, Elsevier, Amsterdam, pp. 449-478.

Ellis, R. and M. Miller (2008), "Provider Payment Methods and Incentives", in H. Kris (ed.), *International Encyclopaedia of Public Health*, Oxford Academic Press, Oxford.

Elzinga, K. and D. Mills (1997), "The Distribution and Pricing of Prescription Drugs", *International Journal of the Economics of Business*, Vol. 4, No. 3, Taylor and Francis, pp. 287-299.

Emmerson, C. et al. (2001), "Should Private Medical Insurance Be Subsidised?", *Health Care UK*, pp. 49-65.

Ess, S. et al. (2003), "European Healthcare Policies for Controlling Drug Expenditure", *PharmacoEconomics*, Vol. 21, No. 2, Springer International Publishing, pp. 89-103.

Forgione, D. et al. (2004), "The Impact of DRG-based Payment Systems on Quality of Health Care in OECD Countries", *Journal of Health Care Finance*, Vol. 31, No. 1, Researchgate, Berlin, pp. 41-54.

Forrest, C. (2003), "Primary Care Gatekeeping and Referrals: Effective Filter or Failed Experiment?", *British Medical Journal*, Vol. 326, No. 7391, British Medical Association, London. pp. 692-695.

Gaynor, M. et al. (forthcoming), "Death by Market Power: Reform, Competition and Patient Outcomes in the National Health Service", *American Economic Journal: Economic Policy*, American Economic Association, Pittsburgh.

Gerdtham, U.-G. and B. Jönsson (2000), "International Comparisons of Health Expenditure: Theory, Data and Econometric Analysis", in A. Culyer and J. Newhouse (eds.), *Handbook of Health Economics*, Vol. 1, Elsevier, Amsterdam.

Gerdtham, U.-G. et al. (1999), "The Impact of Internal Markets on Healthcare Efficiency: Evidence from Healthcare Reforms in Sweden", *Applied Economics*, Vol. 31, No. 8, Taylor and Francis, pp. 935-945.

Gerdtham, U.-G. et al. (1998), "The Determinants of Health Expenditure in the OECD Countries: A Pooled Data Analysis", in P. Zweifel (ed.), *Health, the Medical Profession, and Regulation*, Klewer, Dordrecht.

Giannoni, M. and T. Hitiris (2002), "The Regional Impact of Healthcare Expenditure: The Case of Italy", *Applied Economics*, Vol. 34, No. 14, Taylor and Francis, pp. 1829-1836.

Goldman, D. et al. (2007), "Prescription Drug Cost Sharing: Associations with Medication and Medical Utilization and Spending and Health", *Journal of the American Medical Association*, Vol. 298, No. 1, American Medical Association, Chicago, pp. 61-69.

Griliches, Z. and I. Cockburn (1994), "Generics and New Goods in Pharmaceutical Price Indexes", *American Economic Review*, Vol. 84, American Economic Association, Nashville, pp. 1213-1232.

Gruber, J. (2006), *The Role of Consumer Co-payments for Health Care: Lessons from the RAND Health Insurance Experiment and Beyond*, Henry J. Kaiser Family Foundation, Menlo Park, California.

Haviland, A. et al. (2011), "How Do Consumer-directed Health Plans Affect Vulnerable Populations?", *Forum for Health Economics & Policy*, Vol. 14, No. 2, Walter de Gruyter GmbH, Berlin, pp. 1-23.

Hellinger, F. and W. Encinosa (2006), "The Impact of State Laws Limiting Malpractice Damage Awards on Healthcare Expenditures", *American Journal of Public Health*, Vol. 96, No. 8, American Public Health Association, Washington, DC, pp. 375-381.

Jemiai, N. et al. (2004), "An Overview of Cost Sharing for Health Services in the European Union", *Euro Observer*, Vol. 6, No. 3, London School of Economic and Political Science, University of London, pp. 1-4.

Jones, A. (2000), "Health Econometrics", in A. Culyer and J. Newhouse (eds.), *Handbook of Health Economics*, Elsevier, Amsterdam.

Joumard, I. et al. (2010), "Healthcare Systems: Efficiency and Institutions", *OECD Economics Department Working Papers* No. 627, OECD Publishing, Paris, *http://dx.doi.org/10.1787/5kmfp51f5f9t-en*.

Kenkel, D. and J. Sindelar (2011), "Economics of Health Behaviours and Addictions: Contemporary Issues and Policy Implications", in S. Glied and P. Smith (eds.), *The Oxford Handbook of Health Economics*, Oxford University Press, Oxford.

Kenneally, M. and V. Walshe (2012), "Pharmaceutical Cost-containment Policies and Sustainability: Recent Irish Experience", *Value in Health*, Vol. 15, No. 2, International Society for Pharmacoeconomics and Outcomes Research, Elsevier, Amsterdam, pp. 389-393.

Kibicho, J. and S. Pinkerton (2012), "Multiple Drug Cost Containment Policies in Michigan's Medicaid Program Saved Money Overall, Although Some Increased Costs", *Health Affairs*, Vol. 31, No. 4, Project HOPE: The People-to-People Health Foundation, Bathesda, United States, pp. 816-826.

Kim, J. et al. (2005), "The Effects of Patient Cost Sharing on Ambulatory Utilization in South Korea", *Health Policy*, Vol. 72, No. 3, Elsevier, Amsterdam, pp. 293-300.

Kralewski, J. et al. (2000), "The Effects of Medical Group Practice and Physician Payment Methods on Costs of Care", *Health Services Research*, Vol. 35, No. 3, AcademyHealth, Health Research & Educational Trust, Chicago, pp. 591-613.

Kwon, S. (2003), "Payment System Reform for Healthcare Providers in Korea", *Health Policy and Planning*, Vol. 18, No. 1, Oxford University Press, Oxford, pp. 84-92.

Langenbrunner, J. et al. (2005), "Purchasing and Paying Providers", in J. Figueras, R. Robinson and E. Jakubowski (eds.), *Purchasing to Improve Health Systems Performance*, Open University Press, Maidenhead, United Kingdom.

López Nicolás, Á. and M. Vera-Hernández (2008), "Are Tax Subsidies for Private Medical Insurance Self-financing? Evidence from a Microsimulation Model", *Journal of Health Economics*, Vol. 27, No. 5, Elsevier, Amsterdam, pp. 1285-1298.

Louis, D. et al. (1999), "Impact of a DRG-based Hospital Financing System on Quality and Outcomes of Care in Italy", *Health Services Research*, Vol. 34, No. 1 (Pt 2), AcademyHealth, Health Research & Educational Trust, Chicago, pp. 405-415.

Lundberg, L. et al. (1998), "Effects of User Charges on the Use of Prescription Medicines in Different Socio-economic Groups", *Health Policy*, Vol. 44, No. 2, Elsevier, Amsterdam, pp. 123-134.

Magnussen, J., T. Hagen and O. Kaarboe (2007), "Centralized or Decentralized? A Case Study of Norwegian Hospital Reform", *Social Science & Medicine*, Vol. 64, No. 10, Elsevier, Amsterdam, pp. 2129-2137.

Magnussen, J. et al. (2006), "Effects of Decentralization and Recentralization on Economic Dimensions of Health Systems", in R. Saltman, V. Bankauskaite and K. Vrangbaek (eds.), *Decentralization in Health Care*, Open University Press, Maidenhead.

Manning, W. et al. (1987), "Health Insurance and the Demand for Medical Care – Evidence from a Randomized Experiment", *American Economic Review*, Vol. 77, No. 3, American Economic Association, Nashville, United States, pp. 251-277.

Moreno-Serra, R. and A. Wagstaff (2010), "System-wide Impacts of Hospital Payment Reforms: Evidence from Central and Eastern Europe and Central Asia", *Journal of Health Economics*, Vol. 29, No. 4, Elsevier, Amsterdam, pp. 585-602.

Moreno-Torres, I. et al. (2011), "The Impact of Repeated Cost Containment Policies on Pharmaceutical Expenditure: Experience in Spain", *European Journal of Health Economics*, Vol. 12, No. 6, Springer International Publishing, pp. 563-573.

Morgan, S. et al. (2004), "Seniors' Prescription Drug Cost Inflation and Cost Containment: Evidence from British Columbia", *Health Policy*, Vol. 68, No. 3, Elsevier, Amsterdam, pp. 299-307.

Mosca, I. (2007), "Decentralization as a Determinant of Healthcare Expenditure: Empirical Analysis for OECD Countries", *Applied Economics Letters*, Vol. 14, No. 7-9, Taylor and Francis, pp. 511-515.

Mossialos, E. and J. Le Grand (1999), "Cost Containment in the EU: An Overview", in E. Mossialos and J. Le Grand (eds.), *Health Care and Cost-Containment in the European Union*, Ashgate, Aldershot, United Kingdom.

Mossialos, E. and S. Thomson (2002), "Voluntary Health Insurance in the European Union", in E. Mossialos et al. (eds.), *Funding Health Care: Options for Europe*, Open University Press, Buckingham.

Mossialos, E. et al. (eds.) (2002), *Funding Health Care: Options for Europe*, Open University Press, Buckingham.

Nguyen, N. (1996), "Physician Volume Response to Price Controls", *Health Policy*, Vol. 35, No. 2, Elsevier, Amsterdam, pp. 189-204.

OECD (2013), *OECD.Stat Extracts*, available at: *http://stats.oecd.org*, accessed 11 March, 2013.

Oliveira Martins, J. et al. (2006), "Projecting OECD Health and Long-term Care Expenditures: What are the Main Drivers?", *OECD Economics Department Working Papers* No. 477, OECD Publishing, Paris, *http://dx.doi.org/10.1787/736341548748*.

Orszag, P. (2007), *The Long-Term Outlook for Healthcare Spending*, Congressional Budget Office, Congress of the United States, Washington, DC.

Oxley, H. and M. MacFarlan (1995), "Healthcare Reform: Controlling Spending and Increasing Efficiency", *OECD Economic Study* No. 24, OECD Publishing, Paris, *http://dx.doi.org/10.1787/338757855057*.

Palangkaraya, A. et al. (2009), "The Income Distributive Implications of Recent Private Health Insurance Policy Reforms in Australia", *European Journal of Health Economics*, Vol. 10, No. 2, Springer International Publishing, pp. 135-148.

Palmer, K. (2011), *Reconfiguring Hospital Services: Lessons from South East London*, King's Fund, London.

Propper, C. et al. (2008), "Competition and Quality: Evidence from the NHS Internal Market 1991-1999", *Economic Journal*, Vol. 118, No. 525, Royal Economic Society, Wiley Blackwell, pp. 138-170.

Robinson, R. (2002), "User Charges for Health Care", in E. Mossialos, A. Dixon, J. Figueras and J. Kutzin (eds.), *Funding Health Care: Options for Europe*, Open University Press, Buckingham.

Rubin, R. and D. Mendelson (1996), "A Framework for Cost-sharing Policy Analysis", *PharmacoEconomics*, Vol. 10, No. 2. Springer International Publishing, pp. 56-67.

Saltman, R. et al. (eds.) (2006), *Decentralization in Health Care*, Open University Press, Maidenhead.

Savedoff, W. et al. (2012), "Political and Economic Aspects of the Transition to Universal Health Coverage", *The Lancet*, Vol. 380, No. 9845, Elsevier, Amsterdam, pp. 924-932.

Schneider, P. (2007), "Provider Payment Reforms: Lessons from Europe and America for South Eastern Europe", *HNP Discussion Paper*, October, The World Bank, Washington, DC.

Schöffski, O. and J. von der Schulenburg (1997), "Unintended Effects of a Cost-Containment Policy: Results of a Natural Experiment in Germany", *Social Science & Medicine*, Vol. 45, No. 10, Elsevier, Amsterdam, pp. 1537-1539.

Schokkaert, E. and C. van de Voorde (2011), "User Charges", in S. Glied and P. Smith (eds.), *The Oxford Handbook of Health Economics*, Oxford University Press, Oxford.

Schut, F. and W. van de Ven (2011), "Effects of Purchaser Competition in the Dutch Health System: Is the Glass Half Full or Half Empty?", *Health Economics Policy and Law*, Vol. 6, No. 1, Cambridge University Press, Cambridge, United Kingdom, pp. 109-123.

Sood, N. et al. (2009), "The Effect of Regulation on Pharmaceutical Revenues: Experience in Nineteen Countries", *Health Affairs*, Vol. 28, No. 1, Project HOPE: The People-to-People Health Foundation, Bathesda, United States, pp. w125-w137.

Swartz, K. (2010). Cost-sharing: effects on spending and outcomes, *Research Synthesis Report*.

Thomas, J. et al. (2010), "Low Costs of Defensive Medicine, Small Savings from Tort Reform", *Health Affairs*, Vol. 29, No. 9, Project HOPE: The People-to-People Health Foundation, Bathesda, United States, pp. 1578-1584.

van de Ven, W. and F. Schut (2009), "Managed Competition in the Netherlands: Still Work-in-Progress", *Health Economics*, Vol. 18, Oxford University Press, Oxford, pp. 253-255.

van Doorslaer, E. et al. (1999), "The Redistributive Effect of Healthcare Finance in Twelve OECD Countries", *Journal of Health Economics*, Vol. 18, No. 3, Elsevier, Amsterdam, pp. 291-313.

Volpp, K. et al. (2003), "Market Reform in New Jersey and the Effect on Mortality from Acute Myocardial Infarction", *Health Services Research*, Vol. 38, AcademyHealth, Health Research & Educational Trust, Chicago, pp. 515-533.

Wagstaff, A. (2009), "Social Health Insurance vs. Tax-Financed Health Systems - Evidence from the OECD", *World Bank Policy Research Working Paper* No. 4821, The World Bank, Washington, DC.

Wagstaff, A. and R. Moreno-Serra (2009), "Europe and Central Asia's Great Post-Communist Social Health Insurance Experiment: Aggregate Impacts on Health Sector Outcomes", *Journal of Health Economics*, Vol. 28, Elsevier, Amsterdam, pp. 322-340.

Wanless, D. (2002), *Securing Our Future Health: Taking a Long-Term View*, HM Treasury, London.

White, C. (2007), "Healthcare Spending Growth: How Different is the United States from the Rest of the OECD?", *Health Affairs*, Vol. 26, No. 1, Project HOPE: The People-to-People Health Foundation, Bathesda, United States, pp. 154-161.

Zwanziger, J. et al. (2000), "The Effect of Selective Contracting on Hospital Costs and Revenues", *Health Services Research*, Vol. 35, No. 4, AcademyHealth, Health Research & Educational Trust, Chicago, pp. 849-867.

Zwanziger, J. et al. (1994), "How Hospitals Practice Cost Containment with Selective Contracting and the Medicare Prospective Payment System", *Medical Care*, Vol. 32, No. 8, Journal of the Medical Care Section of the American Public Health Association, Lippincott, Williams and Wilkins, pp. 1153-1162.

Zweifel, P. and W. Manning (2000), "Moral Hazard and Consumer Incentives in Health Care", in A. Culyer and J. Newhouse (eds.), *Handbook of Health Economics*, Elsevier, Amsterdam.

Fiscal Sustainability of Health Systems
Bridging Health and Finance Perspectives

Chapter 6

Country experiences in dealing with fiscal constraint following the 2008 crisis

by
Mark Blecher*

This chapter presents a synthesis of OECD and non-OECD countries' experiences in responding to the global financial crisis, on what concerns the health sector. Many countries initially followed counter-cyclical fiscal policies and tried to sustain social sector expenditure, in particular in health. However, many countries were also soon forced to develop and implement strategies to control or reduce spending, and the health sector was often a target. The country responses to the crisis presented in this chapter provide important examples to other countries facing similar challenges, as well as interesting insights into how longer-term fiscal sustainability of the health sector might be enhanced.

* Mark Blecher is the Chief Director for Health and Social Development in the National Treasury, South Africa.

The statistical data for Israel are supplied by and under the responsibility of the relevant Israeli authorities. The use of such data by the OECD is without prejudice to the status of the Golan Heights, East Jerusalem and Israeli settlements in the West Bank under the terms of international law.

6.1. Introduction

Ongoing increases in health expenditure above inflation have been noted in OECD countries over decades, and questions around the sustainability and trajectory of health expenditure have existed for many years. The global financial and economic crisis which started in 2008 began as a mortgage loan and banking crisis, but rapidly turned into low growth, revenue shortfalls and serious fiscal challenges in many countries. Many countries initially followed counter-cyclical fiscal policies and tried to sustain social sector expenditure. However, many OECD countries were soon forced to develop and implement strategies to control or reduce spending. Countries, whose deficit and debt levels had risen substantially in an effort to stabilise public finances, followed a range of policies. Average fiscal consolidation in OECD countries was 5.5% of GDP by 2012 (OECD, 2012). Often, the fiscal consolidation efforts focused on the expenditure side, although in a third of OECD countries, revenue enhancements were also undertaken (OECD, 2012). In about half OECD countries, health expenditure was affected by fiscal consolidation strategies (OECD, 2012). In some cases, the amounts to be saved were substantial, and the lead times very short. Rapid decisions therefore had to be made. Some countries such as Greece and Ireland experienced particularly large fiscal problems and strong adjustments, international bailouts and difficult consolidation experiences.

The OECD Senior Budget Officials-Health Officials Joint Network on the Fiscal Sustainability of Health Systems (OECD SBO-Health Joint Network) meetings allowed OECD and non-OECD countries to share experiences on how they responded to the crisis as it concerned the health sector. These discussions provided important examples to other countries facing similar challenges, as well as interesting insights into how longer-term fiscal sustainability of the health sector might be enhanced.

One of the main conclusions of this exercise is that some countries' strategies appear to have been useful in finding greater value for money, lowering input costs, improving productivity and setting a basis for more efficient service configurations. However, other interventions appear to have been hurried decisions made with the aim of reducing costs, but which may prove harmful in the longer term. This is the case, for example, with reductions of population coverage and service, or significant increases in user fees. There is certainly scope for improving efficiency in certain areas of the health sector. The *World Health Report* of 2010, for example, not only called for "more money for health" but documented areas where countries could potentially get "more health for the money" (WHO, 2010). The OECD has published a book on various strategies for value-for-money in health spending (OECD, 2010). Amongst others, this looked at evidence-based medicine, health technology assessment, pay for performance, gatekeeping, improved co-ordination of care and the role of ICT. In health, as in other areas, the ability to make sensible choices and decisions is enhanced by having good management tools and governance structures. However, it is always difficult to make tough decisions around how to deal with large funding reductions within short periods.

The duration of the economic slowdown has been longer than originally anticipated in many countries, and several OECD countries still face relatively stagnant health budgets. Often, some of the key solutions to greater efficiency call for more long-term and structural reforms, and short-term expenditure controls might have limited – and in some cases potentially harmful – effects. Will a positive effect of the recession be a greater understanding on longer-term solutions on fiscal sustainability? Dealing with declining budgets and making tough decisions on cuts, efficiency savings and rationalisation are often extremely difficult tasks for health sector managers. Indeed, in addition to their own aspirations for the health system, they face pressures from strongly felt views from the public and from professional stakeholders, as well as from many experts who warn of dire long-term consequences. Given this, attempting to genuinely involve various key stakeholders in building some consensus around decisions, alternate service configurations and structural reforms may help to better shape and improve implementation of reform proposals (Ellins et al., 2014).

The country experiences presented in this chapter are based on country case studies presented to peers within the context of the OECD SBO-Health Joint Network. More information is available in a recent joint study by the WHO and the European Observatory on health systems and policies (Thomson et al., 2014) and in a range of recent country publications as various affected parties have tried to analyse and comment on what have in many cases been the harshest budgets cuts to the health sector in decades (Ellins et al., 2014). This chapter focuses on how national health sectors responded to fiscal constraints represented by lower budgets. It does not enter into debates over whether fiscal constraints were appropriate or too austere, or whether fiscal pressures on social services were or were not appropriate government responses to banking, housing mortgage and other financial crises.

6.2. Results

A summary of some of the available policy tools for dealing with fiscal constraints is shown in Table 5.1 in Chapter 5. Discussions during the 2013 and 2014 OECD SBO-Health Joint Network meetings showed that countries developed four main types of policy responses to the crisis: targeting pharmaceutical prices, personnel expenditure, hospital expenditure and across-the-board cuts (Figure 6.1).

Figure 6.1. **Key policy responses in Europe**

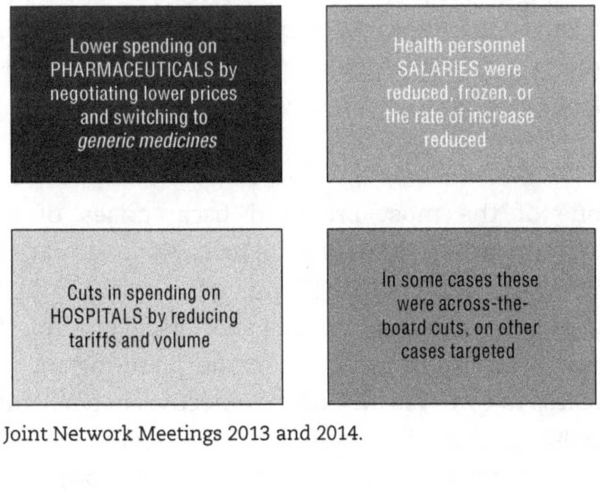

Lower spending on PHARMACEUTICALS by negotiating lower prices and switching to *generic medicines*

Health personnel SALARIES were reduced, frozen, or the rate of increase reduced

Cuts in spending on HOSPITALS by reducing tariffs and volume

In some cases these were across-the-board cuts, on other cases targeted

Source: OECD SBO-Health Joint Network Meetings 2013 and 2014.

The instruments available and used to achieve these objectives varied from country to country. The most widely used instruments were cutting prices, payments and fees (pharmaceuticals, hospitals and physicians) and increasing private participation (cutting pharmaceutical reimbursements or increasing patients' costs) (Figure 6.2).

Figure 6.2. **Budget tools available if health spending exceeds targets, by option**

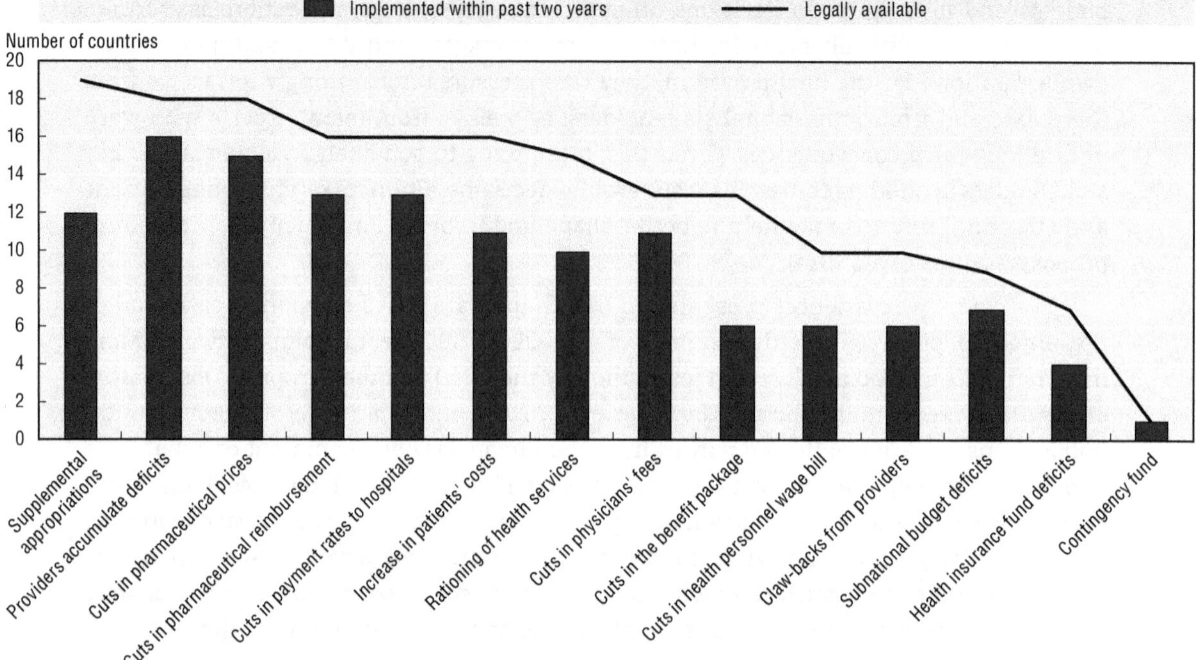

Source: Morgan, D. and R. Astolfi (2014), "Health Spending Continues to Stagnate in Many OECD Countries", *OECD Health Working Papers*, No. 68, OECD, Paris, *http://dx.doi.org/10.1787/5jz5sq5qnwf5-en*.

StatLink http://dx.doi.org/10.1787/888933218942

This chapter presents four brief summary case studies, based on information presented at the OECD SBO-Health Joint Network's meetings. Greece and Ireland are probably the two OECD countries which experienced the largest and most difficult fiscal consolidation. They experienced large financial crises where national debt levels rose markedly and their ability to service it was questioned. They received bailouts from the EU/IMF/World Bank, which were linked to fiscal consolidation programmes. On the other hand, countries including the United Kingdom and France also faced protracted budget shortfalls, but have not suffered as severe economic crises and, despite major challenges, have so far been able to plan and implement interventions in a more gradual and sustainable way.

Greece[1]

Greece faced one of the most profound fiscal crises of all OECD countries. Unemployment grew from 8.6% in January 2007 to 26.7% in January 2014 (ELSTAT, 2014), and public debt from 105% to 142% of GDP (Kentikelenis et al., 2011). Greece entered into a financial bailout agreement with conditions of strict fiscal controls. Fiscal consolidation plans required large and fast savings, which made planning more difficult. However, ensuring universal access to care was an explicit objective, in particular, the commitment to ensure the accessibility of health services for the uninsured. The main strategies followed by Greece were: hospital rationalisation and consolidation, savings in personnel (both numbers and wage rates) and pharmaceutical expenditures and better expenditure management and oversight (Figure 6.3). There has also been some consolidation in social security pools.

Figure 6.3. **Contribution to the evolution of health care expenditure by function of care**

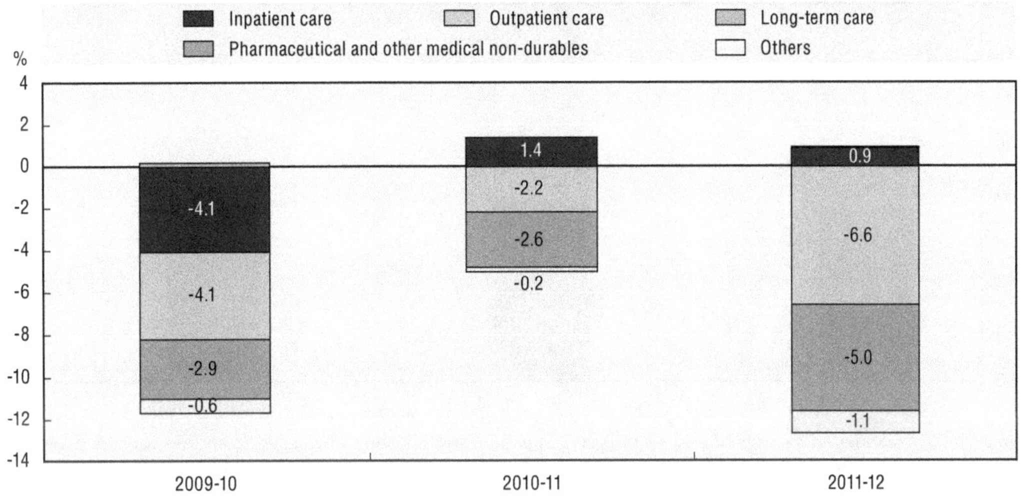

Source: OECD Health Data, 2014.

StatLink http://dx.doi.org/10.1787/888933218953

Regarding hospitals, a new health map was introduced in 2013 as a management tool for the rationalisation of the decision-making process. This map is based on the needs of the population for health care services and human and material resources. The result was extensive mergers of NHS hospitals, the reduction of their number from 127 to 89, beds being reduced by around 2 000. This policy was expected to produce savings of EUR 36 million for 2013, EUR 38 million for 2014 and EUR 38 million for 2015 (Figure 6.4). Budgetary transfers to hospitals have been significantly reduced from EUR 1.6 billion in 2011 to EUR 1.1 billion in 2014 (Figure 6.4). On a more positive note, Greece also introduced a new output-based hospital funding system (Kentikelenis et al., 2014).

Significant attention was given to containing or reducing the public sector wage bill through: rationalisation of the doctors' special wage regime, elimination of seasonal bonuses, hiring restrictions and a reduction in the number of fixed-term contracts by 20%. Numbers of staff were reduced: 1 453 doctors and 1 926 nurses and paramedical staff resigned or retired during 2011-12 (Ministry of Health data), while there were approximately 550 recruitments. The wage bill was reduced from EUR 2.4 billion in 2011 to EUR 1.9 billion in 2013 and approximately the same amount in 2014. Overtime payments for doctors were also reduced, from EUR 356 million in 2011 to EUR 237 million in 2013. OECD publications have previously reported that Greece has amongst the highest number of doctors in the OECD, but amongst the lowest numbers of nurses – it is not clear that in the haste of fiscal consolidation these kinds of variations have been addressed.

Efforts also concentrated on pharmaceutical spending. The share of pharmaceutical spending to GDP was amongst the highest in OECD countries. Prior to the crisis, Greece did not have monitoring of prescriptions and dispensing, a clear pricing or reimbursement mechanisms, nor economic evaluation of the medicines to be reimbursed or circulated in the market. Recent reforms introduced an e-prescription system, a better monitoring and assessment and pricing and reimbursement tools. This allowed substantive cuts to expenditure on pharmaceuticals.

Figure 6.4. **Estimated savings from hospital consolidation: Greece**

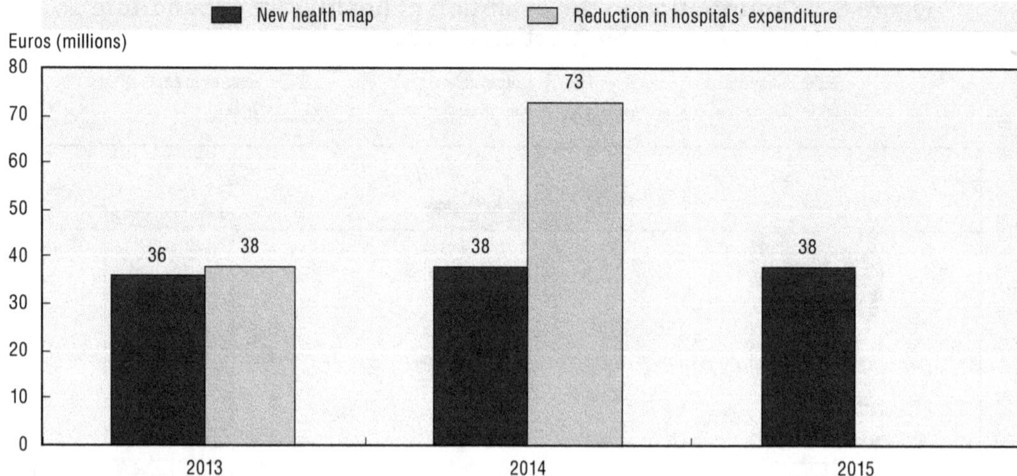

Note: In 2014, estimated savings of EUR 44 million in public hospitals were envisaged from fees for inpatient care. However, this fee was not applied, with the equivalent increase coming from state grants to hospital.

Source: Andrianopoulou, E. (2013), "Health Spending on the Road to Fiscal Consolidation", Presentation to the Joint Network on the Fiscal Sustainability of Health Systems, OECD, Paris, March 2013.

StatLink http://dx.doi.org/10.1787/888933218962

Various co-payments of EUR 25 per inpatient visit were initially envisaged, but these were not applied. Funding came instead from a EUR 45 million equivalent increase of state grants to hospitals, funded by an increase in tobacco taxes.

Efforts were made to improve financial management. An arrears clearance programme for the clearance of government entities' arrears to third parties was launched in November 2012, updated in October 2014. Both programmes were closely monitored by the MOH and GAO. Various fiscal rules and practice mechanisms were put in place. All line ministries and government entities set quarterly budget targets and drew up a monthly budget execution programme closely monitored by the respective Accounting Officer and the General Accounting Office. A Social Budget Committee (SBC) was established with the participation of the Ministries of Finance, Labour and Health to improve spending oversight. An administrative reform in 2011 established the National Organization for the Provision of Healthcare Services (EOPYY), consolidating health branches of eight major social security funds. This allowed for the long-awaited separation between the administration of pensions and health care. However, significant administrative and financial management problems hamper the organisation's effective and efficient operation, although significant efforts have been realised.

While some of the directions of reform appear reasonable, Greek attempts to deal with fiscal constraint in the health sector have received considerable criticism in the literature (Kentikilenis et al., 2011; Infanti et al., 2013). In particular, they are criticised for their magnitude and lack of protection for groups at risk. Vulnerable populations, with high unemployment and lower incomes following the recession, faced increased user charges, reductions in service access, fewer health employees and health workers sometimes not being present as they attempted to supplement their reduced incomes through doing private work. Self-reported unmet need has risen, as has the proportion of the population reporting "bad health". Suicides rose by 17% (which is a common feature in periods of economic and financial crisis), mental health problems have been widely described and HIV infection rates have risen, especially among intravenous drug abusers (partly due to reductions in drug rehabilitation and needle exchange programmes) (WHO, 2010). There is some evidence of the re-emergence of malaria cases for the first time in decades, given reductions in preventive spraying programmes, and the slowing or reversal of the declining trend in child mortality (Karanikolos et al., 2013). Some of these negative outcomes may have been due to the large size and magnitude of the adjustment, which made planning and implementation difficult and the scope of the cuts made being more widespread and unfocussed (Kentikelenis et al., 2014).

Ireland[2]

Following the global economic crisis of 2008, Ireland experienced a severe banking crisis, negative GDP growth, a rise in unemployment, revenue reductions and a substantial fiscal imbalance. Departmental expenditure which had peaked in 2009 at around 39% of GDP has been reduced very substantially to 31% of GDP by 2014. This was a reduction of EUR 10 billion. In this context, health expenditure declined by 8.6% (from EUR 15.5 billion to EUR 14.2 billion) in two years and had not recovered by 2013 (EUR 14.1 billion). Public debt grew to over 120% of GDP, and Ireland received a EUR 85 billion bail-out package.

There were few interventions that could achieve this magnitude of savings. Given that personnel tends to be the largest area of health spending, in an unprecedented step, social partners agreed to a reduction in public sector wages in addition to downsizing personnel numbers (12 000 were downsized according to OECD, 2010). Gross pay in the Irish health sector declined by 16.2% (from EUR 7.5 billion to EUR 6.3 billion) (Figure 6.5). Capital projects were delayed and capital budgets reduced by 26% (OECD, 2012). Ireland also increased co-payments for medicines and hospital accident and emergency visits. Hospital beds were consolidated leading to a reduction of 941 beds (OECD, 2012).

Figure 6.5. **Gross pay in the Irish health sector**

In million EUR

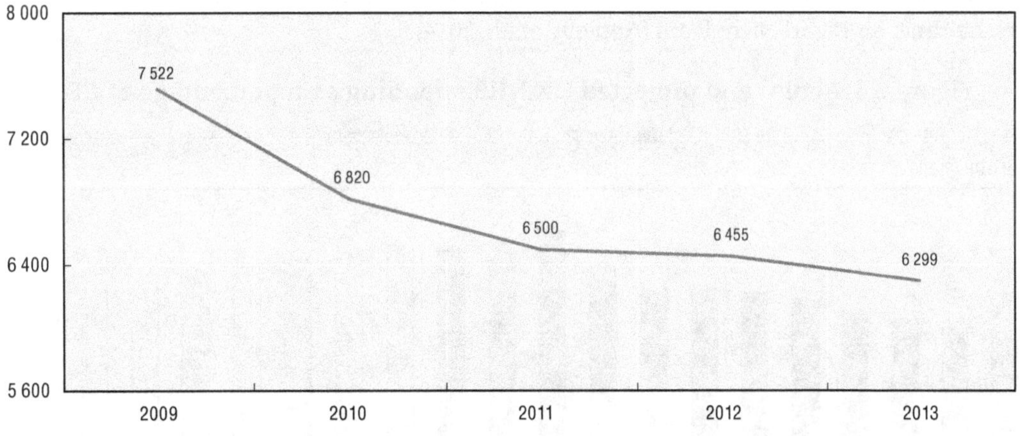

Source: Moloney, D. (2013), "Irish Health Reforms", Presentation to the Joint Network on the Fiscal Sustainability of Health Systems, OECD, Paris, April 2014.

StatLink http://dx.doi.org/10.1787/888933218979

However, the hardships and increased vulnerability of the recession also provoked a different response: to deepen the social security system to improve social protection, moving forward with the Universal Health Insurance (UHI) system. The existing system is somewhat fragmented between the tax-funded public system with user fees, and the voluntary private health insurance (over 50% of population have some form of VHI), which is tax-subsidised. The delivery of a single-tier, largely free health system, supported by Universal Health Insurance is a pillar of the government's health reform programme. It aims at a health system where access is determined by need and costs are borne fairly. The model under consideration involves competing insurers subsidised by government.

A recent assessment of the Irish health response to the fiscal crisis (Burke et al., 2014) suggests that in the first years of the crisis (2008-12) Ireland was able to achieve "more with less" (e.g. big uptake in persons covered with health cards; almost 1 million people who could no longer afford voluntary insurance became reliant on the state; increase in day cases). Part of this improvement was attributed to several years of sustained budget rises in the years before 2008. But as the crisis continued into 2013, the assessment found that a pattern of "less for less" began to emerge in terms of declining numbers in hospital cases, discharges, homecare hours and those receiving free care, alongside increased wait-times. Costs have shrunk in the Drugs Payment Scheme, partly because fewer people are coming for their medicines due to higher co-payments. The authors suggest a limited window of benefit from austerity, beyond which cuts and rationing prevail, which is costly in both human and financial terms. A detailed review of the Irish health system response to the fiscal crisis drew similar conclusions (Thomson et al., 2014).

United Kingdom[3]

From 2000 to 2009, government spending on health care in the United Kingdom grew steadily. Although the Wanless Commission had recommended additional funding for strengthening prevention and for particular services, a fairly significant share of the increases ended up going into wage increases and higher costs of infrastructure projects. When the effects of the banking and fiscal crisis hit the health budget, spending declined by GBP 3 billion in real terms between 2009-11 and budgets were capped until 2015 (Figure 6.6). Long-term sectoral pressures including pay rises, rising chronic diseases and population growth are estimated to cost GBP 13 billion by 2015 and GBP 30 billion by 2021. This has sometimes been called the Nicholson challenge (after the chief executive of England NHS at the time, Sir David Nicholson) (Appleby et al., 2014).

Figure 6.6. **Actual and projected UK NHS spending as a percentage of GDP**

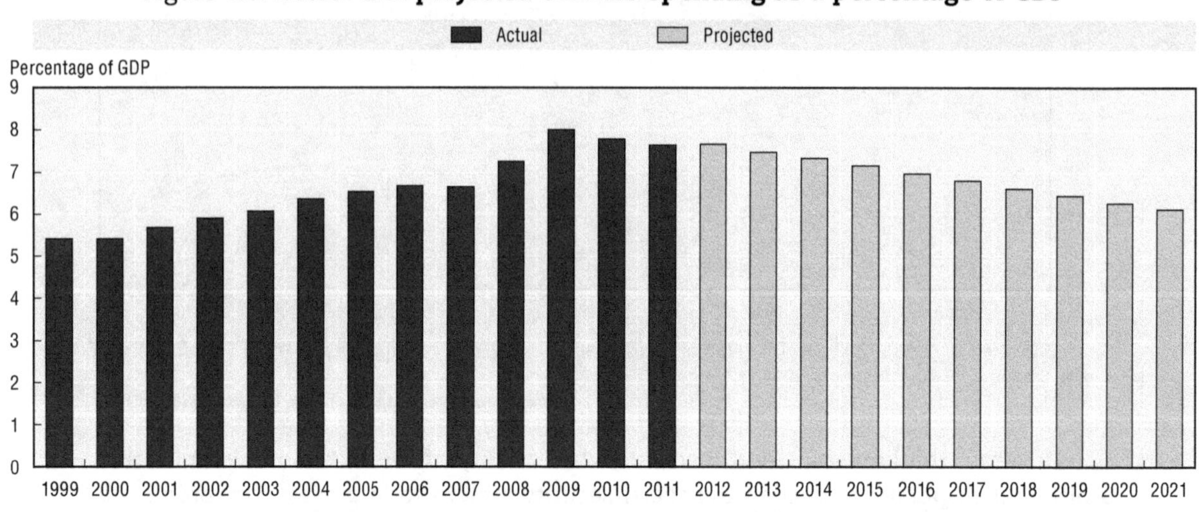

Source: Appleby, J., A. Galea and R. Murray (2014), *The NHS Productivity Challenge: Experience from the Front Line*, King's Fund, London.

The United Kingdom has certain inbuilt stabilisers which help to partially protect against the economic slowdown. Health is particularly political: it is consistently expressed as a key issue by voters and is widely covered in media and public debates. The United Kingdom has a very strong set of institutions and supporting institutions such as the Care and Quality Commission (checking adherence with quality standards), Monitor (overseeing foundation trusts and monitoring their deficits; Monitor, 2014), the King's Fund (policy support and analysis) and NICE (health technology assessment).

There have been a range of processes to look at how to make efficiency and productivity gains (Figure 6.7). The Quality, Innovation, Productivity and Prevention (QIPP) initiative is one major set of proposals to close this gap. Nicholson explained to the Public Accounts Committee of the UK House of Commons that around 40% of the four-year GBP 20 billion funding gap would be generated at local level through "traditional efficiency" gains and incentivised through the payment by results (PbR) system by building tough efficiency factors into the tariff (hospitals in the United Kingdom are paid through a variant of the DRG system called HRG). A further 40% would be found from "central initiatives" – cutting some central budgets, reducing management staff (centrally and at intermediate tiers of the NHS), but significantly, through restricting NHS staff pay as part of the UK Chancellor's public sector pay policy announced in the 2010 budget. Monitor (regulator for foundation trusts) has collected a wide array of analyses of ways to deal with the fiscal consolidation (Monitor, 2013). The King's Fund reported on potential areas for productivity improvement in six hospital foundation trusts (Appleby et al., 2014).

The NHS has attempted to deal with tight budgets by reducing input costs, including through national public sector pay policy and reducing administrative costs (e.g. consolidating various administrative levels and reducing administrative personnel). It has attempted to improve technical efficiency by: reductions in the tariff unit prices paid for hospital care; improved medicine management; improving allocative efficiency, such as shifting care from hospital to community settings (backed by larger budget shifts to this area); and better integration of care and demand management. Some attempts have been made to strengthen GP budget holding, including through Care Commissioning Groups. Hospital bed numbers have been reduced as has length of stay, but total hospital discharges have largely been maintained, suggesting some efficiency gains.

Between 2010 and 2012, staff numbers in the NHS were reduced by 19 669, mainly in the areas of NHS infrastructure and support to clinical staff. However, the NHS has successfully prioritised clinical staff, and doctor and nurse numbers have increased. Wage policies have been kept tightly in check and the combination of staff reductions and pay freezes have led to reduced spending on personnel. Pharmaceutical expenditure has been reduced.

Although service volumes have been largely maintained, there are growing public complaints about longer waiting lists for procedures. The King's Fund reports a waiting list of 3 million people for hospital treatment, the highest level in six years (Appleby et al., 2014). A quarter of hospital trusts have deficits and there are major debates between stakeholders around aspects of NHS reform. Research from the Nuffield Institute and the King's Fund suggests that there are opportunities for further productivity and efficiency improvement, and that it is important that savings are targeted appropriately. The Quality Care Commission monitors deficits in foundation trusts and quality standards, and steps have been taken against poorer performers. However, a range of stakeholders – including the King's Fund – express concerns about the outcomes in the health sector from continued fiscal austerity, and some stakeholders warn of a pending crisis as larger numbers of trusts go into deficit. Although bringing in a new management team may sometimes help to turn around a trust in deficit, the King's Fund warns that major structural reforms are difficult, and repeated management changes can also become part of the problem. At a political level, various proposals are being discussed for revenue increases to bolster the NHS.

Figure 6.7. **Savings in the United Kingdom under the Quality, Innovation, Productivity and Prevention programme (QIPP)**

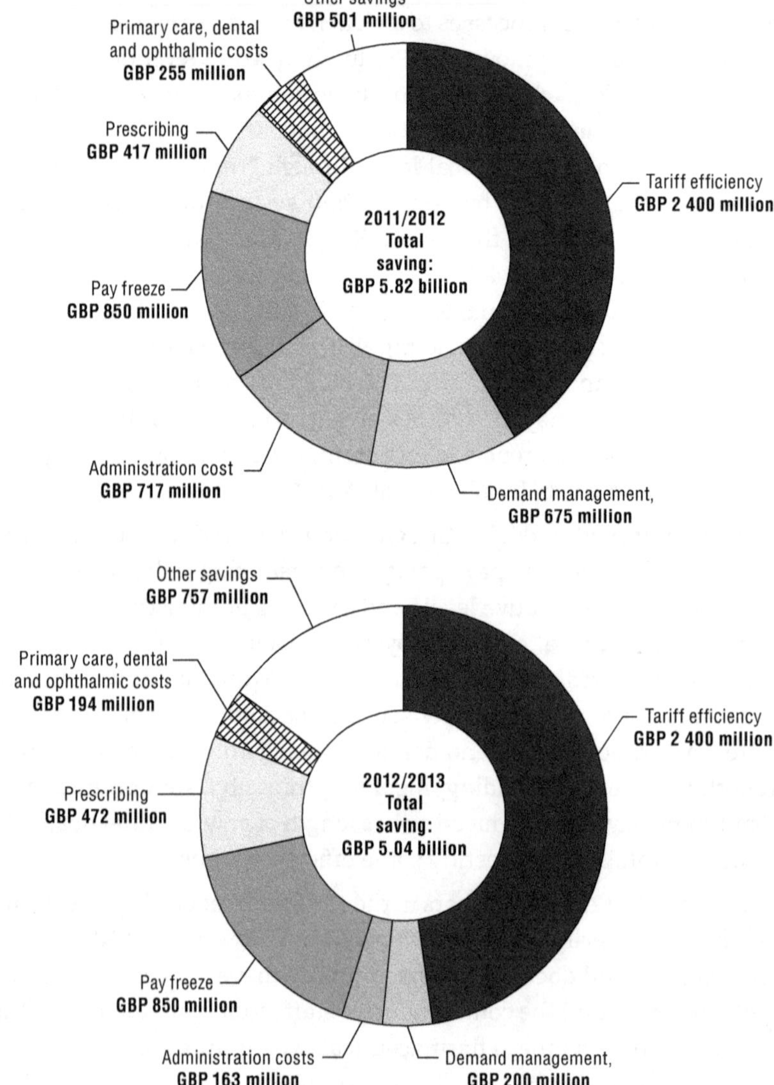

Source: Appleby, J., A. Galea and R. Murray (2014), *The NHS Productivity Challenge: Experience from the Front- Line*, King's Fund, London.

South Africa[4]

When the global economic crisis reached South Africa in 2008, growth slowed and national revenue decreased markedly in 2009/10. A sharp gap has arisen between spending and revenue in the context of low economic growth barely exceeding 2% over the past two years (Figure 6.8). In the fiscal year 2014/15, a deficit of 4% of GDP is projected, with revenue at 29% of GDP and expenditure at 33% of GDP. National debt has risen from

ZAR 526 billion in 2008/09 (22.8% of GDP) to ZAR 2 trillion by 2016/17 (44.3% of GDP). Public debt is not particularly high in international terms as a proportion of GDP (and below the EU fiscal rule of 60% of GDP). However, South Africa pays higher interest rates than high-income countries, and interest on debt has increased as a share of the budget over the same period from 7.6% to 10% (ZAR 54 billion to ZAR 145 billion per annum). It is now approaching the level of health spending (3.2% of GDP for interest vs 3.8% for health care, similar to many OECD countries with larger debt, but lower interest rates). In an attempt to reduce the deficit (to 2.8% of GDP by 2016/17) the government intends to reduce spending as a share of GDP from 33% to 31.9% of GDP by 2016/17, while still maintaining spending levels in real terms. Through this approach, the government hopes to bring down the deficit while protecting social spending.

Figure 6.8. **South Africa fiscal position: Consolidated revenue and expenditure as a percentage of GDP**

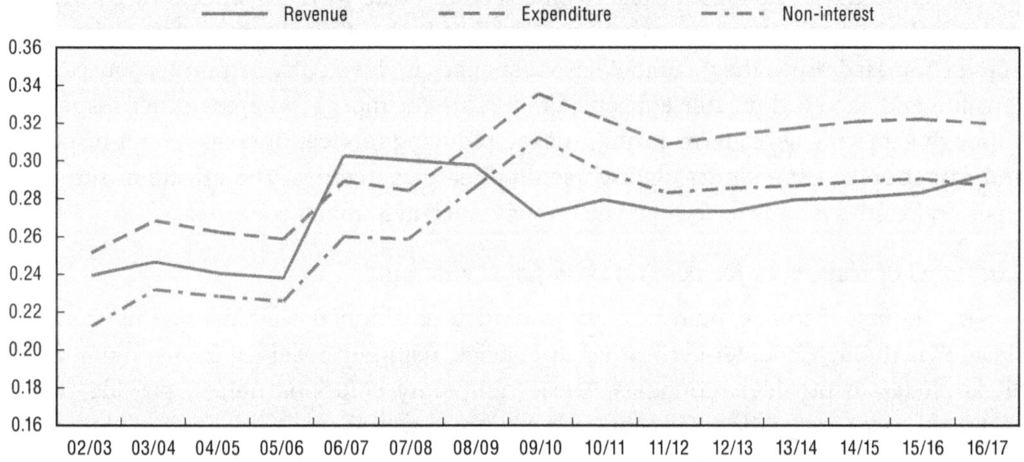

Revenue
Expenditure
Non-interest
0.36
0.34
0.32
0.30
0.28
0.26
0.24
0.22
0.20
0.18
0.16
02/03 03/04 04/05 05/06 06/07 07/08 08/09 09/10 10/11 11/12 12/13 13/14 14/15 15/16 16/17

Source: National Treasury, South Africa.

StatLink http://dx.doi.org/10.1787/888933219007

In the early years following 2008, the government used a counter-cyclical fiscal policy to protect social expenditure. However, as recovery time has become protracted, annual budget increases have become very constrained, impacting on health spending which comprises 12.6% of government spending. Non-interest spending growth is anticipated to slow to 2.2% in 2015/16 and 1.9% in 2016/17. Over the medium term, government health budgets grow only 1.6% per annum (in real terms), a far cry from the 5% per annum of previous years. This low growth is a problem, particularly because of the large HIV/AIDS epidemic which requires an additional 400 000 new persons to be put on treatment each year (costing USD 160 million additional per annum) and the continuing growth of compensation expenditure.

The government has put in place a cross-cutting savings exercise, which involves savings in non-core areas in all sectors, e.g. entertainment, catering, and business class air-travel. Health Departments have responded to the slowdown by freezing posts (which is difficult to reconcile with increasing numbers of patients on HIV/AIDS treatment), reducing investment in facilities and capital equipment, and trying to focus expenditure on protecting a set of "non-negotiable" spending areas prescribed by the Health Minister. Savings have been achieved in medicine expenditure, especially for antiretroviral medicines for

HIV/AIDS (procured centrally) through a better negotiating strategy, informed by international benchmarking. Despite this, the low budget growth aggravates the risk of harm from poor budgeting, supply chain and other practices, and reports of stock-outs of basic essential medicines are not uncommon.

Besides the medium-term to long-term prospect of improved economic growth, the main opportunity for increasing revenue for health lies in the planned introduction of a system of National Health Insurance. This is proposed to increase public health funding from 4% to 5% of GDP. Without this, public health funding would be declining as a proportion of GDP. This potentially creates a disjuncture where certain structural savings made now (e.g. for some provinces reductions in personnel numbers) might need to be reversed as the NHI comes into effect.

6.3. Discussion

In reflecting on how countries' health sectors dealt with the effects of their fiscal crises and budget limitations, what is striking first is the difficulty many countries faced in the short lead times they had to devise responses to deep cuts. Certain responses were sensible and achieved greater efficiency and value for money, whereas other responses, although achieving short-term savings, risked reducing services, increasing out-of-pocket and catastrophic expenditure, and worsening health outcomes. The effects of the fiscal crisis on health systems have been vociferous criticism in many countries.

Examples of responses for dealing with fiscal restraint

In the first instance, many countries tried to cushion the effects of the economic slowdown through counter-cyclical fiscal policies, using up reserves in insurance funds or surpluses in provider groupings. These temporary solutions helped provide partial protection, especially where the economic downturn was short.

Most countries strengthened their expenditure (and often performance) monitoring, reporting and oversight systems. Many put in place enhanced parliamentary and other committees to improve oversight of spending. This has also helped to identify potential areas of waste, improve budgeting and in some cases introduce new approaches to budgeting such as performance-based budgeting.

Several countries tried to find ways to increase revenues for health. Around half of OECD countries increased excise tax on alcohol or tobacco. Alcohol taxes were increased in England and Finland, and taxes on soft drinks introduced in Finland, France and Hungary (Karanikolos et al., 2013). A recent study (Thomson et al., 2014) reports increasing contribution rates (Bulgaria, Greece, Netherlands), raising ceilings on contributions (Bulgaria, Netherlands and Czech Republic) and broadening the revenue base by extending contributions to non-wage income such as dividends (Slovakia), pensions (Croatia for wealthier pensioners) or the self-employed (Slovenia). Some countries introduced new taxes earmarked for social security (France, Denmark and Hungary). The case of National Health Insurance in South Africa was mentioned above.

User charges or co-payments were increased in almost 50% of OECD countries, as reported in responses to the OECD survey on budgeting practices in health (e.g. Ireland, Greece). In general, a range of experts advised the OECD Joint SBO-Health Network that this was not a preferred response, because of the risk of poorer patients not accessing needed care as well as the risk of increasing catastrophic health expenditure by households. In contrast, some countries reduced user charges to assist vulnerable populations through the economic downturn (OECD, 2012).

In most countries, governments had to take steps to control expenditure in the health sector, in the context of falling or restrained budgets, even though many health sectors are likely to have had major misgivings about consolidation [*The Lancet* reports that in Iceland, there was such strong public opposition to health sector cuts that implementation was near impossible, and the overall negative effect on health outcomes less apparent (Infanti et al., 2013)].

Many countries have relied on interventions on pharmaceutical policy to make savings and appear to have been fairly successful with this. There have been a range of seemingly successful interventions in different countries, including centralised purchasing (thus leveraging greater buying power), greater use of essential drug lists, use of health technology assessment to assess new medicines (NICE in the United Kingdom, HITAP in Thailand), use of generics, price benchmarking and reference price setting both internally and internationally and lower reimbursement tariffs. Other interventions used in some countries include better stock management and pricing controls.

Spending on personnel is by far the single largest input cost in health systems and it is difficult to make substantial efficiency savings in this sector without attention to this area. The easy but potentially harmful solution many countries have followed is simply not to fill posts emptied through resignation (Greece), etc. More sophisticated solutions have been to better match personnel to workloads, improve productivity in areas where this makes sense, review staff mix (e.g. task-shifting such as use of nurses to share workload with doctors at primary care level) and use of norms and standards for staffing. UK research suggests there is potential for productivity gains. In many countries, controlling wage costs has been a major challenge in the sector. Israel shared with the OECD SBO-Health Joint Network experiences with negotiating doctors' salaries which led to a large national doctors' strike (Afek, 2014). South Africa, similarly, has a substantial problem of controlling significant real wage increases at a time of substantial fiscal deficits. In this context, the ability of Ireland (and Greece) to negotiate low wages was a remarkable social compromise. Nevertheless, it is important to recognise that fewer personnel with lower salaries are now managing a more vulnerable population.

Hospitals are the largest functional area of expenditure and it is difficult to achieve substantial efficiencies in the sector without hospital reforms. The United Kingdom appears to have had positive experiences with demand management interventions to keep unnecessary admissions out of hospital. These include telephone hotlines, self-care, strengthening primary care gatekeeping, and referral systems. There are huge variations in admission rates and hospital beds across OECD countries (Figures 6.9 and 6.10), which suggest that some countries are performing relatively inefficiently compared to their peers (OECD, 2013). Some countries have relatively low bed occupancies (Netherlands, the United Sates, Turkey) (WHO, 2010). Similarly, there is a great deal of medical practice variability in a wide range of medical procedures such as caesarean sections, coronary bypass, cholesterol lower drugs, hip and knee replacement etc. across OECD countries (OECD, 2010). These medical practice variations suggest over-use by some countries and under-use in others. The general pattern across OECD countries though is of gradually reducing bed numbers and length of stay, and increasing day surgery. This trend suggests some moves to greater efficiency.

Figure 6.9. **Variability in hospital beds by country in OECD**

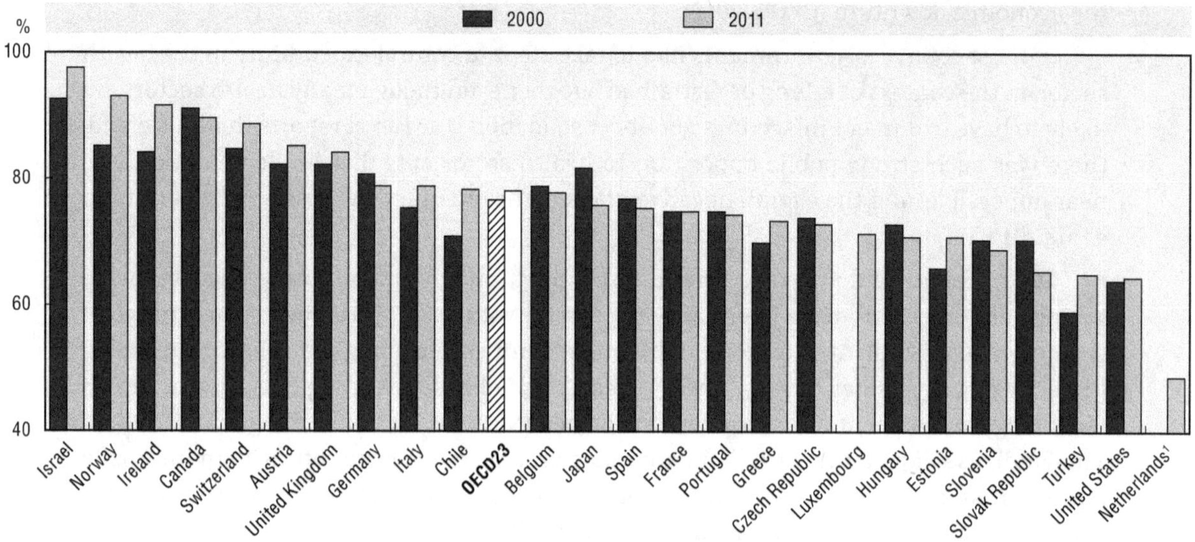

1. In the Netherlands, hospital beds include all beds administratively approved rather than those immediately available for use.

Source: OECD Health Statistics, http://dx.doi.org/10.1787/health-data-en.

StatLink http://dx.doi.org/10.1787/888933219010

Figure 6.10. **Variation in hospital discharges by country in OECD**

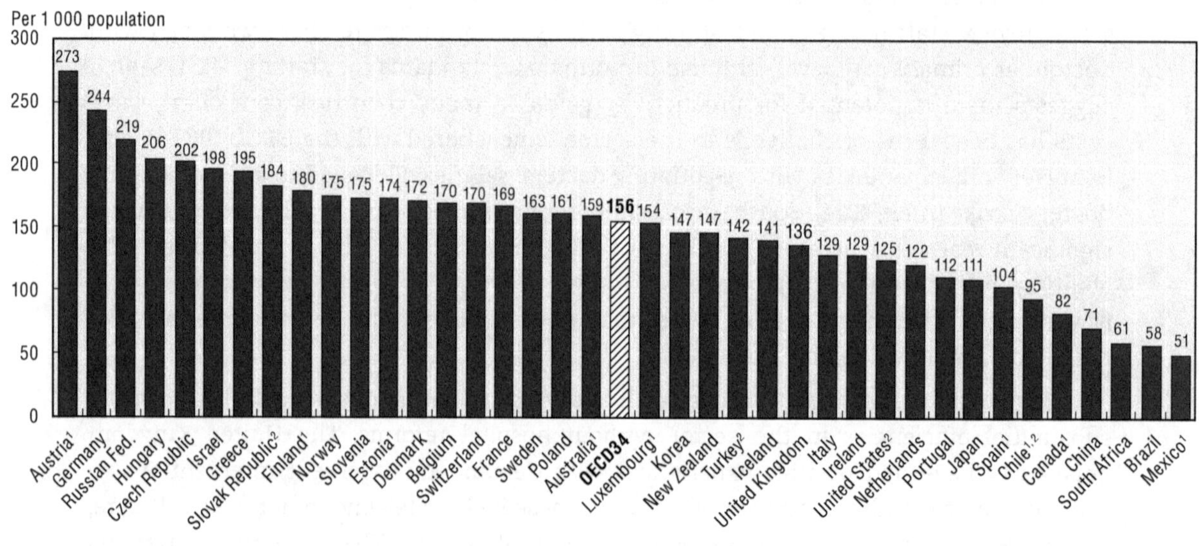

1. Excludes discharges of healthy babies born in hospital (between 3-10% of all discharges).

2. Includes same-day separations.

Source: OECD Health Statistics, http://dx.doi.org/10.1787/health-data-en.

StatLink http://dx.doi.org/10.1787/888933219025

In this context, some countries have consolidated hospitals (e.g. Greece). This can be a rational response to underutilised and inefficient supply capacity. However, if poorly planned and communicated, or if implemented too radically, such interventions can lead – and have led – to reductions in service provision and rejection by affected communities and stakeholders. Several countries, including Canada, have reported increased waiting times for cancer treatment, which appears an unwanted outcome (Ellins et al., 2014). The Netherlands made some modifications in their hospital reimbursement system, simplifying and consolidating the number of diagnostic and treatment categories (DTCs) in their payment system to allow for more streamlined price negotiations. Thailand caps payments on their DRG system to limit total hospital expenditure.

Strengthening primary care and prevention is certainly an appropriate long-term strategy to building efficient supply-side systems. Many interventions can be performed more cost-effectively at the primary care level, and treatment at inappropriate levels of care is a common cause of technical inefficiency in health systems. Several countries, such as the United Kingdom and the Netherlands, have tried to strengthen co-ordination across levels of care to streamline care and support appropriate level of care interventions (Ellins et al., 2014). Similarly, many key disease areas, such as chronic disease, can be substantially reduced through appropriate prevention programmes. While some countries made positive steps in this direction, others questionably cut these aspects of public health budgets (the Czech Republic, Denmark, Estonia, Ireland, Italy, the Netherlands) (Ellins et al., 2014). In some cases, this may have been inappropriate short-term cost-cutting responses to what could have been long-term solutions.

Redefining health benefit packages, in particular using health technology assessments may be useful. Universal health coverage is sometimes pictorially represented as a cube with three axes: population coverage; benefit package and proportion of fees paid by the insurer. Several experts advised that in the context of fiscal constraint, the axis of coverage and financial protection should as far as possible be protected. However, they suggested there is potential to modify benefit packages, particularly in considering cost-effectiveness of new technologies to be introduced, through health technology assessments. The Netherlands for example reduced benefits such as for sleep disorders, erectile dysfunction, or in-vitro fertilisation (IVF). Several countries have technology assessment agencies such as NICE in the United Kingdom and HITAP in Thailand, and these can help to provide a logical and acceptable basis for incorporating or rejecting new technologies. They also sometimes assist in acquiring new technologies at lower cost, by providing cut-offs for cost-effectiveness.

Administration costs should be a preferred target of efficiency savings rather than patient care. The United Kingdom has consolidated administrative levels and reduced administrative personnel numbers; Greece has pooled several fragmented funds, Thailand has extremely low administrative expenditure in the UC Fund (only 1.2%).

Purchasing and reimbursement reforms may also assist in achieving greater value for money. The United Kingdom has built efficiency savings into tariffs. Thailand uses capitation to control primary care expenditure and caps hospital DRG payments. Several new provider payment models are emerging that seek explicitly to align payment incentives with health system objectives related to quality, care co-ordination, health improvement, and efficiency by rewarding achievement of targeted performance measures. Many OECD countries therefore are experimenting with these methods of paying health care providers to improve the quality of health care and coverage of priority services (Table 6.1). The results of a study of several pay for performance programmes in OECD countries shows only modest impacts on quality measures and mixed results for efficiency and equity (direct incentives for efficiency have not been effective and direct incentives for equity have mixed results) (Cashin et al., 2014). However, these programmes set a new matrix for discussion between providers and purchasers, which open the door to discussion of provider payment reform, quality measurement, and accountability for outcomes.

Table 6.1. **Pay for performance programme in several OECD countries**

Programme focus	Country	Programme		Year programme began
Primary care	Australia	PIP	Practice Incentives Programme	1998
	Estonia	PHC QBS	Primary Health Care Quality Bonus System	2005
	France	ROSP*	Payment for Public Health Objectives	2009
	Germany	DMP	Disease Management Programmes	2002
	New Zealand	PHO Performance Programme	Primary Health Organization Performance Programme	2006
	Turkey	FM PBC	Family Medicine Performance Based Contracting Scheme	2003
	United Kingdom	QOF	Quality and Outcomes Framework	2004
	United States – California	IHA*	Integrated Healthcare Association Physician Incentive Program	2002
Hospital	Korea	VIP	Value Incentive Programme	2007
	United States – Maryland	MHAC	Maryland Hospital Acquired Conditions Program	2010
	United States – National	HQID	Hospital Quality Incentive Demonstration	2004

Source: Cashin, C. et al. (eds.) (2014), "Paying for Performance in Healthcare: Implications for Health System Performance and Accountability", European Observatory on Health Systems and Policies Series, Open University Press.

Potential consequences

Each country must examine its own needs and supply systems and determine where the best options for them potentially lie for short and long-term efficiencies and optimal service configuration. However, comparing against peer countries and learning from other country experience can potentially assist country governments. Members of the OECD Joint Network on the Fiscal Sustainability of Health Systems have valued being able to share experiences.

Part of the difficulty of managing fiscal constraints in health systems is the difficulty in projecting the duration of the period of the downturn. Short-term declines can be addressed by short-term efficiencies, looking for wastage and short-term savings, efficiencies, postponing of capital projects. However, longer-term reductions tend to require longer-term structural changes such as: shifting of chronic care from hospitals to primary care, reviewing hospital bed configurations, changing reimbursement mechanisms, modifying patient demand patterns and building up decentralised day surgery capacity. These long-term configurations can also entail their own transitional costs.

Ellins argues that short-term quick-fix responses have been dominant and may well not have long-term effects, and that many countries have not sufficiently used the opportunity to look seriously at long-term structural reforms (Ellins et al., 2014). They argue that periods of fiscal crisis provide opportunities to make structural changes to the health sector, but that this requires a good overall strategic vision from sectoral leaders. At the same time, they and other authors point out that the health sector has in some cases pursued substantial savings initiatives, reductions in services, increases in user charges, etc., but without a strong evidential base and insufficient monitoring and evaluation of the effects on quality of care and patient outcomes (OECD, 2010; OECD, 2012; Ellins et al., 2014).

There is evidence that in some countries, responses to the fiscal crisis have led to negative implications for quality of care, for health outcomes or for access (Infanti et al., 2013). The effects of health service reductions, if not well targeted, can aggravate the negative effects of the economic crisis itself on unemployment, poverty and health outcomes (Van Gool and Pearson, 2014).

The challenge for governments is to try to devise a set of interventions which as far as possible do not have these effects. This requires a focus on looking for areas of greater efficiency, restructuring to more cost-effective care pathways and service configurations (e.g. treating at appropriate level). Structural changes take time and may require bridging finance to build up alternate care pathways.

Rushed reforms and large cuts may go beyond achieving greater efficiency and better patterns to care and become blunderbuss cuts in services, prevention and public health. There is emerging evidence in several countries of poor health outcomes of such policies, with an increase in unmet need and a shifting of the financial burden to the most vulnerable. It is increasingly emerging that major structural reforms for consolidation take time, require strong management and governance, often require bridging finance (if new patterns of care are being developed to replace the old) and require substantial and difficult negotiations with stakeholder groups such as community and health professionals.

In contrast to the savings interventions described above, many countries have also made specific attempts to improve coverage and benefits and to reduce user fees to assist and protect increasing numbers of unemployed, poorer and more vulnerable populations during periods of recession. Countries have often introduced mixed responses – trying to achieve savings in some areas while improving services and protecting vulnerable groups in others.

6.4. Conclusion

The discussions within the OECD SBO-Health Joint Network on the Fiscal Sustainability of Health Systems has helped to share experiences across countries, and between Ministries of Health and of Finance, complementing a growing literature on the effects of the fiscal crisis on health.

Several countries have found sensible strategies which increase technical or allocative efficiency or aim to restructure services to a more sustainable path. Ideally, such strategies should help the health sector not only to cope in difficult periods of fiscal crisis, but potentially also to chart a longer-term sustainable fiscal path. Some patterns of care in the health sector are inherently expensive and inappropriate, e.g.: excessive hospitalisation at the expense of primary care, inappropriate use of medicines, widespread use of fee-for-service with its incentive for over-supply and over-use of procedures such as caesarean section, etc. However, in some cases, reforms can provide both better care, and more efficiency.

Some of the interventions used, while achieving some cost containment, are likely to have harmful effects over the medium to long term. Interventions that have tended to have negative effects on quality, outcomes and access include those that have raised user fees, cut services or personnel across the board and reduced coverage and benefits for essential services, including prevention and public health. Increasingly, researchers and policy makers are asking whether sufficient attention is being given to evaluation of the responses to fiscal constraint with respect to effects on quality, outcomes and access.

Structural reforms take time, strong governance, consultation and communication and may require bridging finance to build up alternate care pathways. Overly rushed reforms and cuts that are too large may go beyond being a challenge to achieve greater efficiency and better patterns to care to become blunderbuss cuts in services, prevention and public health. For these, there is emerging evidence in several countries of poor health outcomes, service delivery failures, an increase in unmet need and shifting of financial burden to the most vulnerable.

Notes

1. Based on a presentation by Evdoxia Andianopolou, March 2013, to then OECD Joint Network on the Fiscal Sustainability of Health Systems, supplemented by selected additional references.
2. Based on a presentation by David Maloney, April 2014, to the OECD Joint Network on the Fiscal Sustainability of Health Systems , supplemented by several additional references.
3. Based on presentations by Anita Charles, March 2013, to the OECD Joint Network on the Fiscal Sustainability of Heath Sytems, and selected additional references.
4. Based by a presentation by Mark Blecher, March 2013, to the OECD Joint Network on the Fiscal Sustainability of Health Systems, and selected additional references.

References

Afek, A. (2014), "Challenges with Wage Negotiations in Israel", April 2014 presentation to the Joint Network on the Fiscal Sustainability of Health Systems, OECD, Paris.

Andrianopoulou, E. (2013), "Health Spending on the Road to Fiscal Consolidation", March 2013 presentation to the Joint Network on the Fiscal Sustainability of Health Systems, OECD, Paris.

Appleby, J., A. Galea and R. Murray (2014), *The NHS Productivity Challenge: Experience from the Front-line*, King's Fund, London.

Berwick, D.M. and A.D. Hackbarth (2014), "Eliminating Waste in US Health Care", *Journal of American Medical Association*, Vol. 307, No. 14, American Medical Association, Chicago, pp. 1513-1516.

Burke, S., S. Thomas, S. Barry and C. Keegan (2014), "Indicators of Health System Coverage and Activity in Ireland During the Economic Crisis 2008-2014 – From 'More with Less' to 'Less with Less'", Health Policy, Vol. 117, Elsevier, Amsterdam, pp. 275-278.

Cashin, C. et al. (eds.) (2014), "Paying For Performance in Healthcare: Implications for Health System Performance and Accountability", European Observatory on Health Systems and Policies Series, Open University Press, United Kingdom.

Ellins, J., S. Moore, M. Lawrie et al. (2014), "International Responses to Austerity", *Evidence Scan* No. 22, Health Foundation, Birmingham.

Infanti, A., A. Andryou, H. Kalofonou et al. (2013), "Financial Crisis and Austerity Measures in Greece: Their Impact on Health Promotion Policies and Public Health Care", *Health Policy and Planning*, Vol. 113, Oxford University Press, Oxford, pp. 8-12.

Karanikolos, M., P. Mladovsky, J. Cylus, S. Thomson, S. Basu, D. Stuckler, J. Mackenbach and M. McKee (2013), "Financial Crisis, Austerity, and Health in Europe", *The Lancet*, Vol. 381, Elsevier, Amsterdam, pp. 1323-1331.

Kentikelenis, A., M. Karanikolos, A. Reeves, M. McKee and D. Stuckler (2014), "Greece's Health Crisis: From Austerity to Denialism", *The Lancet*, Vol. 383, No. 9918, 22 February 2014, Elsevier, Amsterdam, pp. 748-753, *http://dx.doi.org/10.1016/S0140-6736(13)62291-6*.

Kentikelenis, A., M. Karamakalos et al. (2011), "Health Effects of Financial Crisis, Omens of a Greek Tragedy", *The Lancet*, Vol. 378, Elsevier, Amsterdam, pp. 1457-1458.

Moloney, D. (2013), "Irish Health Reforms", April 2014 presentation to the Joint Network on the Fiscal Sustainability of Health Systems, OECD, Paris.

Monitor (2014), "Consolidated Financial Statements 2013/14", London, *www.gov.uk/monitor*.

Monitor (2013), "Improvement Opportunities in the NHS: Quantification and Evidence Collection". National Archives, London, *http://webarchive.nationalarchives.gov.uk/20140306143136/http://www.monitor-nhsft.gov.uk/sites/all/modules/fckeditor/plugins/ktbrowser/_openTKFile.php?id=37844.*

Morgan, D. and R. Astolfi (2014), "Health Spending Continues to Stagnate in Many OECD Countries", *OECD Health Working Papers*, No. 68, OECD Publishing, Paris, *http://dx.doi.org/10.1787/5jz5sq5qnwf5-en.*

OECD (2013), *Health at a Glance 2013: OECD Indicators*, OECD, Paris, *http://dx.oi.org/10.1787/health_glance-2013-en.*

OECD (2012), *Restoring Public Finances, 2012 Update*, OECD, Paris.

OECD (2010), *Value for Money in Health Spending*, OECD, Paris, *http://dx.doi.org/10.1787/9789264088818-en.*

Thomson, S., M. Jowett and P. Madlovsky (eds) (2012), "Health System Responses to Financial Pressures in Ireland. Policy Options in an International Context", Copenhagen: World Health Organisation Regional Office for Europe and European Observatory on Health Systems and Policies *www.euro.who.int/en/about-us/partners/observatory/publications/studies/health-system-responses-to-financial-pressures-in-ireland.*

Thomson, S., J. Figueras, T. Evetovits et al. (2014), "Economic Crisis, Health Systems and Health in Europe: Impact and Implications for Policy", Copenhagen: WHO Regional Office for Europe, European Observatory on Health Systems and Policies *www.euro.who.int/en/about-us/partners/observatory/publications/policy-briefs-and-summaries/economic-crisis,-health-systems-and-health-in-europe-impact-and-implications-for-policy.*

Van Gool, K. and M. Pearson (2014), "Health, Austerity and Economic Crisis: Assessing the Short-term Impact in OECD Countries", *OECD Health Working Papers*, No. 76, OECD, Paris, *http://dx.doi.org/10.1787/5jxx71lt1zg6-en.*

WHO – World Health Organization (2010), "Health Systems Financing: The Path to Universal Coverage", *World Health Report* 2010, WHO, Geneva.

ANNEX 6.A1

Menu of policy options

Table 6.A1.1. **Menu of policy options**

Area	Intervention	Concept	Country	Comment
Fiscal cushion	Counter-cyclical fiscal policy			
	Use-up accumulated surpluses in insurance fund/hospitals		Estonia	
Improve budget management and expenditure oversight	Improve expenditure monitoring, controls and oversight; Management; Improved budgeting eg. better links to outputs; Value for money monitoring			
	Performance based budgeting; performance monitoring; value for money monitoring			
Revenue	New increase taxes; earmarked or not			
	Increase insurance contributions, or broaden base, change limits, etc.			
	User fees introduce, increase or change		Ireland, Greece	Generally not favoured as make discourage necessary use; May have role for bipassing or specific demand modification
Hospitals	Rationalisation	Consolidate low use beds/hospitlas		
	More day surgery; shorter LOS			
	Increasing productivity eg doctor: patient ratio			
	Standardisation eg great variability in procedures, beds, admissions across countries			
Level of care	PHC gatekeeping			
	Try to shift balance of work to treat at appropriate level eg more at PHC, lower level hospitals	Demand management tools; referral chains		
	Self care; demand management tools, call-lines			
Reimbursement reform	Capitation for PHC	Supply side reform which helps to contain price and quantity	Thailand, United Kingdom	
	DRG; capped DRG			
	Budget holding eg to control referrals			
Medicines	Central procurement			Medicines intervention have been amongst the most widely used and successful during the post 2008 recession
	Tougher negotiation, benchmarking international and local			
	Generic policy			
	Essential drug lists (EDLs), treatment guidelines, appropriate use of medicines			

Table 6.A1.1. **Menu of policy options** *(cont.)*

Area	Intervention	Concept	Country	Comment
Benefit package	Use of HTA to exclude less cost-effective new interventions			
Capital equipment	Delay projects; don't over-capitalise; use of standardised designs; competitive purchasing and dealing with cartels			
Medical equipment	Delay purchase; essential lists EEL; servicing; appropriate technologies			
Personnel	Retrenchment; staff mix; lower level cadre substitution			
	Technically efficient allocation to match workloads			
	Freeze or reduce wage levels, benefits, salary freeze			
Laboratory	Protocols; cheaper inputs			Personnel costs are often largest cost driven in health systems
Administration	Consolidate; review multi-level administrations			
Funding pool consolidation		Reduce duplication		
Information systems		May help avoid duplicate tests, improve efficiency		
Coverage	Exclusion of certain groups eg wealthier			Generally discouraged priority to UHC
Prevention and public health		Rather prevent eg chronic dieases	United Kingdom (wanless)	In some cases countries reduced funding, which is likely to be counter-productive

Fiscal Sustainability of Health Systems
Bridging Health and Finance Perspectives

Chapter 7

The effects of ageing on the financing of social health provision

by
Chris Heady*

This chapter discusses how population ageing might affect the way that social health provision is financed, and the importance of favouring taxes that minimise their adverse impact on economic performance, both out of concern for general well-being, and in order to maintain popular support for social health provision.

* Chris Heady is Economics Professor at the University of Kent and was the OECD Head of Tax Policy and Statistics Division from 2000 to 2009.

The statistical data for Israel are supplied by and under the responsibility of the relevant Israeli authorities. The use of such data by the OECD is without prejudice to the status of the Golan Heights, East Jerusalem and Israeli settlements in the West Bank under the terms of international law.

7.1. Introduction

This chapter considers how population ageing might affect the way that social health provision is financed. It is well known that total (public and private) health expenditure as a share of GDP has been increasing across the OECD (Figure 7.1 and Table 7.1) and that this is expected to grow further, in part because of population ageing (De la Maisonneuve and Oliveira Martins, 2013). This implies that the governments of most OECD countries will have to increase their tax[1] financing of health care faster than the growth of GDP or reduce expenditure on other sectors if they are to maintain or increase the government's share of health expenditure. Figure 7.2 and Table 7.2 show that the OECD average has experienced a modest increase in this share in recent times, but that several governments have reduced their share since 2000. In this situation of growing pressure on government health expenditure, it is important that the taxes used to generate this financing minimise their adverse impact on economic performance, both out of concern for general well-being and in order to maintain popular support for social health provision.

Figure 7.1. **Total expenditure on health**

Percentage of gross domestic product

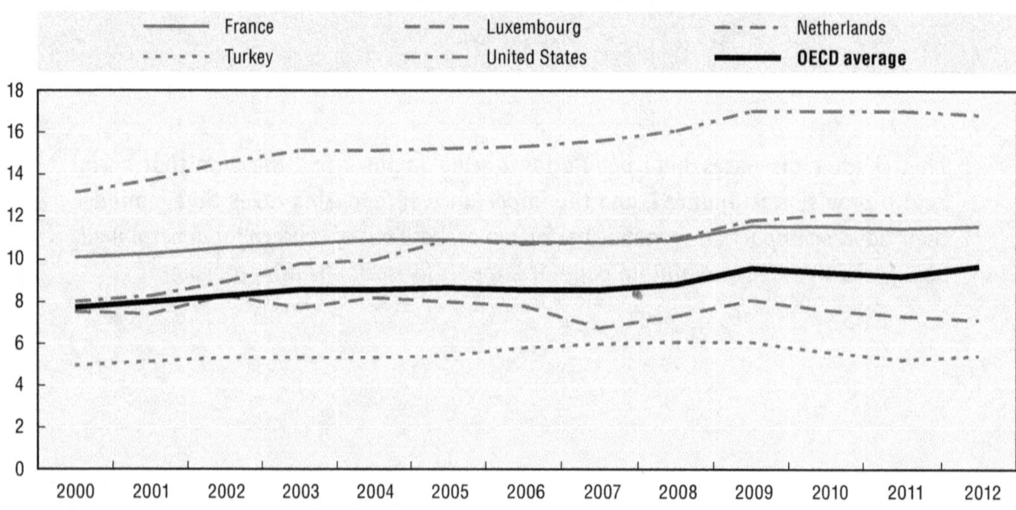

Note: OECD average in 2012 calculated from 31 countries with available data. Individual countries chosen to illustrate range of experiences.

Source: OECD National Accounts Statistics, http://dx.doi.org/10.1787/na-data-en.

StatLink http://dx.doi.org/10.1787/888933219039

As many OECD countries specifically earmark a portion of social security contributions to fund public health care, the possible long-term consequences of this policy are the main focus of this chapter, particularly as it can be argued that the base for such contributions (labour incomes) may decline as the population ages. However, the analysis presented here is wider than this in two respects. First, some countries have used increased social security contributions to generate additional finance for public health care even if they do not formally earmark the revenue. Second, the chapter

Table 7.1. **Total expenditure on health**

Percentage of gross domestic product

Country	1960	1970	1980	1990	2000	2001	2002	2003	2004	2005	2006	2007	2008	2009	2010	2011	2012	2013
Australia	3.7	..	6.1	6.7	8.1	8.2	8.4	8.3	8.6	8.5	8.5	8.5	8.7	9.0	8.9	9.1	..	..
Austria	4.3	5.2	7.4	8.4	10.0	10.1	10.1	10.3	10.4	10.4	10.2	10.3	10.5	11.2	11.1	10.9	11.1	..
Belgium[1]	..	3.9	6.3	7.2	8.1	8.3	8.5	9.6	9.7	9.6	9.6	9.6	9.9	10.7	10.6	10.6	10.9	..
Canada	5.4	6.9	7.0	8.9	8.7	9.1	9.4	9.5	9.6	9.6	9.7	9.8	10.0	11.1	11.1	10.9	10.9	..
Chile	..	..	..	..	6.4	6.5	6.5	7.4	7.0	6.8	6.3	6.5	7.0	7.6	7.1	7.2	7.3	7.4
Czech Republic	..	..	..	4.5	6.3	6.4	6.8	7.1	6.9	6.9	6.7	6.5	6.8	7.8	7.4	7.5	7.5	..
Denmark	..	..	8.9	8.3	8.7	9.1	9.3	9.5	9.7	9.8	9.9	10.0	10.2	11.5	11.1	10.9	11.0	..
Estonia	..	..	..	..	5.3	4.9	4.8	4.9	5.1	5.0	5.0	5.2	6.1	6.9	6.3	5.8	5.9	..
Finland	3.8	5.5	6.3	7.7	7.2	7.4	7.8	8.2	8.2	8.4	8.3	8.0	8.3	9.2	9.0	8.9	9.1	9.4
France	3.8	5.4	7.0	8.4	10.1	10.2	10.6	10.8	10.9	10.9	10.9	10.8	10.9	11.6	11.6	11.5	11.6	..
Germany	..	6.0	8.4	8.3	10.4	10.5	10.7	10.9	10.7	10.8	10.6	10.5	10.7	11.8	11.6	11.2	11.3	11.3
Greece	..	5.5	5.9	6.7	8.0	8.9	9.2	9.0	8.8	9.7	9.7	9.8	10.1	10.2	9.5	9.8	9.3	..
Hungary	..	..	..	..	7.2	7.2	7.6	8.6	8.2	8.4	8.3	7.7	7.5	7.7	8.1	8.0	8.0	..
Iceland	3.0	4.7	6.3	7.8	9.5	9.3	10.2	10.4	9.9	9.4	9.1	9.1	9.1	9.6	9.3	9.0	9.0	9.1
Ireland	3.7	5.0	8.2	6.0	6.2	6.8	7.1	7.3	7.6	7.6	7.5	7.9	9.0	9.9	9.2	8.7	8.9	..
Israel	..	..	7.7	7.1	7.3	7.8	7.7	7.6	7.5	7.5	7.3	7.3	7.3	7.3	7.3	7.3	7.3	..
Italy	..	..	..	7.7	7.9	8.1	8.2	8.2	8.5	8.7	8.8	8.5	8.9	9.4	9.4	9.2	9.2	9.1
Japan	3.0	4.4	6.4	5.8	7.6	7.8	7.9	8.0	8.0	8.2	8.2	8.2	8.6	9.5	9.6	10.1	10.3	..
Korea	..	..	3.7	4.0	4.4	5.0	4.9	5.2	5.2	5.7	6.1	6.4	6.6	7.2	7.3	7.4	7.6	7.8
Luxembourg	..	3.1	5.2	5.4	7.5	7.4	8.3	7.7	8.2	7.9	7.7	6.7	7.3	8.1	7.6	7.3	7.1	..
Mexico	..	..	..	4.4	5.0	5.4	5.5	5.9	6.0	5.9	5.7	5.8	6.0	6.5	6.3	5.9	6.2	..
Netherlands	..	..	7.4	8.0	8.0	8.3	8.9	9.8	10.0	10.9	10.7	10.8	11.0	11.9	12.1	12.1	..	..
New Zealand	..	5.2	5.8	6.8	7.6	7.7	8.0	7.8	8.0	8.3	8.7	8.4	9.3	9.8	10.0	10.0	..	..
Norway	2.9	4.4	7.0	7.6	8.4	8.8	9.8	10.0	9.6	9.0	8.6	8.7	8.6	9.7	9.4	9.3	9.3	9.6
Poland	..	..	..	4.8	5.5	5.9	6.3	6.2	6.2	6.2	6.2	6.3	6.9	7.2	7.0	6.9	6.8	..
Portugal	..	2.4	5.1	5.7	9.3	9.3	9.3	9.7	10.0	10.4	10.0	10.0	10.2	10.8	10.8	10.2	..	..
Slovak Republic	..	..	..	..	5.5	5.5	5.6	5.8	7.2	7.0	7.3	7.8	8.0	9.2	8.5	8.0	8.1	..
Slovenia	..	..	..	..	8.3	8.6	8.6	8.8	8.5	8.5	8.4	8.0	8.5	9.4	9.1	9.1	9.4	..
Spain	1.5	3.5	5.3	6.5	7.2	7.2	7.3	8.2	8.2	8.3	8.4	8.5	8.9	9.6	9.6	9.4	9.3	..
Sweden	..	6.8	8.9	8.2	8.2	8.9	9.2	9.3	9.1	9.1	8.9	8.9	9.2	9.9	9.5	9.5	9.6	..
Switzerland	4.9	5.5	7.4	8.2	9.9	10.3	10.6	10.9	11.0	10.9	10.4	10.2	10.3	11.0	10.9	11.1	11.4	..
Turkey	..	..	2.4	2.7	4.9	5.2	5.4	5.3	5.4	5.4	5.8	6.0	6.1	6.1	5.6	5.3	5.4	..
United Kingdom	3.9	4.5	5.6	5.9	6.9	7.2	7.5	7.8	7.9	8.1	8.3	8.4	8.8	9.7	9.4	9.2	9.3	..
United States	5.1	7.1	9.0	12.4	13.1	13.8	14.6	15.1	15.2	15.2	15.3	15.6	16.1	17.1	17.0	17.0	16.9	..
OECD average	**3.8**	**5.0**	**6.6**	**6.9**	**7.7**	**8.0**	**8.2**	**8.5**	**8.6**	**8.6**	**8.6**	**8.6**	**8.9**	**9.6**	**9.4**	**9.2**	**9.2**	**9.1**

1. Excluding investments.

Source: OECD Health Statistics, http://dx.doi.org/10.1787/health-data-en.

StatLink http://dx.doi.org/10.1787/888933219443

includes a discussion of which taxes might best be used to finance increases in health care costs that is applicable to all OECD countries, regardless of whether they earmark social security contributions.

The main findings are as follows. First, in terms of economic efficiency, most OECD countries would benefit from looking at the use of less distortionary and broader-based taxes. Second, increasing social security contributions to support health care could worsen labour market performance. Third, public support for public expenditure on health care would not be helped by the use of earmarked social security contributions, but would be helped by the use of taxes with broader bases that bear more heavily on the older population. Fourth, financing from social security contributions could be at risk from both a declining labour share of income and an increase in income inequality, and the use of broader-based taxes would reduce these risks. Fifth, the earmarking of sin taxes to help finance health care could make a contribution, but this is always likely to be fairly small and cannot be expected to be a significant source of funds to meet increasing needs.

The chapter also considers what light the recent experiences of OECD countries shed on the likelihood of some of the possible threats to social security funding being realised. The analysis shows that countries with heavy reliance on social security contributions are more likely to have a high tax wedge on labour,[2] and hence an increased likelihood of poor labour market performance. However, there was no evidence yet that countries which rely heavily on social security contributions have been less able to maintain public support for health expenditure.

In brief, the implications of this chapter are that:

- Broader-based and less distortionary taxes are likely to be the best means of meeting any increasing financing needs for public health care.
- The use of social security contributions should be moderated, especially for those countries that rely on them heavily.
- Sin taxes can have a modest role to play but will not solve the financing problems created by population ageing.

The analysis in the chapter is set out as follows. Section 7.2 analyses the choice between different types of tax to help finance the expected increase in government health expenditures, including the arguments for and against using social security contributions to finance social expenditures. Section 7.3 examines the political economy of support for social health care and how it might be affected by the distortionary effects of the taxes used to finance it. Section 7.4 then considers whether population ageing might threaten the sustainability of using social security contributions as a major source of finance. Section 7.5 considers the earmarking of "sin taxes" for health care. Finally, Section 7.6 looks at the experience of OECD countries, considering the effects of the differing extents to which they rely on social security contributions.

7.2. The choice between different types of tax

In much economic policy discussion of financing public services, the emphasis is on the total amount of taxation and its distribution between different groups of taxpayers, without regard to how the choice among different types of taxes can affect economic performance. This effect of taxation on economic performance, often referred to by economists as a tax's "distortionary cost", differs between different taxes, for example between personal income tax and value added tax (VAT). This implies that governments should not simply choose the taxes that finance health expenditures according to their distribution effects or some other aspect of political acceptability. They should also take account of these distortionary costs.

A recent OECD study of tax and economic growth (OECD, 2010) examined the effects of tax structure, rather than simply the total amount of tax raised, on the rate of economic growth in OECD countries. Shortly afterwards, the two-volume Mirrlees report (Mirrlees et al., 2010 and 2011) looked at how tax systems in the United Kingdom and other countries could be reformed in a way that improved the more general concept of "social welfare" without altering the total size of government. The findings of the two studies are broadly consistent and so nothing of importance to the discussion in this chapter is lost by concentrating on the OECD study with its stronger OECD-wide focus.

The main conclusions of the OECD study relevant to this chapter are that:

- A shift from income taxes (particularly corporate but also personal) towards consumption taxes and recurrent taxes on residential property[3] would probably, in most OECD countries, increase economic growth.
- Reforms to the design of individual taxes could be expected to improve economic performance. Beneficial reforms mostly consist of those that broaden the base of the tax and lower its rate. In particular, moves towards a single rate of VAT would be preferable to an increase in the main VAT rate.

The report recognised that growth-enhancing reforms would be likely to increase inequality, a reflection of the general conflict between equity and efficiency in much of economic policy. However, it can be argued that the resulting increased inequality could be offset by measures that would be likely to be less harmful to economic growth than current tax systems (Arnold et al., 2011). For example, the distributional consequences of moving to a single rate of VAT could be largely offset by changes to social benefits at a cost that would be significantly less than the additional revenue raised (particularly as it is those on higher earnings that benefit most in absolute terms – not as a percentage of income – from reduced tax rates). Also, there are several ways in which recurrent taxes on residential property can be reformed to remove the apparent regressive nature of these taxes in some countries. These views are also present in the Mirrlees report.

The general implication of the OECD tax and growth study for this chapter is that, to minimise adverse effects on economic performance while protecting those on lower incomes, additional requirements for finance of health spending should be met mainly by moving towards less distortionary and broader based taxes.

Turning to the issue of financing health care through social security contributions, the OECD tax and growth study could not find robust evidence of a difference between social security contributions and personal income tax in their effects on economic growth. Thus, the conclusion that growth could be increased by shifting the balance of taxation away from personal income applies equally to social security contributions. This finding was surprising as it has been argued by Disney (2004) and others that social security contributions have a smaller distortionary effect than personal income tax because an individual's social security contributions have an effect on the pension that the worker will receive upon retirement.

It is possible that this unexpected finding results from the fact that OECD countries differ widely in the extent to which an individual worker's contributions over their lifetime affect their retirement pension. This implies that it is still possible that Disney is correct and that, in countries with a strong link between contributions and pensions, social security contributions are less distortionary. However, it should be noted that Disney's argument related specifically to pensions and that it cannot be expected to apply to social security contributions that are earmarked for health care. This is because the health care that workers will receive, both before and after retirement, is only related to their health condition and not to the amount of social security contributions that they have paid.

This final point implies that social security contributions earmarked for health care are no less distortionary than personal income tax. In fact, it can be argued that they will be more distortionary as most social security contributions have an upper income limit, after which additional contributions are at a reduced (possibly zero) rate. This means that the costs of social security contributions bear more heavily on workers with low or middle income than the more progressive personal income tax. In addition to the obvious distributional impact of this fact, there is a distortionary impact as it means that any given amount of additional revenue from social security contributions will increase the tax burden on low-income and middle-income workers (as measured in the OECD by the tax wedge) than a corresponding revenue increase from personal income tax. This is important as the reassessment of the *OECD Jobs Study* (OECD, 2005) found that increases in the tax wedge have a substantial negative effect on the employment rate – a clear distortionary impact.

7.3. The political economy of support for social health care

In addition to the question of which taxes to use to finance social health provision, there is the question of how much total tax citizens are prepared to pay to preserve the level of public service provision. There does not appear to be any literature on the effect of ageing specifically on support for public health provision; but there is literature on the welfare state in general with interesting implications for the health sector. This section briefly reviews some key aspects of this literature.

Until fairly recently, the general view in the literature was that population ageing would increase support for the welfare state as the older members of society are the main beneficiaries of these expenditures and so support their maintenance or even their increase. However, Razin, Sadka and Swagel (2002) developed a theoretical political economy model of the size of the welfare state that raised the possibility that population ageing could result in a reduced level of social provision. They also presented some statistical analysis that suggested that the size of the welfare states in many countries had been reduced by population ageing.

The theoretical model was based on the standard "median voter" model of democracy, under which the actual size of the welfare state would be given by the views of the person whose preference for it was in the middle of the population's distribution of views. Razin, Sadka and Swagel (2002) argued that the median person would be somebody who had not yet retired from work, unless ageing had become very extreme. Such a person would decide the size of the welfare state by balancing its cost (in terms of that person's tax bill) and the benefits that person would receive. As population ageing would increase the cost of any given level of provision, this could result in the median person's costs increasing without any increase in benefits to that person, reducing the level of provision for which the median person would vote. This analysis was used to explain their statistical findings. Razin, Sadka and Swagel (2002) also note a further conclusion from their theoretical model: the (partial) financing of the welfare state from a tax on capital income could reverse their result as this would bear more heavily on the retired than the working population and so increase the level of expenditure for which the median person would vote.

This article produced a vigorous debate (Disney, 2007; Galasso and Profeta, 2007; Simonovits, 2007; Razin and Sadka, 2007; and Disney et al., 2007) about both the statistical analysis and the theoretical model. One key assumption of Razin, Sadka, and Swagel (2002) that was identified was that the payments by the working median person had no influence on the benefits that (s)he would receive after retirement. This was criticised on two grounds: that in many countries increased social security contributions result in higher benefits after retirement, and that even if they don't, many working people would vote for higher benefits in the belief that the larger welfare state would survive until after their retirement. However, none of the critics attacked the idea that greater use of taxes on capital income to finance the welfare state would reduce the chances of population ageing resulting in less support for the welfare state, because some of the burden of such taxes would fall on retired people.

It is possible to draw some conclusions from this debate without taking a position on the more detailed points. First, the best statistical evidence currently available suggests that population ageing has increased rather than reduced the size of the welfare state as a whole. Second, any possible future threat to political support for the welfare state is more likely if the link between the amount that workers pay towards it and the size of their benefits in retirement is weakened. Third, a shift of funding towards taxes paid partly by retired people would reduce any threat to political support.

Turning to the specific case of public health care, the situation does not seem to be as secure as for the welfare state as a whole. Starting with the data, while many OECD countries have maintained or increased the proportion of health expenditure financed by the public sector in recent years, several have not (Figure 7.2 and Table 7.2). However, there has been no careful statistical analysis of whether this is due to population ageing or to other factors, such as the recent economic crisis.

Turning to the theoretical considerations, there is not as strong a link between a working taxpayer's contributions to the health system (whether in the form of social security contributions or other taxes) and that person's future health care as there is in a public pension system in which benefits are linked to contributions. This makes it all the more important that the distortionary cost of financing increased public health care expenditures should be kept to a minimum, along the lines discussed in Section 7.2, and that consideration be given to increasing the contribution to this financing from people above retirement age by making use of broader based taxes.

Figure 7.2. **Public expenditure on health**

Percentage of total expenditure on health

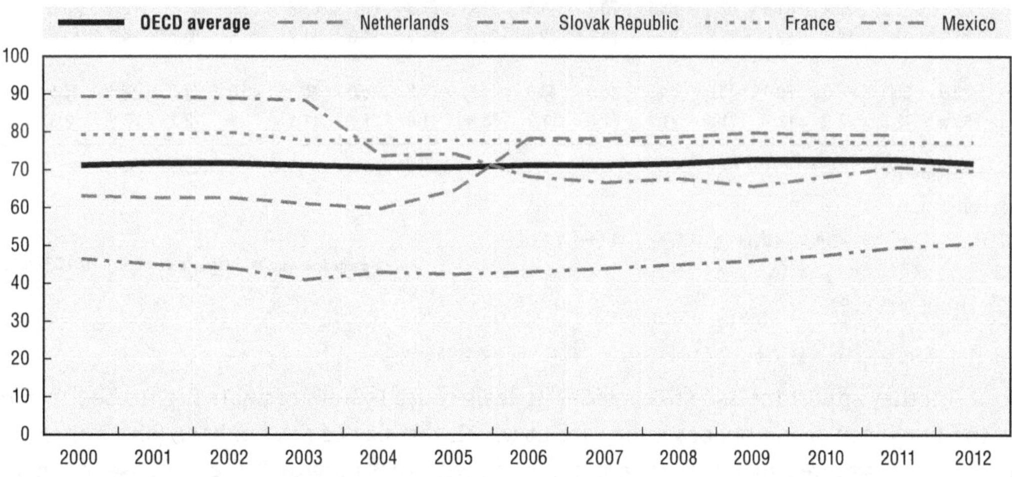

Note: Individual countries chosen to illustrate range of experiences. Netherlands' expenditure data presented by public expenditure as share of current total health expenditure from 2002 to 2012. OECD average calculation for 2012 based on 31 countries with available data.

Source: OECD National Accounts Statistics, *http://dx.doi.org/10.1787/na-data-en*.

StatLink http://dx.doi.org/10.1787/888933219042

Table 7.2. **Public expenditure on health**

Percentage of total expenditure on health

	1960	1970	1980	1990	2000	2001	2002	2003	2004	2005	2006	2007	2008	2009	2010	2011	2012	2013
Australia	50.3	..	62.6	66.2	66.8	66.3	66.9	66.1	66.7	66.9	66.6	67.5	67.9	68.5	67.8	68.4	..	..
Austria	69.4	63.0	68.8	72.9	75.6	75.1	74.8	74.5	74.7	75.3	75.7	75.8	76.3	76.4	75.5	76.5	75.9	..
Belgium[1]	..	..	..	..	74.6	75.4	73.8	74.5	75.8	75.8	73.6	73.2	74.7	76.1	75.0	75.7	75.2	..
Canada	42.6	69.9	75.6	74.5	70.4	70.0	69.5	70.2	70.2	70.2	69.8	70.2	70.5	70.9	70.8	70.6	70.1	..
Chile	..	..	..	..	52.1	53.5	54.5	38.8	39.9	40.0	42.1	43.2	44.1	47.7	48.6	48.8	49.2	46.0
Czech Republic	..	96.6	96.8	97.4	90.3	89.8	90.5	89.8	89.2	87.3	86.7	85.2	82.5	84.0	83.8	84.2	84.0	..
Denmark	..	..	87.8	82.7	83.9	84.2	84.5	84.5	84.3	84.5	84.6	84.4	84.7	85.0	85.1	85.3	85.8	..
Estonia	..	..	..	..	77.2	78.6	77.1	77.0	75.5	76.7	73.3	75.6	77.8	75.3	78.9	79.3	78.7	..
Finland	54.1	73.8	79.0	80.9	71.3	72.0	72.5	74.6	75.0	75.4	74.8	74.4	74.5	75.2	74.2	74.6	75.0	75.3
France	62.4	75.5	80.1	76.6	79.4	79.4	79.7	78.9	78.8	78.8	78.7	78.3	76.7	76.9	77.5	77.3	77.4	..
Germany	..	72.8	78.7	76.2	79.5	79.3	79.0	78.5	76.8	76.6	76.5	76.4	76.6	76.9	76.7	76.5	76.7	76.8
Greece	..	42.6	55.6	53.7	60.0	60.8	58.0	59.8	59.1	60.1	62.0	60.3	59.9	61.7	66.7	67.4	67.1	..
Hungary	..	..	..	..	70.7	69.0	70.2	71.1	69.6	70.0	69.8	67.3	67.1	65.7	64.8	63.8	62.6	..
Iceland	66.7	66.2	88.2	86.6	81.1	81.0	81.9	81.7	81.2	81.4	82.0	82.5	82.6	82.0	80.4	80.4	80.5	80.5
Ireland	76.0	81.7	82.0	71.7	75.1	75.7	76.3	76.7	77.0	75.9	75.1	75.5	75.1	72.0	69.6	67.8	67.6	..
Israel	..	..	..	..	62.6	62.0	63.2	61.7	60.9	59.3	59.8	59.0	59.5	60.5	61.8	60.8	59.8	..
Italy	..	..	..	79.5	72.5	74.6	74.5	74.5	76.0	76.2	76.6	76.6	78.9	79.6	78.9	77.1	77.3	78.0
Japan	60.4	69.8	71.3	77.6	80.8	81.4	81.3	80.4	80.8	81.6	79.4	80.4	80.8	80.5	82.1	82.6	82.1	..
Korea	..	..	21.6	38.4	48.6	54.9	53.7	52.4	52.6	52.9	55.3	55.8	55.9	58.2	56.6	55.5	54.5	53.4
Luxembourg	..	88.9	92.8	93.1	85.1	84.3	85.5	84.2	84.8	84.9	85.1	84.1	84.1	84.0	85.9	85.3	83.5	..
Mexico	..	..	..	40.4	46.6	44.8	43.9	44.2	45.2	45.0	45.2	45.4	46.9	48.3	47.5	49.6	50.6	..
Netherlands[2]	..	..	73.2	71.2	66.4	65.8	65.5	66.5	65.6	65.8	82.4	84.1	84.8	85.4	79.6	79.4	79.5	
New Zealand	..	80.3	88.0	82.4	78.0	76.4	77.9	78.3	79.6	79.7	80.1	82.4	82.8	83.0	83.2	82.7	..	..
Norway	77.8	91.6	85.1	82.8	82.5	83.6	83.5	83.7	83.6	83.5	83.8	84.1	84.4	84.6	84.7	84.8	85.0	85.5
Poland	..	..	..	91.7	70.0	71.9	71.2	69.9	68.6	69.3	69.9	70.4	71.8	71.6	71.2	70.3	69.2	..
Portugal	..	59.0	64.3	65.5	66.6	67.0	68.6	68.7	68.1	68.0	67.0	66.7	65.3	66.5	65.9	65.0	..	..
Slovak Republic	..	..	..	..	89.4	89.3	89.1	88.3	73.8	74.4	68.3	66.8	67.8	65.7	68.1	70.9	69.7	..
Slovenia	..	..	..	..	74.0	73.3	73.4	71.6	73.1	72.7	72.3	71.8	73.9	73.2	74.2	73.5	71.5	..
Spain	58.7	65.4	79.9	78.7	71.6	71.2	71.3	70.4	70.6	71.0	71.6	71.9	73.2	74.7	74.4	73.4	71.7	..
Sweden	..	86.0	92.5	89.9	84.9	81.1	81.4	82.0	81.4	81.2	81.1	81.4	81.5	81.5	81.5	81.7	81.3	..
Switzerland	..	..	..	52.4	55.4	56.9	57.7	58.3	58.4	59.5	59.1	59.1	65.2	65.5	65.2	65.4	65.8	..
Turkey	..	..	29.4	61.0	62.9	68.1	70.7	71.9	71.2	67.8	68.3	67.8	73.0	..	78.6	79.6	76.8	..
United Kingdom	85.2	87.0	89.4	83.6	78.8	79.5	79.6	79.8	81.2	81.7	81.3	81.2	82.5	83.4	84.0	83.4	84.0	..
United States	22.9	36.1	41.0	39.4	43.0	44.0	43.9	43.8	44.1	44.2	45.0	45.2	46.0	47.3	47.4	47.5	47.6	..
OECD average	**60.5**	**72.6**	**73.0**	**72.7**	**71.3**	**71.7**	**71.8**	**71.2**	**70.8**	**71.0**	**71.1**	**71.1**	**71.9**	**72.2**	**72.5**	**72.5**	**71.9**	**70.8**

1. Excluding investments.

2. Current expenditure.

Source: OECD Health Statistics, http://dx.doi.org/10.1787/health-data-en.

StatLink http://dx.doi.org/10.1787/888933219459

7.4. The sustainability of social security revenues

Another important issue to consider in designing a system of financing for health care is the buoyancy of the tax base, the rate at which the size of the tax base (and hence the revenues if tax rates stay unchanged) increases with GDP growth. If the tax base increases at the same rate as GDP, the only necessary increases in tax rates will be those that reflect the increasing share of public health care expenses in GDP. If the tax base grows at a higher rate than GDP, it is possible that no tax rate rises will be necessary. However, if the tax base grows at a slower rate than GDP, tax rate rises are inevitable and could lead to ever-increasing distortionary costs.

This consideration argues for a tax base that is as broad as possible, representing as high a proportion of GDP as possible, so that it is likely to grow at a similar rate to GDP. One of the possible difficulties with social security contributions, in addition to the distortionary cost discussed in Section 7.2, is that (in most OECD countries) their tax base is a part of labour income and labour income could fall as a share of GDP. This possibility needs to be taken seriously as the labour share in GDP did fall for most OECD countries (Figure 7.3) by an average (of countries for which data are available) of about 2.0 percentage points since 1980, with some countries experiencing larger falls and a few experiencing increases. The question therefore arises of whether a declining share of labour income can be a continuing result of population ageing.

Figure 7.3. **Compensation of employees**

Percentage of gross value added

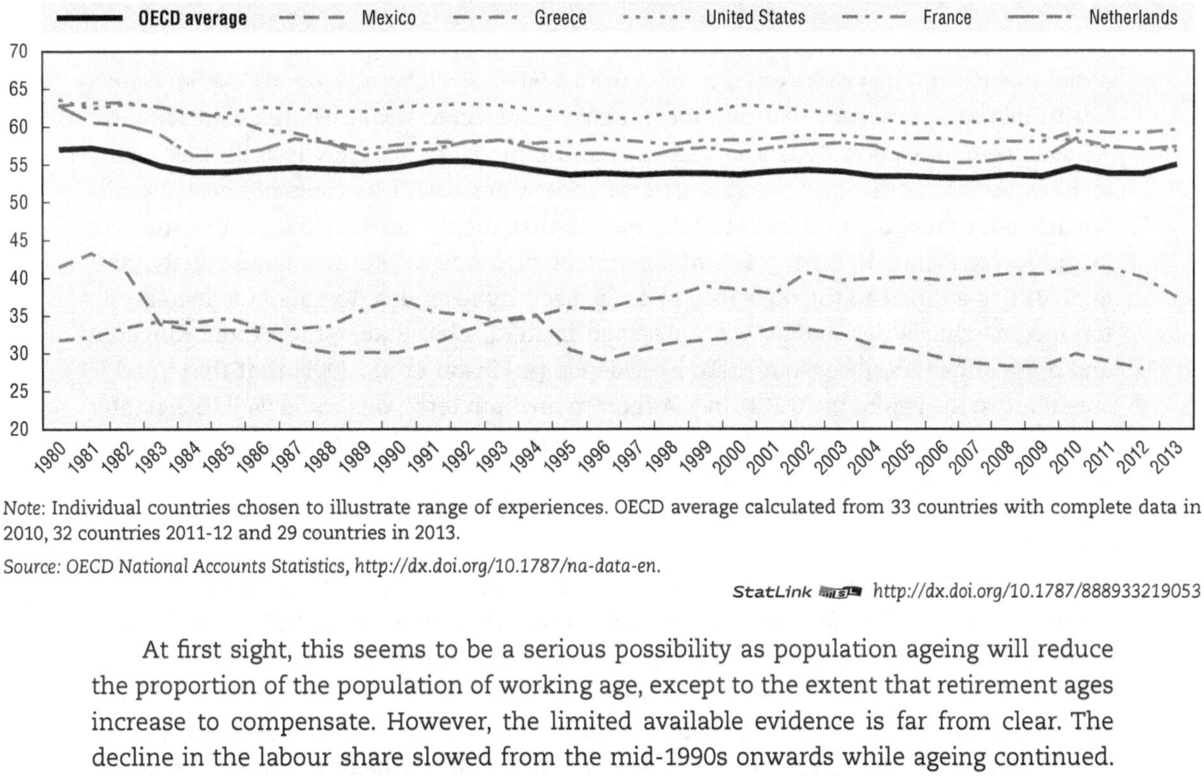

Note: Individual countries chosen to illustrate range of experiences. OECD average calculated from 33 countries with complete data in 2010, 32 countries 2011-12 and 29 countries in 2013.

Source: OECD National Accounts Statistics, http://dx.doi.org/10.1787/na-data-en.

StatLink http://dx.doi.org/10.1787/888933219053

At first sight, this seems to be a serious possibility as population ageing will reduce the proportion of the population of working age, except to the extent that retirement ages increase to compensate. However, the limited available evidence is far from clear. The decline in the labour share slowed from the mid-1990s onwards while ageing continued. It therefore seems likely that there is another explanation of at least part of the decline, with the effects of globalisation and the increased competition from low wage economies a plausible explanation.

In addition, the theoretical argument is not as strong as it seems at first. If the supply of labour relative to capital is reduced by population ageing, the labour market can be expected to respond by increasing wages. Whether this results in an overall reduction or increase in labour's share of GDP depends on the relative sizes of the labour force reduction and the wage increase. In a simple macro-economic growth model this depends on whether the elasticity of substitution between labour and capital is greater than or less than one. As the consensus amongst economists is that this elasticity is close to one, it seems that any effect of population ageing on the labour share is likely to be small.

However, it is possible that there are forces that reduce or even eliminate the predicted increase in wages discussed in the previous paragraph. One example of this is the period of rapidly increasing global competition, referred to above, in which the wages of relatively unskilled workers were kept down by the low global prices with which OECD firms had to compete. Another possibility is that wages could be kept down by an increase in immigration. However, even if immigration did have this effect, it should be noted that immigration would also be increasing the domestic labour force and so increasing the base of social security contributions.

Thus, the fact that the labour share has fallen significantly at times does raise concerns and it would be prudent to broaden the range of taxes used to finance health care to include taxes with broader bases, not only for reasons of political support and economic efficiency but also as an insurance against future falls in the labour share of GDP.

The importance of doing this can be illustrated by a growing threat to revenues from social security funding that does not come from a fall in the labour share of GDP but from a likely fall in the proportion of labour income that is subject to social security contributions. As discussed in Section 7.2, social security contributions do not usually collect as high a share of the labour incomes of high earners as of low and middle earners because of limits on the main rates of contribution. This means that the recent increase in the share of labour income going to the top 10% of the income distribution (Atkinson and Piketty, 2007 and 2010) is a threat to the buoyancy of social security revenues. To date, this increase in top income shares has mainly been observed in the United States, the United Kingdom and a few other countries; but there is evidence (Atkinson et al., 2009) that this trend is spreading to the rest of the OECD. In the short to medium term, this could well be a greater threat to health care funding from social security than population ageing and it reinforces the value of using broad-based taxes.

7.5. Sin taxes

Some OECD countries have earmarked tax revenues from excise duties on alcohol and tobacco ("sin taxes") to financing the public contribution to health care. To some extent, there is a good case that can be made for this practice. First, these excise duties can be justified (at least to some extent) by the effects on the community at large (externalities) that can follow from the consumption of these products. Second, a substantial part of these externalities take the form of increased requirements for health expenditure to care for effects of this consumption. Third, the standard arguments against earmarking specific tax revenues (that it can lead to excessive expenditures on the area to which the taxes are earmarked, if revenues increase substantially) clearly does not apply as the level of health expenditure is generally substantially higher than the revenue from these taxes. Finally, there is an obvious political argument for making people who consume harmful products contribute to the costs of dealing with this harm.

However, it is unlikely that sin taxes will ever raise enough money to cover the expected increases in health expenditure. As Table 7.3 shows, the revenue from specific consumption taxes (a category that includes sin taxes) has been falling as a share of tax revenues in

Table 7.3. **Revenue shares of the main tax categories in the OECD area**[1]

	1965	1975	1985	1995	2005	2010
Personal income tax	26	30	30	26	24	24
Corporate income tax	9	8	8	8	10	9
Social security contributions[2]	18	22	22	25	25	26
(employee)	*(6)*	*(7)*	*(7)*	*(9)*	*(9)*	*(9)*
(employer)	*(10)*	*(14)*	*(13)*	*(14)*	*(14)*	*(15)*
Payroll taxes	1	1	1	1	1	1
Property taxes	8	6	5	5	6	5
General consumption taxes	12	13	16	19	20	20
Specific consumption taxes	24	18	16	13	11	11
Other taxes	2	2	2	3	3	3
Total	**100**	**100**	**100**	**100**	**100**	**100**

1. Percentage share of major tax categories in total tax revenue. Data are included from 1965 onwards for Australia, Austria, Belgium, Canada, Denmark, Finland, France, Germany, Greece, Iceland, Ireland, Italy, Japan, Luxembourg, the Netherlands, New Zealand, Norway, Portugal, Spain, Sweden, Switzerland, Turkey, the United Kingdom and the United States; from 1972 for Korea; from 1980 for Mexico; from 1990 for Chile; from 1991 for Hungary and Poland; from 1993 for the Czech Republic; and from 1994 for Estonia, Israel, the Slovak Republic and Slovenia.

2. Including social security contributions paid by the self-employment and benefit recipients (heading 2300) that are not shown in the breakdown over employees and employers?

Source: OECD Revenue Statistics, http://dx.doi.org/10.1787/tax-data-en.

StatLink http://dx.doi.org/10.1787/888933219467

OECD countries. This is probably partly due to consumption of these items growing at a different rate from GDP and partly due to the fact that these taxes tend to become a smaller part of the purchase price over time unless the government explicitly increases the tax rates on them.[4] Also, the rate at which these taxes are levied should reflect the externalities that they create, and so should not increase unless the extent of their damage increases. If, instead, they are increased to reflect the demands on publicly financed health care, these taxes will become further and further removed from their optimal values and create substantial distortions.

Overall, therefore, the part that sin taxes play in financing health care is likely to stay small and it would be unwise to try to regard them as a major source of additional funding to meet population ageing.

7.6. The experience of OECD countries

This section examines the extent to which OECD countries make use of social security contributions to finance health care and examines recent trends in those countries that make the greatest use of them. One important consideration is the possible distortionary effects of these contributions. Since 1965, there has been a general increase across the OECD in the share of tax revenue that is attributed to social security contributions as a whole; but this trend has slowed markedly since 1995 (Table 7.3). This slowdown will have contributed to the fact that the OECD average tax wedge has reduced over the last ten years, and so countries are generally keeping their labour market distortions in check (Table 7.4).

OECD countries which use social security contribution to finance more than half of the government's health care expenditures are (Table 7.5): Austria, Belgium, the Czech Republic, Estonia, France, Germany, Hungary, Israel, Japan, Korea, Luxembourg, the Netherlands, Poland, the Slovak Republic, Slovenia, Switzerland, Turkey and the United States.

Table 7.4. **Trends in the tax wedge**

Income tax plus employee contributions less cash benefits, single persons, 100% of average earnings as a percentage of labour costs

	2000	2003	2004	2005	2006	2007	2008	2009	2010	2011
Australia	31.0	28.2	28.2	28.5	28.3	27.7	26.9	26.7	26.8	26.7
Austria	47.3	47.4	48.3	48.1	48.5	48.8	49.0	47.9	48.2	48.4
Belgium	57.1	55.7	55.4	55.5	55.5	55.6	55.9	55.3	55.4	55.5
Canada	33.2	32.0	32.0	31.9	31.9	31.2	31.3	30.6	30.5	30.8
Chile	7.0	7.0	7.0	7.0	7.0	7.0	7.0	7.0	7.0	7.0
Czech Republic	42.6	43.2	43.5	43.7	42.5	42.9	43.4	42.0	42.1	42.5
Denmark	44.1	42.4	41.0	40.9	41.0	41.1	40.9	39.5	38.3	38.4
Estonia	41.3	42.3	41.5	39.9	39.0	39.0	38.4	39.2	40.1	40.1
Finland	47.8	45.0	44.5	44.6	44.0	43.9	43.8	42.5	42.5	42.7
France	49.6	49.8	49.9	50.1	50.2	49.3	49.3	49.3	49.3	49.4
Germany	52.9	53.2	52.2	52.1	52.3	51.9	51.5	50.9	49.2	49.8
Greece[1]	35.2	35.2	35.8	35.2	35.8	37.0	37.0	38.2	38.2	..
Hungary	54.6	50.8	51.8	51.1	52.0	54.5	54.1	53.1	46.6	49.4
Iceland	28.8	31.5	31.9	32.1	31.8	30.5	30.9	30.5	33.4	34.0
Ireland	28.9	24.4	24.1	23.5	23.0	22.2	22.3	24.7	25.8	26.8
Israel	29.0	27.1	25.3	24.9	23.5	24.1	21.7	20.2	19.4	19.8
Italy	47.1	46.0	46.3	45.9	46.1	46.4	46.6	46.8	47.2	47.6
Japan	24.7	27.4	27.3	27.7	28.8	29.3	29.5	29.2	30.2	30.8
Korea	16.3	16.3	17.0	17.3	18.1	19.7	19.9	19.5	20.1	20.3
Luxembourg	37.1	33.5	33.9	34.7	35.3	36.3	34.7	33.9	34.3	36.0
Mexico	12.4	16.7	15.2	14.7	15.0	15.9	15.1	15.3	15.5	16.2
Netherlands	40.0	37.2	38.8	38.9	38.4	38.8	39.2	38.0	38.1	37.8
New Zealand	19.4	19.5	19.7	20.0	20.4	21.1	20.5	18.1	17.0	15.9
Norway	38.6	38.1	38.1	37.2	37.4	37.5	37.5	37.2	37.2	37.5
Poland	38.2	38.2	38.4	38.7	39.0	38.2	34.7	34.1	34.2	34.3
Portugal	37.3	37.4	37.4	36.8	37.1	37.7	37.6	37.5	37.6	39.0
Slovak Republic	41.9	42.5	42.2	38.0	38.3	38.4	38.8	37.7	37.9	38.9
Slovenia	46.3	46.2	46.3	45.6	45.3	43.3	42.9	42.2	42.5	42.6
Spain	38.6	38.6	38.8	39.0	39.1	39.0	38.0	38.3	39.7	39.9
Sweden	50.1	48.2	48.4	48.1	47.8	45.3	44.8	43.2	42.8	42.8
Switzerland	21.6	21.2	20.9	20.9	20.9	21.1	20.6	20.7	20.7	21.0
Turkey[2]	40.4	42.2	42.8	42.8	42.7	42.7	39.9	37.4	37.9	37.7
United Kingdom	32.6	33.8	33.9	33.9	34.0	34.1	32.8	32.4	32.6	32.5
United States	30.4	29.9	29.8	29.8	29.9	30.0	29.6	30.1	30.4	29.5
Unweighted average										
OECD average	**36.6**	**36.1**	**36.1**	**35.9**	**35.9**	**35.9**	**35.5**	**35.0**	**35.0**	**35.2**
OECD-EU21	**43.4**	**42.4**	**42.5**	**42.1**	**42.1**	**42.1**	**41.7**	**41.3**	**41.1**	**41.7**

..: Not available.

1. The 2011 average earnings figure for Greece was not available at the final compilation stage.

2. Wage figures are based on the old definition of average worker (ISIC D, Rev. 8).

Source: OECD Taxing Wages 2011, http://dx.doi.org/10.1787/tax_wages-2011-en.

StatLink http://dx.doi.org/10.1787/888933219471

Those countries that identify a share of social security contributions that is less than half are: Canada, Chile, Finland, Iceland, Norway, Portugal and Spain. Of the others, Australia and New Zealand[5] do not have government social security schemes and Denmark does not use them at all to finance health care. Greece, Ireland, Italy, Mexico, Sweden and the United Kingdom all have social security contributions but do not report their share to the OECD.[6] In the case of some of these countries, the reason for not reporting is that the government's budget is operated on a consolidated basis without earmarking social security contributions.

Table 7.5. **Use of social security contributions to finance health care**

Country	Year	General government excluding social security as % of total health care expenditure	Social security funds as % of total health care expenditure	Social security as % of general govenment funding
Australia	2011	64.33	0.00	0.00
Austria	2012	30.60	41.81	57.74
Belgium	2012	10.88	64.33	85.54
Canada	2012	64.96	1.34	2.03
Chile	2012	39.26	6.53	14.26
Czech Republic	2012	4.45	77.87	94.59
Denmark	2012	82.20	0.00	0.00
Estonia	2012	10.40	68.15	86.76
Finland	2012	56.91	14.35	20.14
France	2012	3.76	70.95	94.96
Germany	2012	6.61	68.01	91.14
Greece	2012	28.33	38.82	57.81
Hungary	2012	7.89	52.14	86.85
Iceland	2012	51.72	28.81	35.77
Israel	2010	16.42	43.82	72.74
Japan	2011	9.54	72.19	88.33
Korea	2012	10.92	42.39	79.52
Luxembourg	2012	8.07	69.80	89.64
Netherlands	2011	7.72	71.80	91.23
New Zealand	2011	74.89	7.80	9.43
Norway	2012	70.49	10.89	13.38
Poland	2012	6.01	59.64	90.84
Portugal	2011	60.63	1.26	2.20
Slovak Republic	2012	6.51	62.66	90.59
Slovenia	2012	3.02	65.17	95.57
Spain	2012	66.00	4.63	6.56
Sweden	2012	76.87	...	0.00
Switzerland	2012	20.29	45.52	69.17
Turkey	2008	24.22	41.65	63.23
United States	2012	5.10	41.51	89.07

Source: OECD Health Statistics, http://dx.doi.org/10.1787/health-data-en.

StatLink http://dx.doi.org/10.1787/888933219486

Do countries relying heavily on social security contributions have a tax wedge on labour higher than the OECD average,[7] raising concerns about the discouragement of labour force participation? Figure 7.4 shows that countries with a higher reliance on social security contributions for financing health care tend to have a higher tax wedge on labour. This suggests that the extent of reliance on social security contributions in the financing of health care could be a factor in determining the size of the wedge and thus the distortion of labour markets.

Also, have countries had difficulty maintaining support for public funding of health care when they rely heavily on social security contributions to support it? Figure 7.5 shows that there is no relationship between the increases in the government share of health care and the reliance on social security contributions. Governments with a high reliance on social security contributions are no more likely to have reduced their share of health care expenditure as those with a lower reliance, suggesting that they are just as able to maintain support for public funding of health care.

Figure 7.4. **Reliance on social security contributions and the tax wedge**

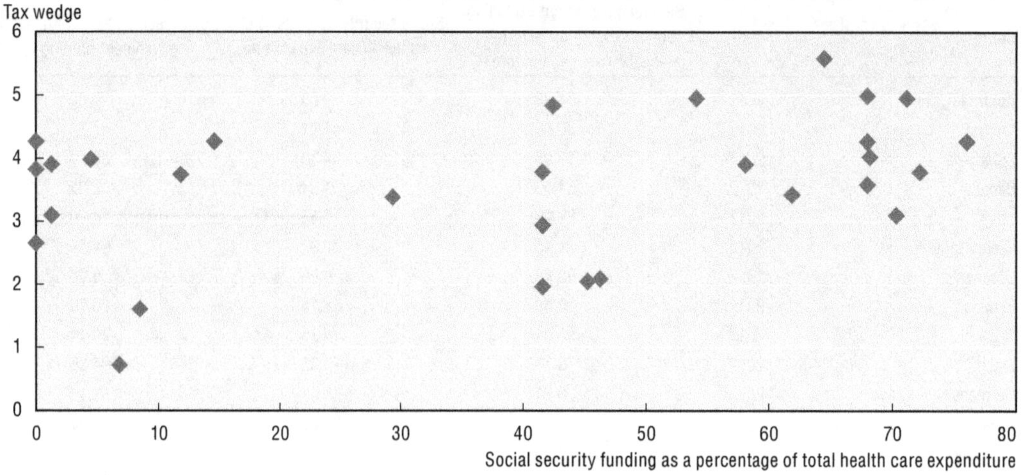

Tax wedge

Social security funding as a percentage of total health care expenditure

Source: OECD National Accounts Statistics, http://dx.doi.org/10.1787/na-data-en.

StatLink http://dx.doi.org/10.1787/888933219064

Figure 7.5. **Reliance on social security contributions and the increase in the government share of health care expenditure since 2000**

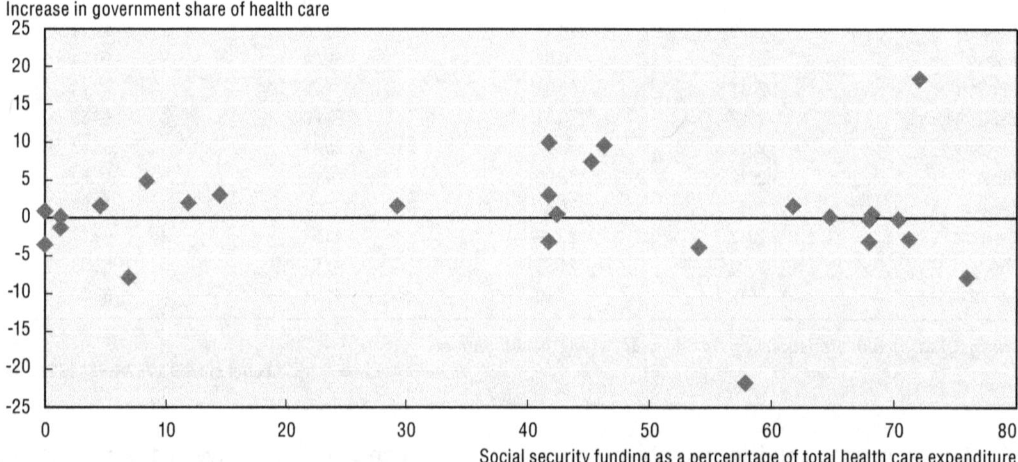

Source: OECD National Accounts Statistics, http://dx.doi.org/10.1787/na-data-en.

StatLink http://dx.doi.org/10.1787/888933219075

The conclusion of this analysis is that the data analysed here support the idea that social security funding of health care increases labour market distortions but do not support the idea that it reduces support for public funding.

Notes

1. Throughout this chapter, "tax" is meant to include compulsory social security contributions unless they are specifically excluded.
2. The level of revenue obtained from recurrent taxes on residential property varies widely across the OECD. This recommendation applies particularly to those countries with relatively low revenues from this source.
3. The level of revenue obtained from recurrent taxes on residential property varies widely across the OECD. This recommendation applies particularly to those countries with relatively low revenues from this source.

4. This is because these taxes are only partly (if at all) based on the value of the product but also on the physical quantity sold.
5. The social security contributions for New Zealand in the table are organised outside government.
6. For Sweden, the share financed by social security is either zero or very small.
7. Those countries that provide more than 50% of health care finance from social security and also have a tax wedge on labour higher than the OECD average are: Austria, Belgium, the Czech Republic, Estonia, France, Germany, Hungary, the Netherlands, the Slovak Republic, Slovenia and Turkey. Those countries that rely less on social security contributions but have a tax wedge on labour higher than the OECD average are: Denmark, Finland, Norway, Portugal and Spain.

References

Arnold, J.M., B. Brys, C. Heady, A. Johansson, C. Schwellnus and L. Vartia (2011), "Tax Policy for Economic Recovery and Growth", *Economic Journal*, Vol. 121, Royal Economic Society, Wiley-Blackwell, pp. F59-F80.

Atkinson, A.B. and T. Piketty (2010), "Top Incomes over the Twentieth Century: A Global Perspective", Oxford University Press, Oxford.

Atkinson, A.B. and T. Piketty (2007), "Top Incomes over the Twentieth Century: A Contrast between Continental European and English-Speaking Countries", Oxford University Press, Oxford.

Atkinson, A.B., T. Piketty and E. Saez (2009), "Top Incomes in the Long Run of History", *NBER Working Paper*, No. 15408, National Bureau of Economic Research, Cambridge, United States.

De la Maisonneuve, C. and J. Oliveira Martins (2013), "Public Spending on Health and Long-term Care: A New Set of Projections", *OECD Economics Department Working Paper*, OECD Publishing, Paris, *http://dx.doi.org/10.1787/5k44t7jwwr9x-en.*

Disney, R. (2007), "Population Ageing and the Size of the Welfare State: Is there a Puzzle to Explain?" in *European Journal of Political Economy*, Vol. 23, Elsevier, Amsterdam, pp. 542–553.

Disney, R. (2004), "Are Contributions to Public Pension Programmes a Tax on Employment?" in*Economic Policy*, Centre for Economic Policy Research, the Centre for Economic Studies of the University of Munich and the Paris School of Economics, Wiley-Blackwell, pp. 269-311.

Disney, R., V. Galasso and P. Profeta (2007), "A Further Comment on Ageing and the Welfare State", *European Journal of Political Economy*, Vol. 23, Elsevier, Amsterdam, pp. 576–577.

Galasso, V. and P. Profeta (2007), "How Does Ageing Affect the Welfare State?', *European Journal of Political Economy*, Vol. 23, Elsevier, Amsterdam, pp. 554–563.

Mirrlees, J. et al. (2011), "Tax by Design", Oxford University Press, Oxford.

Mirrlees, J. et al. (2010), "Dimensions of Tax Design", Oxford University Press, Oxford.

OECD (2010), *Tax Policy Reform and Economic Growth*, OECD Publishing, Paris, *http://dx.doi.org/10.1787/9789264091085-en.*

OECD (2005), "OECD Jobs Strategy: Lessons from a Decade's Experience", Main Report, OECD Economics Department, Working Party No. 1 on Macroeconomic and Structural Policy Analysis, OECD, Paris, *http://olisweb.oecd.org/vgn-ext-templating/ECO-CPE-WP1(2006)1-ENG.pdf?docId=JT00196265&date=1135083728000&documentId=345792&organisationId=1&fileName=JT00196265.pdf.*

Razin, A. and E. Sadka (2007), "Ageing Population: The Complex Effect of Fiscal Leakages on the Politico-economic Equilibrium", *European Journal of Political Economy*, Vol. 23, Elsevier, Amsterdam, pp. 564–575.

Razin, A., E. Sadka and P. Swagel (2002), "The Ageing Population and the Size of the Welfare State", *Journal of Political Economy*, Vol. 110, No. 4 (August), Elsevier, Amsterdam, pp. 900-918.

Simonovits, A. (2007), "Can Population Ageing Imply a Smaller Welfare State?', *European Journal of Political Economy*, Vol. 23, Elsevier, Amsterdam, pp. 534–541.

Fiscal Sustainability of Health Systems
Bridging Health and Finance Perspectives

Chapter 8

Health care budgeting in France

by
Ankit Kumar, Grégoire de Lagasnerie, Delphine Rouilleault and Camila Vammalle*

This chapter presents the evolution of the institutions and policies developed in France to ensure the fiscal sustainability of the French health care system. Particularly notable was the introduction of the National Objective for Healthcare Spending (ONDAM) targets in 1996. This was later improved with the introduction of an early warning system, which allows payments to be withheld from health providers, and the official validation of targets by the Parliament. On the revenue side, this chapter examines how the introduction of the Contribution Sociale Généralisée (CSG) has successfully reduced reliance on wage-based contributions for health insurance.

* The main authors of this chapter are Ankit Kumar (OECD Health Division), Grégoire de Lagasnerie (OECD Health Division), Delphine Rouilleault (École nationale d'administration) and Camila Vammalle (OECD Budgeting and Public Expenditures Division). The draft of this chapter has been undertaken with the benefit of discussions and feedback from French officials in the Ministry of Health and the Ministry of Finance. We are particularly grateful to Dominique Polton and Marie-Camille Lenormand for their time and for helping identify key officials. The authors wish to thank the Chairperson of the Senior Budget Officials – Health Joint Network, Geert van Maanen, and Michael Borowitz, Valérie Paris and Hervé Boulhol of the OECD Secretariat for their suggestions throughout the writing of this chapter. The views and opinions expressed in this chapter are those of the authors and mistakes remain their own.

The statistical data for Israel are supplied by and under the responsibility of the relevant Israeli authorities. The use of such data by the OECD is without prejudice to the status of the Golan Heights, East Jerusalem and Israeli settlements in the West Bank under the terms of international law.

8.1. Introduction

France is of particular interest to policy makers involved in setting health budgets because the health care system was founded on social insurance principles but has evolved to be more like a government-managed health care system over time. A combination of the government and social health insurance institutions seeks to finance a high level of accessibility to health care services, with the financial objective of having a neutral impact on the public budget. As France has traditionally raised funding through a combination of social contributions and taxes that are specifically appropriated for health, it is possible to observe the extent to which deficits in health care financing have contributed to public deficits over time. This is difficult to do in budget-funded health care systems such as the United Kingdom, Australia and Canada, where health care is funded from government revenues at large.

France has struggled to achieve its objective of containing the size of health care deficits over the past two decades. This has seen the French government take on a more active role in setting controls on how much and where funds are spent in the health system. The government has also sought to diversify sources of revenue away from simply wage-based contributions. The combination of these measures has improved the sustainability of health care; but deficits remain a constant feature of health care financing.

This chapter provides an overview of how policy makers seek to manage the impact of health care on France's public budget today. In doing so, it:

- Provides an overview of health spending in France in the context of other OECD countries as well as the contribution of social health insurance to public deficits and debt.
- Describes the key institutions responsible for paying for health care services and demonstrates how the government has come to play a larger role in setting overall controls on how much is spent on health and where it has spent.
- Profiles the progressive shift away from wage-based contributions towards more diversified sources of revenues.
- Analyses the arrangements for managing social security (including health care) debt in France today.

This chapter focuses on macroeconomic control of health care spending and financing. It highlights good practices for budgeting for health care and the likely factors contributing to their success. While Box 8.1 provides a high-level overview of the French health care system to show how health budgets are managed, more details on policies for payments in hospitals, primary care and other forms of health care in France are contained in the WHO/European Observatory Publication profile of the French health care system (Chevreul et al., 2011).

Box 8.1. **Overview of the French health system**

Social health insurance is one of the French government's four "social security" entitlements for its citizens, along with pensions, family benefits and insurance for occupational injuries. In 2013, the total amount of social security expenditures reached EUR 463 billion. Pensions were the largest item of expenditure, accounting for EUR 215 billion. Health came second, with a total of EUR 189 billion.

The social health insurance system covers all residents in France through different social health funds to which people are automatically affiliated according to their occupation. The main one is the *Caisse Nationale de l'Assurance Maladie des Travailleurs Salariés* (CNAMTS) which covers more than 80% of the population including almost all salaried workers and their families, as well as the unemployed and the poorest fringes of the population. A range of other funds provide health insurance coverage for a select few categories of workers. The two main funds are for self-employed workers and agricultural workers. A variety of other smaller funds exist for very specific occupational status (miners, sailors, employees of national railways, etc.).

These funds provide general cover for health care services and medical goods included in a benefit package established at the national level. The public benefit package is considered to be rather generous in terms of services covered but generally imposes co-payments to patients. France is unique amongst OECD countries in that nearly all the population (96% in 2010) resorts to complementary health insurance in addition to their public cover, to help finance rising obligations for out-of-pocket payments. Among the people who have access to complementary insurance, 44% depend on collective agreements associated with their profession or employer, while a further 56% have individual contracts (IRDES, 2010).

Hospital care is delivered by public, private-non-profit and private-for-profit hospitals. France has a relatively high number of hospitals beds per capita, with around 6.4 beds per 1 000 population (compared to the 4.9 OECD average). Among them, private-for-profit hospitals account for 23% of the total number of beds and not-for-profit private hospitals account for 14% of total beds. Both public and private hospitals are mainly financed through a DRG-based system for acute care.

In terms of services providers, with a level of 3.3 doctors per 1 000 population, France ranks in line with the OECD average of 3.2 doctors per 1 000 population. Half of these doctors are GPs, one of the highest levels of GPs among the OECD. French doctors are generally self-employed in ambulatory care (GPs and specialists) and private clinics, but are salaried in public hospitals. Self-employed doctors are mainly paid through fee-for-service, with a small component of pay-for-performance introduced for GPs recently. Furthermore, specific annual lump-sum payment are paid to physician notably for patients with chronic disease (EUR 40 per year per patient) or patients older than 85 years old (EUR 5 per visits). Freedom of choice of doctor is a major feature of the health care system, with patients free to choose which physician (including specialists) they see and how often they see them and then receive reimbursement for these visits from health funds. A "soft gatekeeping" system was also introduced in 2004, which gives the patient a financial incentive to register with a GP and obtain a referral prior to consulting a specialist; however it is not mandatory.

Source: OECD, IRDES.

8.2. Health and the public budget

France spends more on health than most OECD countries

France is the third highest spender on health care relative to its economy among OECD countries. In 2011, France spent 11.6% of its GDP on health care, some 2.3% of GDP more than the OECD average of 9.3%. This placed it behind the United States (at 17.7% of GDP) and the Netherlands at 11.9% (Figure 8.1). France sits alongside the Netherlands and Germany as countries which rely predominately on social-insurance-based financing of health care and have a high level of spending relative to the OECD average.

Figure 8.1. **Total health expenditure as share of GDP, 2011 (or nearest year)**

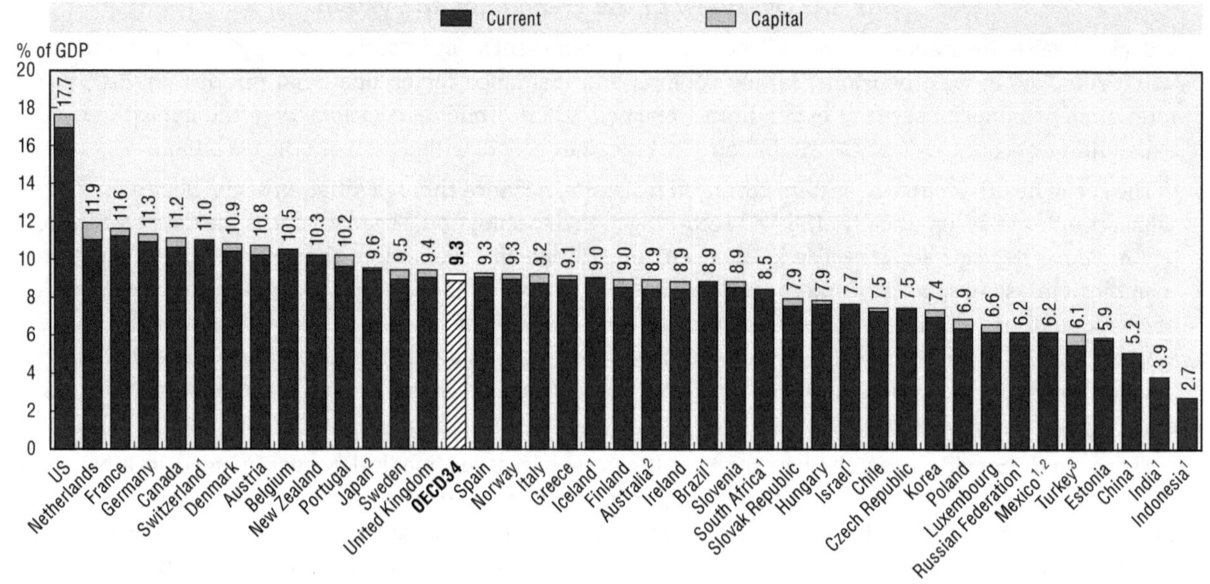

1. Total expenditure only.
2. Data refer to 2010.
3. Data refer to 2008.

Source: OECD Health Statistics, http://dx.doi.org/10.1787/health-data-en; WHO Global Health Expenditure Database.

StatLink http://dx.doi.org/10.1787/888933219082

Public funding for health in France is above the OECD average

France has a slightly higher share of public funding in total health care spending than the OECD average. In 2011, public spending represented 77% of health care expenditure in France, of which 73 percentage points come from social insurance funds and four points from direct government spending. This placed France slightly above the OECD average of 72% of public funding, ranking it 14th on the level of public funds as a proportion of total spending on health.

Private health insurance plays a larger role in France than in many other OECD countries

A particularly interesting feature of France's health care system is the important role of private health insurance. Total private spending on health care in France accounts for 22% of total health care spending; the biggest part of this is private health insurance, which accounts for about 14% of total spending on health care. This places France ahead of all other OECD countries except the United States and Chile. France is followed by Slovenia (14%), Canada (13%), Ireland (12%), Germany (10%) and Switzerland (nine per cent) in this regard (Figure 8.2). Some 96% of the French population subscribes to complementary health insurance. Complementary insurance can either be collective, as part of a labour market convention and financed by employers, or through individual contributions along with some government subsidies.

Health is the second largest area of public spending in France

In 2011, health accounted for 14.7% of total general government spending in France (close to the OECD average 14.5). This made it the second highest public spending area after social protection (42.6% of total government spending) (OECD, 2013). As France has the third highest level of government spending among OECD countries, this also makes it one of the largest shares of public spending on health relative to GDP (Figure 8.3).

Figure 8.2. **Expenditure on health by type of financing, 2011 (or nearest year)**

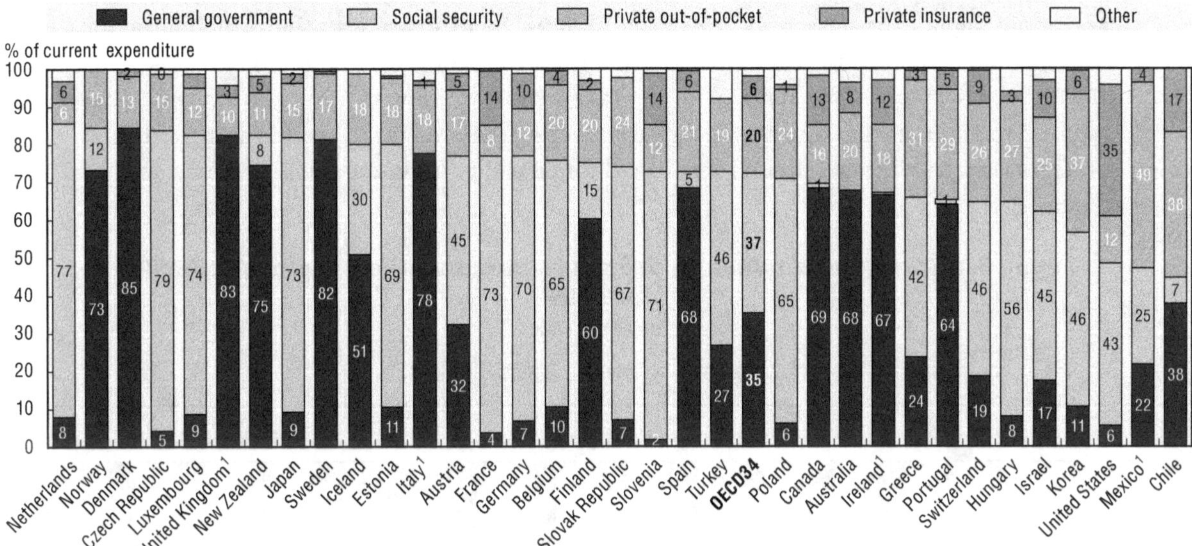

1. Data refer to total health expenditure.

Source: OECD Health Statistics, http://dx.doi.org/10.1787/health-data-en.

StatLink http://dx.doi.org/10.1787/888933219092

Figure 8.3. **General government health spending compared to general government overall spending as a share of GDP, 2009 (or nearest year)**

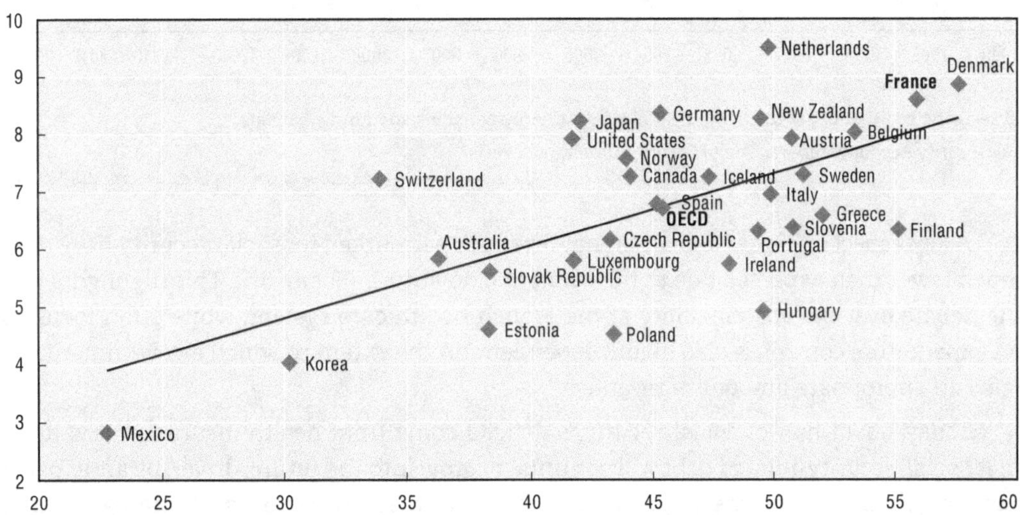

Source: OECD Health Statistics, *http://dx.doi.org/10.1787/health-data-en*; OECD National Accounts Statistics, *http://dx.doi.org/10.1787/na-data-en*. Data for Australia are based on government finance statistics provided by the Australian Bureau of Statistics.

StatLink http://dx.doi.org/10.1787/888933219100

Health deficits represent a large part of overall social security deficits, and France is seeking to deliver a balanced health budget within five years

While for most of the last 40 years social security (which in France includes health, pensions and family benefits) has not been a major contributor to public deficits, this has changed over the past decade. Deficits in social security have become persistent and more significant during the 2000s. Until 2004, health care was the principal factor driving this. While health care deficits have remained significant in monetary terms since 2004, deficits in pensions have also increased substantially, resulting in considerably larger deficits in social security at large. Between 1998 and 2012, health deficits (based on the salaried workers' scheme) accounted for 68% of cumulative social security deficits (Figure 8.4).

Figure 8.4. **Social security/health deficits (salaried workers regime/CNAMTS) since 1998**

In billion EUR

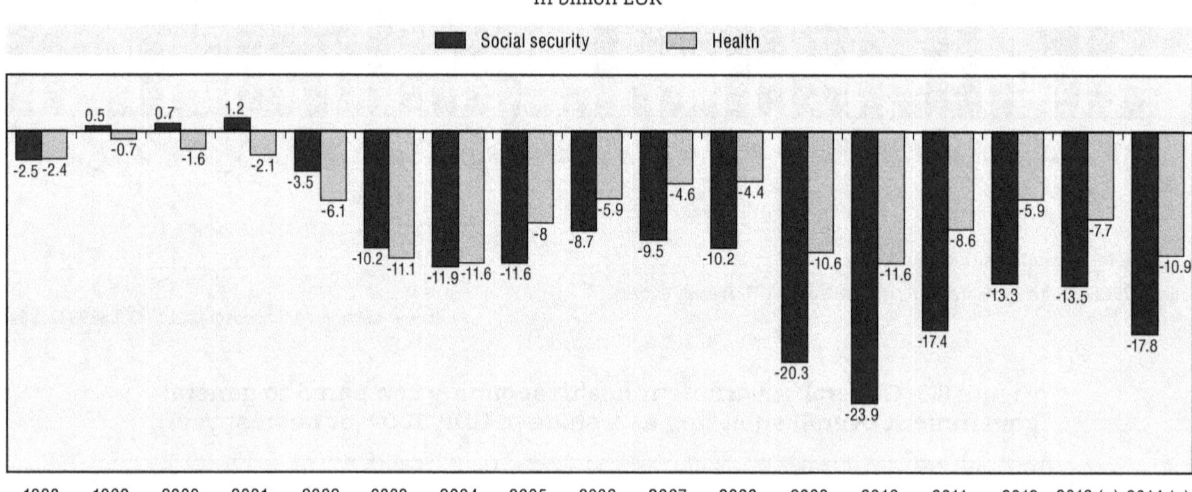

(p): Prevision.

Note: "Social security" represents deficits net of health care, primarily pensions and family benefits.

Source: Social Security Accounts reports, Social Security Directorate, Paris,

StatLink http://dx.doi.org/10.1787/888933219117

A key aspect of higher deficits is that revenues earmarked for social security have been much lower than expected due to the economic downturn (Figure 8.5). This highlights that the debate over the sustainability of the French health care system, while often focusing on expenditure control, is also highly dependent on the extent to which a government can raise an appropriate amount of revenue.

Today, about half of social security's deficits come from health insurance. It is likely that social-security-related debt will continue to grow into the future, driven by anticipated deficits in pensions as the population ages. In its medium-term fiscal strategy, France outlines multi-year ceilings on health expenditures as one of the key measures for bringing public finances back under control. The government has outlined a plan to reduce the deficit on the health care component of its social security system progressively down to EUR 2.7 billion by 2017 (Figure 8.6).

Figure 8.5. **Health branch of total social security revenues and expenditures since 2005**

In billion EUR (2012 and 2013 budgets)

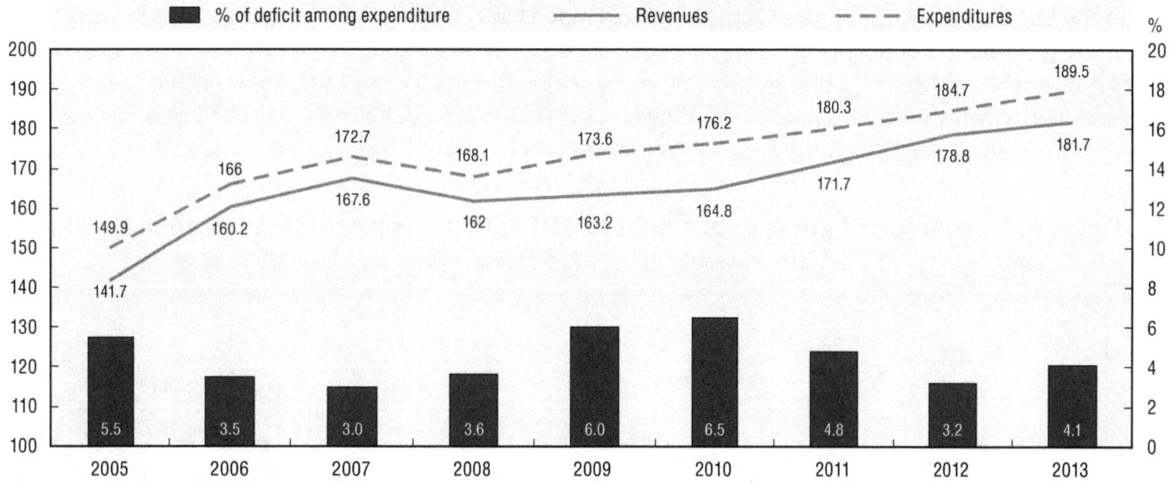

Source: Social Security Accounts reports and Social Security Financial Act, 2014, Social Security Directorate, Paris,

StatLink http://dx.doi.org/10.1787/888933219120

Figure 8.6. **Total social security deficits projections up to 2017**

In billion EUR

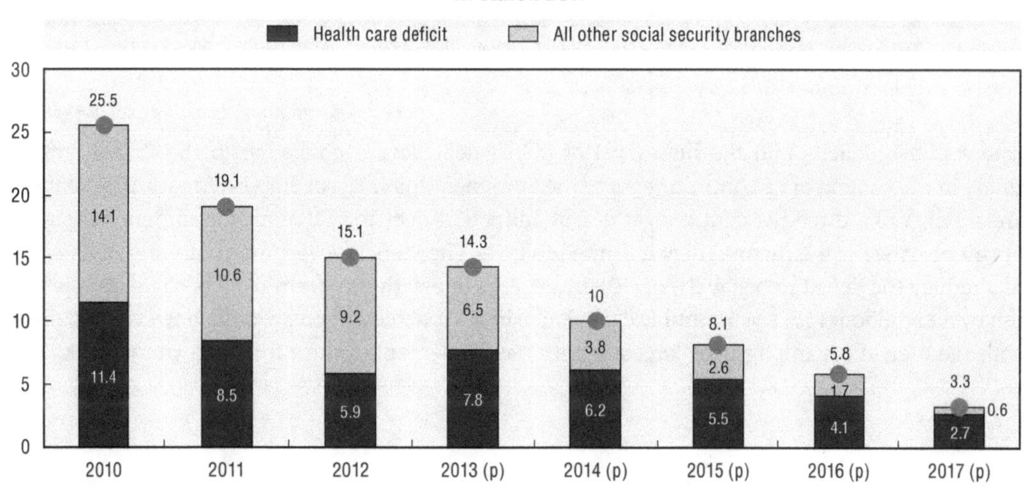

(p): Prevision.

Source: Social Security Financial Act, 2014, Social Security Directorate, Paris,

StatLink http://dx.doi.org/10.1787/888933219134

Box 8.2. **France's broader fiscal consolidation challenges**

The size of health spending has brought this area to the attention of French policy makers as they grapple with the ongoing challenge of fiscal consolidation. France has not recorded a budget surplus in ten years, with the government budget deficit having run at 4.1% of GDP in 2013. In 2013, social security accounted for 18.5% of the total deficit. Gross public debt in France represents 93.5% of GDP in 2013, and the share of social security (which includes health spending and deficits) in total public debt has been growing steadily since the mid-2000s.Social security debt now represents about 10% of GDP (Figure 8.7) and 11% of total debt.

Figure 8.7. **Evolution of gross public debt to GDP ratio (Maastricht definition) in France**

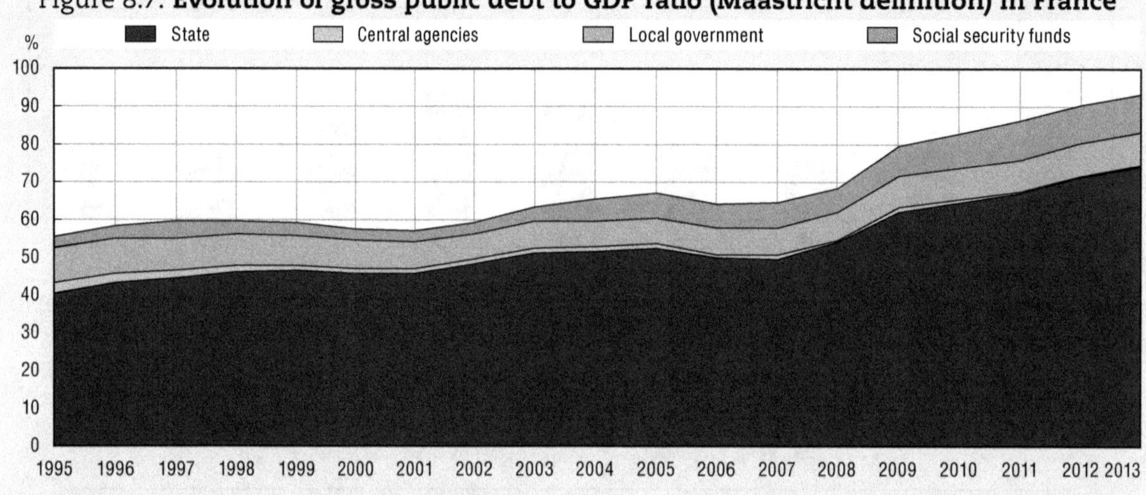

Source: INSEE, *www.insee.fr/fr/themes/indicateur.asp?id=40*.

StatLink http://dx.doi.org/10.1787/888933219145

Persistent public deficits and the high level of public debt pose a challenge to the French government, particularly in the context of its commitments to the European Union Fiscal Stability Treaty. The treaty not only reaffirms a target of a three-per-cent budget deficit and a 60% debt-to-GDP limit for all member states, but it also sets an objective of a structural deficit limited to 0.5%. The French government has stated its objective to gradually reduce the deficit to below 3% of GDP by 2017, in line with its commitments to the European Union, and then by an additional 1% a year until fiscal balance in 2020. Achieving this would, however, require a major fiscal consolidation effort amongst the largest France has implemented since the post-war era (OECD, 2012).

8.3. Institutional framework and budgeting practices

The French health care system has its origins in a social health insurance model whereby a range of independent social institutions financed health care to workers by levying contributions on employers and employees (known as a "Bismarckian" health care system). Over time, the government has come to play a much more influential role in health care financing. It has reformed how social health insurers operate and how they pay for health care providers and more recently it has set limits on overall levels of health spending.

The combination of these changes has seen the progressive transformation of the French health care system to be more like the United Kingdom, Australia and Canada, where the government finances health care from its budget and is generally the major owner and operator of health care services (known as a "Beveridge" health care system). Today, France's health care system lies between the academic typology of Bismarck and Beveridge health care systems, made up of historically inherited institutions that are constrained by a government that has gradually re-asserted control over health care spending.

Governance of the health system

Health care insurance in France was founded as a Bismarckian system, with insurance progressively expanded from those in the salaried labour force to the population at large

When it was established, French social security was similar to other Bismarckian health care systems. Health cover was first provided to those in to the formal labor force, with wage-based contributions granting workers and their families insurance for their essential health care expenses. However, since the founding of social security in 1945, successive governments have pursued reforms to broaden health care insurance well beyond the formal labour force to reach universal entitlement. Today, almost the entire population is covered by social health insurance.

Box 8.3. **The progressive expansion of social health insurance in France**

When health insurance was introduced in 1945, it only covered those workers in the salaried sector, which excluded a large number of people, particularly the poor. During the 1960s and 1970s, significant progress was made towards extending public health care insurance to the majority of the population. This culminated in 1978 with the creation of the *assurance personnelle* (personal insurance) which provided health cover to all those who did not fit into existing public schemes, along with complementary measures to support unemployed people, unmarried couples, dependents and people with insufficient incomes.

However, even the *assurance personnelle* required people to make a financial contribution towards the cost of health insurance, meaning that a small segment of the population (around 0.5%) continued to have no insurance for essential health care costs. These were generally non-working foreigners and the poorest people. It was only with reforms in the late 1990s that France finally achieved universal coverage. This occurred as *assurance personnelle* was extended and replaced by a system called *Couverture Maladie Universelle* (Universal health coverage), which set residency in a French territory as the defining principle for benefiting from health coverage, and provided free insurance to those who did not have the capacity to pay. By 2011, about 2.2 million people (around 3% of the population) benefitted from the *Couverture Maladie Universelle*.

Figure 8.8. **Total public and primary private health insurance**

Percentage of total population covered by social health insurance

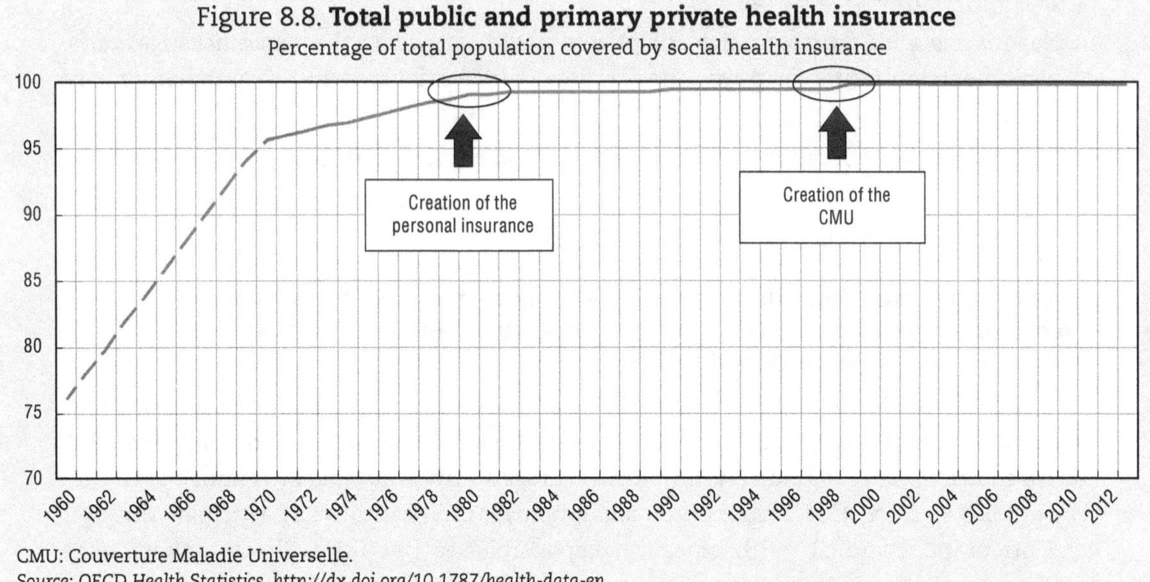

CMU: Couverture Maladie Universelle.

Source: OECD Health Statistics, http://dx.doi.org/10.1787/health-data-en.

StatLink http://dx.doi.org/10.1787/888933219154

Social health insurance funds are the key operational entities that pay health care providers for services delivered to patients. The funds handle 98% of total public health care spending in France (INSEE, 2011). The central government accounts for a further 2% of spending, mainly on prevention policies and agencies that deliver system-wide public health services (drug regulation, blood supply, animal health, etc.). Finally, local governments can provide, on a voluntary basis, some additional financial grants for targeted populations.

The Caisse Nationale d'Assurance Maladie des Travailleurs Salariés is the main institution that manages health insurance

While France has a number of different health insurance funds, the most important of them is the *Caisse Nationale d'Assurance Maladie pour les Travailleurs Salariés* (CNAMTS). The CNAMTS covers 85% of the population, mostly salaried workers and the unemployed. A further 15%, made up of farmers, independent workers, public servants and many others (12 different special regimes) are covered through other funds. At a national level, the CNAMTS is in charge of maintaining a financial balance in health insurance. It does so by monitoring pharmaceutical prescribing and referrals to additional services in order to improve the behaviour of patients and providers to deliver better health outcomes and contain expenditure.

While the CNAMTS is principally run as a national organisation, it oversees a structure of local and regional branches. It directly operates some 101 local branches known as the *Caisses Primaires d'Assurance Maladie* (CPAM), which are mainly in charge of providing reimbursements to patients for medical services, audits of patient claims and other administrative tasks. They also manage a system that was implemented in 2004 that gives incentives to patients to see a general practitioner before seeing a specialist in order to get full reimbursement for their visit.

The President of the CNAMTS chairs a joint body representing all three major social health insurance funds called UNCAM (*Union Nationale des Caisses d'Assurance Maladie)*, which plays a system-wide role in:

- Negotiating with representatives of private health providers the *conventions médicales*, agreements on tariffs for private health providers, particularly in the ambulatory care sector.
- Defining the level of reimbursement for drugs and medical services.
- Defining which medical services are reimbursed (though admitting drugs into public reimbursement is still a government responsibility).

Over time, the administration of the CNAMTS has gone from a decentralised organisation run by trade unions and employer representatives to a more centralised and technocratic institution

The CNAMTS was originally founded as an independent public institution with an administrative structure entirely separate from the state. Initially, it had a management board chaired by labour union and employer representatives; but this has changed over the time (Box 8.4). Since 2004, labour union and employer representatives participate through an "orientation council" with advisory responsibilities but little direct management power.

Box 8.4. **Evolution of the management of the CNAMTS**

While at its creation the management of the CNAMTS included a significant role for labour unions, in 1967 the government changed the composition of the management boards to introduce a "parity principle" involving equal representation from both unions and employers. In 1982, the newly elected socialist government reintroduced elections for CNAMTS board members and reinstated the supremacy of unions over employers' federations in terms of number of board members. But elections only occurred in 1983 and the system then froze due to a lack of motivation from both the government and the unions. This led to a progressive acknowledgment of the failure of the principle of the management of the health insurance by the trade unions and employers representatives.

In 1996, the electoral process for designating the members of the CNAMTS's local and national boards was abolished and the "parity principle" of representation was reintroduced. But this did not lead to better management of the CNAMTS and a new health insurance reform in 2004 replaced the administrative boards of the CNAMTS and CPAM (where unions and employers were also represented) with "orientation boards" with missions reduced to the general direction of health policies. From this point, trade union and employer representatives were no longer considered as the real managers of the CNAMTS.

This loss of power for trade unions and employers representatives in the management of the CNAMTS at large has been followed by the organisation's progressive transformation into a more centralised professional institution with technocratic management. For example, the President of the CNAMTS, nominated every five years by the Council of Ministers, now appoints local branch heads, who were previously appointed by local representatives of unions and employers. In parallel, local branches have also seen their autonomy reduced over time, as there has been a greater harmonisation of internal processes driven from the centre.

While social health insurance funds in France have continued to maintain a professional identity, and remain the payers for health care services, the age of high-level employer and union involvement in its management and daily operations is over. While the President of the CNAMTS holds considerable influence in the administration of the health care system, the state sets the overall fiscal parameters within which the organisation may work through the annual budget process.

Health in the budget process

The government has progressively taken back control of overall health spending through the Social Security Financing Act

Unlike many other social insurance countries which decentralise the control of health spending to health insurance funds to some extent, France has a high degree of government control over health spending. The parliament ultimately sets the fiscal parameters within which the CNAMTS and other social health insurance funds are asked to maintain their spending, and there is a high degree of transparency in health budgeting in France.

This form of health budgeting in France dates back to 1996 when the Plan Juppé reasserted the government's role in determining the level of social security spending. The Plan Juppé established the annual Social Security Financing Act (LFSS – *Lois de Financement de la Sécurité Sociale*) which subjects the expenditure and financing sources of all aspects of French social security to approval by the parliament, a process that is enshrined in the constitution. This makes the parliament a major player responsible for health.

The annual process of creating the Social Security Financing Act requires finance, health and social affairs officials to work together to control social security expenditure, including health

Every year, the Finance Ministry produces a draft Social Security Financing Act, known as the *Projet de Loi de Financement de la Sécurité Sociale* (PLFSS), in collaboration with the Ministry of Health, the Ministry of Labour and other social security entities. The PLFSS provides a detailed review of the social security's accounts and their financial position at the time of publication, an evaluation of the anticipated evolution of social security spending for the forthcoming year and projections for four years ahead. On the basis of these projections, the PLFSS specifies new measures – for both expenditure and revenue – to be introduced to ensure that social security's impact on general government financing meets overall fiscal objectives. Most importantly, it proposes high-level targets for spending in the forthcoming year across different areas of social security, especially health care.

The Social Security Financing Act draft is prepared between June and October by the administration and is initially produced by the *Direction de la Sécurité Sociale* (the Social Security Directorate), an administrative body which is under the joint supervision of the Budget and Health Ministries. Initially, the Social Security Directorate was under the supervision of the Health and Social Affairs Ministry; but after a period of rising deficits, its supervision was also given to the Ministry of Finance. This culminated in 2007 with the creation of the Minister for Finance and Public Accounts who is in charge of drafting the PLFSS. The Social Security Directorate is jointly supervised by both Health and Finance Ministries in order to better integrate both perspectives. Nonetheless, the finalisation of the PLFSS generally involves arbitration by the Prime Minister's Office.

Following the publication of the PLFSS, the document is debated intensively in the parliament, under a specific annual timetable starting no later than 15 October. By law, the parliament must handle the procedure within 50 days (including consideration by both the National Assembly and the Senate). If it does not do so, the government is allowed to bypass the parliament and legislate by an emergency decree. By mid-December, the Social Security Financing Law is therefore always enacted.

Figure 8.9. **Calendar of the Social Security Act**

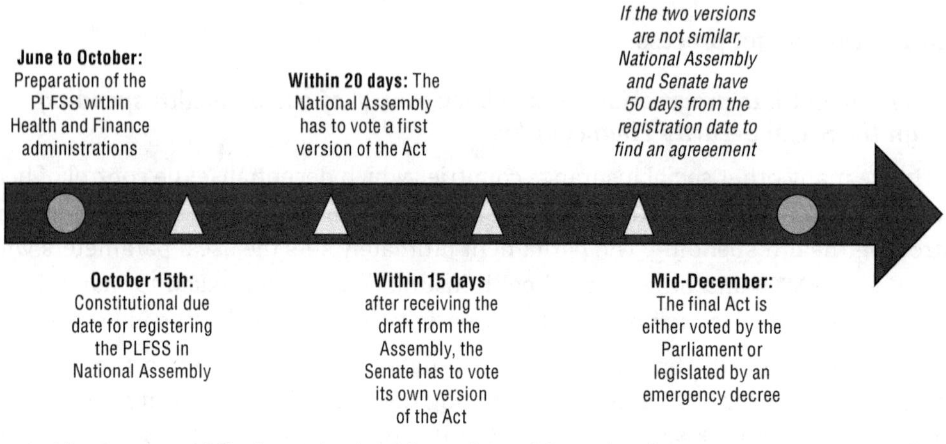

June to October: Preparation of the PLFSS within Health and Finance administrations

October 15th: Constitutional due date for registering the PLFSS in National Assembly

Within 20 days: The National Assembly has to vote a first version of the Act

Within 15 days after receiving the draft from the Assembly, the Senate has to vote its own version of the Act

If the two versions are not similar, National Assembly and Senate have 50 days from the registration date to find an agreeement

Mid-December: The final Act is either voted by the Parliament or legislated by an emergency decree

Source: Article LO111-6 and following, Code of Social Security, Social Security Directorate, Paris,

Setting expenditure levels for health

The National Objective for Healthcare Spending is a detailed target used to monitor health spending in France

The specification of an overall expenditure target for health care, known as the National Objective for Healthcare Spending (*Objectif National de Dépenses de l'Assurance Maladie* – ONDAM), is one of the most significant aspects of the Social Security Financing Law. It represents the total amount of health spending that the parliament sets as an objective for a calendar year. Once published, it gives all stakeholders a precise spending objective and defines specific savings objectives. In 2013, the ONDAM was EUR 174 billion, or 38% of the total EUR 463 billion social security spending. The ONDAM specifies the percentage of health spending growth that the government is willing to accept in any given year. For example, the 2013 global objective is EUR 174.5 billion, or 2.7% growth compared to 2012 (Table 8.1).

The ONDAM overall target is split into three sub-targets for the main types of health service providers (ambulatory care, hospitals and medico-social centres). Ambulatory care and hospitals absorb most of the ONDAM, with 2013 targets of 45.9% and 43.6% of total health expenditures respectively (Table 8.1). Hospitals are further subdivided between health care centres under DRG (diagnosis-related group) payments (hospitals, clinics) and other health care establishments (mostly rehabilitation and psychiatry), while medico-social establishments are split between centres for the elderly and centres for the handicapped.

Table 8.1. **ONDAM sub-categories actuals, predictions and targets for the years 2010, 2011, 2012 and 2013**

	2010	2011	2012 predictions	2013 targets	Growth rates
Ambulatory care	75.2	77.3	78.5	80.5	2.6%
Hospitals	10.9	72.9	74.6	76.5	2.6%
DRG-based establishments	52.6		55.4	56.7	2.4%
Other	18.4		19.2	19.8	3.1%
Medico-social	15.2	15.8	16.5	17.1	4.0%
Elderly care centres	7.3	7.6	8	8.4	4.6%
Handicap centres	7.9	8.3	8.4	8.7	3.3%
Other	1	1.1	1.2	1.3	5.9%
Total	**162.4**	**167.1**	**170.8**	**175.4**	**2.7%**

Source: Data from *Projet de Loi de Financement de la Sécurité Sociale* (PLFSS) 2012, 2013, Annex 7, Social Security Directorate, Paris, *www.securite-sociale.fr/Lois-de-financement-de-la-Securite-sociale-LFSS-par-annee.*

StatLink http://dx.doi.org/10.1787/888933219497

The origin of the French health care system in independent operation by social insurance has meant that there is little tradition of specifying *a priori* (or prospective) global budgets for health care. The French population has been accustomed to free choice of providers for both ambulatory and hospital care, with public insurance obliged to reimburse the amount and kind of care that patients and their doctors choose. Doctors in France do not play a role in "rationing" access to care as they may do on grounds of equity or urgency in the United Kingdom. For most of its history, the French government has not played a proactive role in influencing overall health care spending.

The National Objective for Health Care in 1996 marked a significant break from this tradition and represents the reassertion of the government in controlling health care spending. However, when it was first introduced, the ONDAM did not prove sufficient to contain spending by social health insurance funds within budgetary targets. In part, this may be because there were few mechanisms to ensure compliance when the ONDAM was first introduced. Closer monitoring of the ONDAM and automatic measures that reduce spending in case of overrun have been introduced progressively to improve its effectiveness.

When setting the ONDAM, the government draws a precise list of savings necessary to meet the target

To calculate the ONDAM target, health and finance administrations start by forecasting the trend of health expenditure. This is first done by applying a theoretical growth rate to the forecast expenditure of the current year. The deferred effects of measures implemented in the previous years are then added to this first trend. This results in an indicator known as the "trend ONDAM" (*ONDAM tendanciel*), which is a projection of how health expenditure would evolve if no new expenditures or savings were decided.

The trend ONDAM is then compared to the target suggested by senior ministers. The difference between the natural evolution and the political objective determines the scope of the savings measures the government must propose to reach the target. Final targets for the ONDAM and its sub-categories are then determined, taking into account the financial impact of the new savings measures proposed and, by a regular dialogue between officials and the government's executive on the overall target, the policy measures to be adopted to achieve them.

In 2013, while the trend ONDAM would have implied a 4.1% growth in health spending, the approved ONDAM target was finally set at 2.7% growth, implying that a series of measures were identified to decrease expenditure in all health care areas. The ONDAM for ambulatory care was reduced from a 4.8% trend level to a 2.6% target, mainly by measures on drugs prices and prescription volumes which together reduced spending plans by about EUR 1.5 billion in 2013 (Figure 8.10). As for hospital expenditures, the ONDAM target was set at 2.6% growth rate, 0.6 points below the 3.4% trend ONDAM. In order to reach this objective, savings of almost EUR 600 million were imposed on hospitals through productivity gains.

Figure 8.10. **Main savings included in the ONDAM between 2010 and 2013**

In million EUR

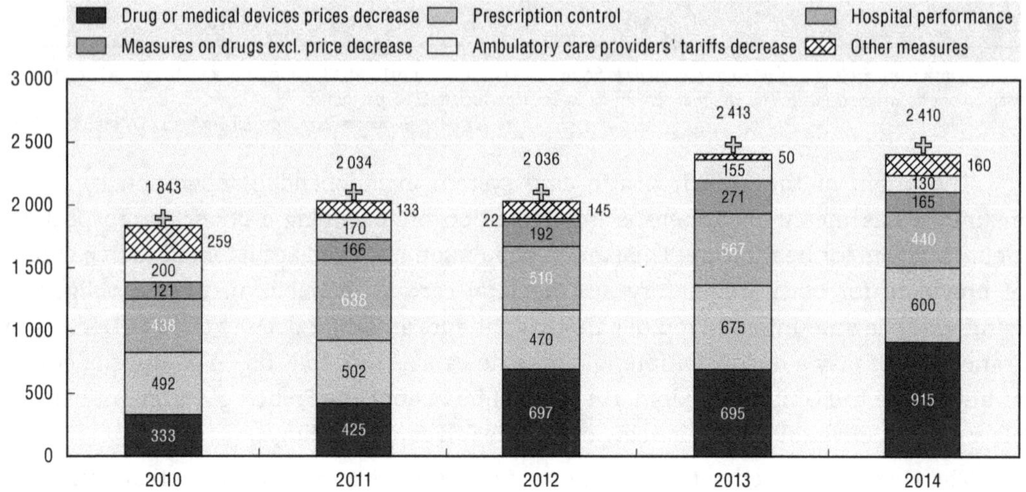

Source: *Loi de Financement de la Sécurité Sociale* (LFSS) 2011, 2012, 2013, Social Security Directorate, Paris, *www.securite-sociale.fr/Lois-de-financement-de-la-Securite-sociale-LFSS-par-annee*.

StatLink http://dx.doi.org/10.1787/888933219164

ONDAM targets were not met until very recently

During the past ten years, ONDAM targets were consistently overrun, leading to large social security deficits. Although the creation of the ONDAM was seen as a useful step towards better monitoring of health spending, its non-binding nature meant no stakeholder had the full responsibility to respect it when it was first put into place. For the majority of the first decade of its operation, actual spending seriously exceeded ONDAM targets (as shown in Figure 8.11). At first, this did not raise much attention, as the better macroeconomic situation saw social security revenues increase, minimising the impact on overall deficits. However, this changed during the economic downturn of 2001-02 as revenues did not keep up with growth in spending, making health the main driver of social security deficits (Figure 8.11). Health spending continued to overrun the ONDAM through 2009, despite efforts to set the ONDAM at a more achievable level and to follow up spending better.

Figure 8.11. **Voted ONDAM vs. achieved health expenditures**

Percentage growth

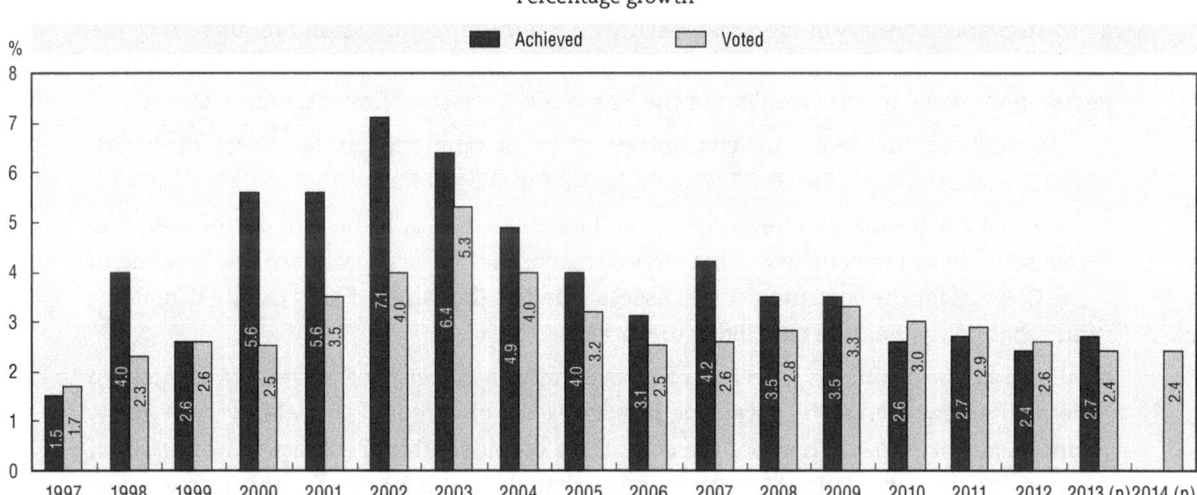

Source: *Projet de Loi de Financement de la Sécurité Sociale* (PLFSS), Social Security Accounts, Social Security Directorate, Paris, *www.securite-sociale.fr/Lois-de-financement-de-la-Securite-sociale-LFSS-par-annee*.

StatLink http://dx.doi.org/10.1787/888933219178

This inability to reach the targets led the administration to conclude they needed closer monitoring of health expenditures and the ONDAM's prospects for realisation within the course of the year. The apparent realisation that the hypotheses on which the targets were set were probably too vague led to the creation of an ONDAM Alert Committee in 2004 (see Section 3.2). ONDAM targets progressively became not vague objectives but real targets to be achieved in order to achieve sustainable health budgets.

While the growth rate of health expenditures has been decreasing for a decade, the ONDAM has only been successfully respected since 2010. The growth rate in health spending has dropped below 3% since 2010, from a high of 7.1% in 2002. However, the French Health Ministry forecasts that France will need to achieve a 2% ONDAM growth rate in the coming years to end health deficits. This would represent on average, an additional annual savings of EUR 10 billion over 2015-17.

8.4. Controlling key elements of health expenditures

Recent years have seen the process for setting budgets through the ONDAM expand from its origins as a political objective to a process for monitoring and responding to changes in health care spending throughout the year. Behind this has been the creation of two key institutions, the Alert Committee and the Steering Committee, each equipped with a number of policy tools.

The role of new institutions in controlling health expenditure

The Alert Committee is responsible for monitoring and reporting progress towards meeting the ONDAM

The Alert Committee on the Evolution of Health Insurance Spending was established in 2004 and its responsibilities have progressively expanded as health spending has continued to grow. The committee's role is to alert the parliament, the government and the national health insurance funds when social health insurance spending is growing too fast and is likely to put the agreed ONDAM for a particular year at risk. The Alert Committee consists of: the General Secretary of the Social Security Accounting Commission (nominated by the Cour des Comptes), the Director General of the French National Statistics Institute and a person nominated by the President of the Economic, Social and Environmental Council.

Throughout the year, the committee provides opinions on the level of health expenditures relative to the ONDAM. In doing so it is obliged to:

- Assess at the beginning of every year (no later than 15 April) the amount of spending realised for the previous year. This allows the committee to re-evaluate the baseline of the ONDAM for the current year and assess whether the targeted growth rate is realistic and that policy measures are likely to work.
- Publish before 1 June an assessment of whether the current year's ONDAM is likely to be realised. By decree, the government fixes a level of accepted ONDAM overrun (0.5 % since 1 January 2013). Whenever the committee considers that there is a "serious risk" of exceeding the voted ONDAM target by more than 0.5%, it has to notify this immediately (through an alert process) to the government, parliament and the health insurance funds. These organisations are then obliged to propose corrective measures within a month, after which the committee is to evaluate the potential impact of the chosen recovery measures.
- Publish before 15 October (i.e. before the parliamentary discussion for the next Draft Social Security Financing Act) an evaluation of both the current year's prospects for realising the ONDAM and the contents and rationale behind the ONDAM target for the following year. At that time, it can raise concerns if it believes that the administrators' growth-rate projections and proposed savings are not realistic.

The establishment of the Alert Committee and its mandate is a sign of the transformation of the ONDAM from a broad political objective to an operational target. The processes initiated by the Alert Committee reinforce efforts to monitor spending regularly and undertake frequent short-term forecasts of health expenditure. Furthermore, the Alert Committee's ability to compel other stakeholders to take corrective action generates permanent pressure which is likely to have contributed to increased efforts to contain spending within the ONDAM in more recent years.

When it was originally founded in 2004, the Alert Committee had fewer mechanisms to oblige the government and the national health insurance funds to taken actions to contain spending. Following the publication of a report on the monitoring of health expenditures in

Figure 8.12. **The year-long process of the Alert Committee**

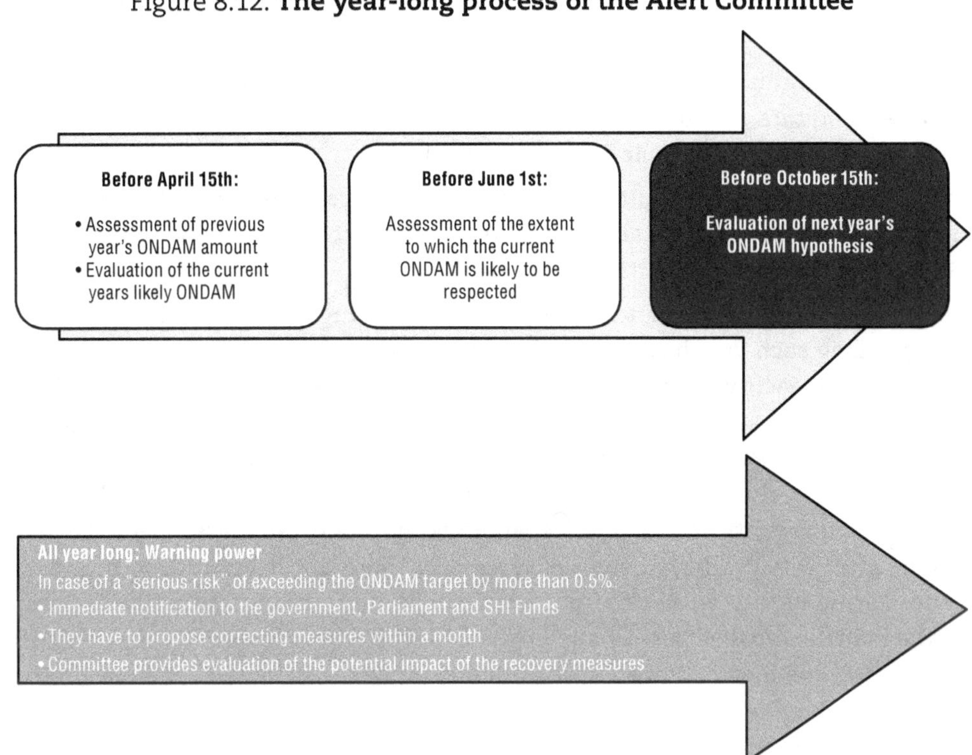

May 2010 (*Rapport Briet*), a number of additional measures were undertaken to strengthen and supplement the role of the committee. In particular, the Alert Committee was provided with the ability to undertake an evaluation of the ONDAM before the Draft of the Social Security Financing Act is submitted to parliament.

A Steering Committee of key government actors and representatives of the health funds has recently been constituted to improve co-operation in meeting the ONDAM

In addition to the Alert Committee, an ONDAM Steering Committee was created in 2010 in the aftermath of the publication of the *Rapport Briet*. This Steering Committee gathers representatives from all Health and Budget Ministries, as well as representatives from all major health funds. The committee's main objective is to foster co-operation amongst each of the key actors to avoid a situation requiring a warning from the Alert Committee. It monitors health expenditures covered by the ONDAM every month, implements all savings that have been decided to help meet the target, and prepares the ONDAM for the following year. This committee works on the basis of the financial information provided by an ONDAM Statistical Committee which reports monthly on health spending for each ONDAM sub-target.

New policies to constrain budgets in order to meet the target

The government has introduced new policies which compel the budget to stay on track

The government has introduced two new measures to ensure that spending remains within the ONDAM in a particular year. It has given the Alert Committee power to reduce payments and to withhold a portion of anticipated spending as a buffer against the risk of a budget overrun. Today, the alert process, which can be triggered by the Alert Committee if the ONDAM target overruns by more than 0.5%, has immediate consequences in terms of health spending:

- If the Alert Committee notifies that ambulatory care is responsible for the overrun of health expenditure, all budgeted increases in providers' fees or reimbursement levels are immediately frozen for a limited period of time.
- Since 2009, if the Alert Committee sends a warning concerning a possible overrun of the current ONDAM due to hospital expenditures, the ministry and the CNAMTS can reduce DRG payments during the course of the year.

Along with these measures, a new policy of withholding a small portion of anticipated health spending each year has recently been introduced. Once the ONDAM is defined at the beginning of each year, it is now mandatory to set aside 0.3% of the total ONDAM of the year as a precautionary measure. This can only apply to health spending which is provided in the form of fixed budgets so it is mostly public hospitals that have been affected by these reforms as they receive part of their overall funding in the form of fixed payments. In contrast, outpatient spending is normally reimbursed by social health insurance after services have been delivered and there are fewer means to influence demand. Payments are withheld from both public and private hospitals in order to share the burden across sectors by applying a 0.3% coefficient to all DRG payments since 2013. In effect, this means that social health insurance funds pay 99.7% of each service. The remaining 0.3% is withheld until the end of the year and only given to health care providers if the ONDAM is not overrun. This has been a critical factor in helping maintain ONDAM targets. As shown in Figure 8.13 below, over 2010 and 2012, the level of health spending has been slightly less than the ONDAM target. When broken down into the key components, inpatient spending has overrun its sub-targets but this has been offset by credits withheld from inpatients at the end of the year and by outpatient spending at less than its sub-targets.

Furthermore, the government has incorporated the ONDAM into its shift towards specifying multi-year budget objectives. Unlike many OECD countries which have a history of publishing projections of key expenditures for the next three or four years, this is a relatively new development in France. While the ONDAM is notionally a spending target for a single year, the government publishes projections with the intended progression of the ONDAM over the next three years. These are intended to act as a constraint for policy makers to maintain growth within the multi-year targets as they go through the annual process of adjusting the ONDAM.

The budgetary processes ushered in by the ONDAM has improved monitoring of health expenditures and working relations between stakeholders, though its true impact on containing spending remains unclear

A unique feature of the Social Security Financing Act is that it outlines the policy measures that must be undertaken to achieve the agreed target in light of short-term projections of health spending. As policy makers must simultaneously think about an overall spending objective (ONDAM) and the policy measures to achieve it, they have the ability to put the necessary actions in place in advance to help ensure spending targets are met. In contrast, other countries that have budget-funded health care systems (the United Kingdom, Australia, New Zealand and Canada, for example) are likely to develop policy measures that meet their health and overall fiscal objectives, but are not necessarily related to a targeted level of spending for health on its own.

Figure 8.13. **Key factors behind actual health spending below the ONDAM, 2010 to 2012**

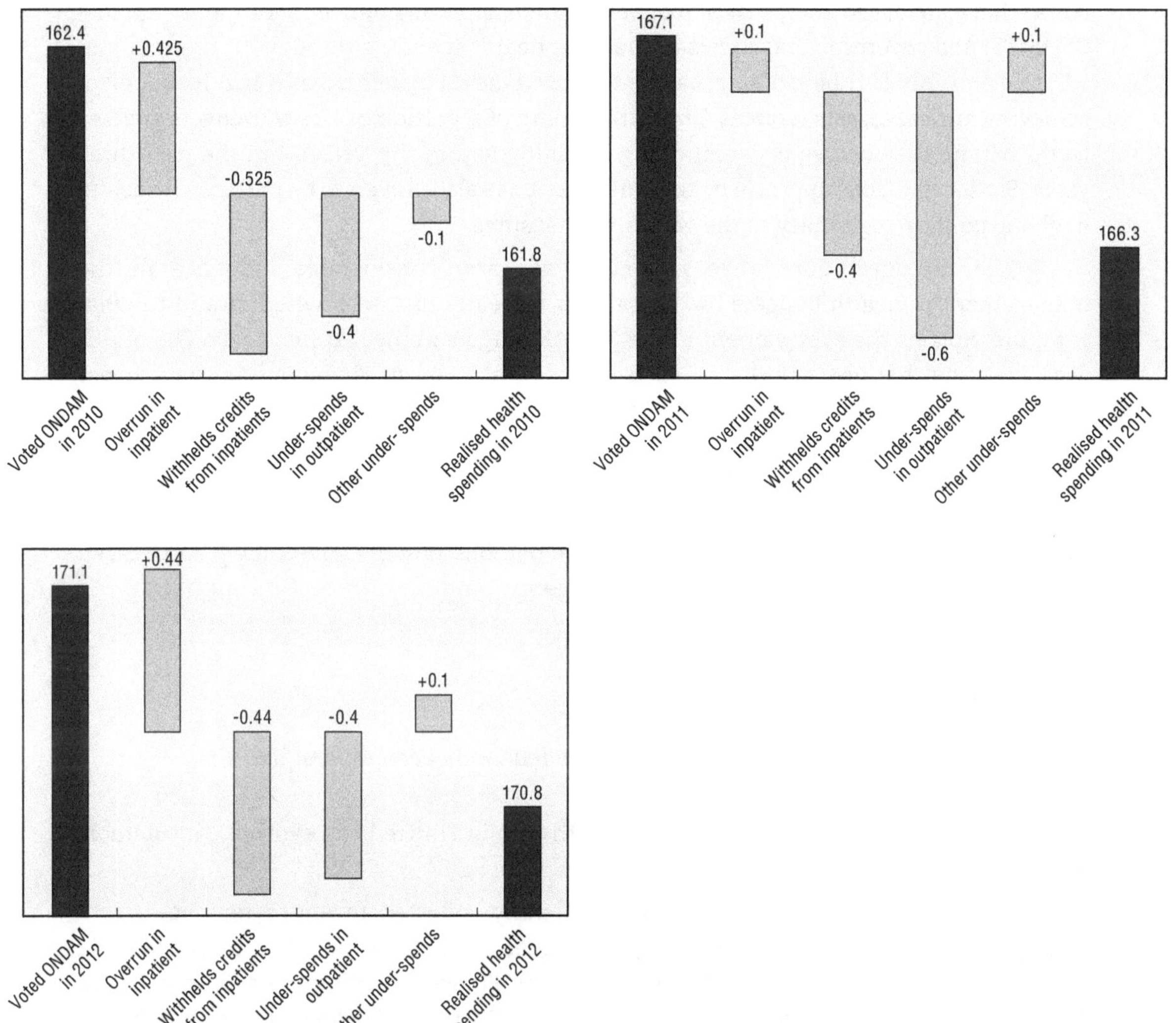

Source: *Loi de Financement de la Sécurité Sociale* (LFSS) 2010, 2011, 2012, Social Security Directorate, Paris, *www.securite-sociale.fr/Lois-de-financement-de-la-Securite-sociale-LFSS-par-annee.*

StatLink http://dx.doi.org/10.1787/888933219182

The Draft Social Security Financing Act appears to be a useful form of goal-setting for France's multiple social security institutions and it appears to have contributed to a greater level of focus on budgetary management of health care spending. Social insurance health care systems are often characterised by more actors involved in the financing of health care. In such a situation, particularly with France's legacy of multiple insurers, setting the Draft Social Security Financing Act provides a tool to oblige major entities in the health care system to discuss how much they plan to spend in the year ahead. In practical terms, this means that the CNAMTS, the other insurers, the Ministries of Finance and of Health, hospital organisations and doctors are all engaged in discussions on overall spending over the course of the year.

By providing a common goal to multiple institutions, the Draft Social Security Financing Act has opened a new dialogue between the main actors of the French health sector and between Ministries of Health and of Finance. This distinguishes France from other OECD countries where the Ministry of Finance, the Ministry of Health or the health insurer tends to be the dominant player in determining the level of health spending and relationships between these entities can often be adversarial. In practical terms, the arrangements in France have increased co-operation between independent insurance institutions (e.g., the CNAMTS) and government agencies on tracking health spending throughout the year and creating a means to trigger policy makers to undertake further changes if the likelihood of achieving annual targets reduces. The withholding of a portion of health budgets is a key factor behind the success in maintaining spending within the ONDAM in the past three years. Similarly, official approval by the Parliament has also proven to be particularly useful in giving political legitimacy to the goals and measures.

While the Alert Committee has come to carry considerable influence in the management of health budgets in France, it is too early to assess whether and to what extent it explains the achievement of the ONDAM targets in the last two years. The multi-year forecasts that are included in each Draft Social Security Financing Act have never been respected, nor has the objective of balancing health insurance finances been met. The 2005 Draft Social Security Financing Act forecast a balanced health budget by 2007. The 2013 Draft Social Security Financing Act forecasts that this will not happen before 2017. Nonetheless, the very creation of institutions which have the ability to enforce policy measures that could reduce health expenditure demonstrate the government's increased commitment to delivering on its budgetary targets.

8.5. Financing health care

Sources of funds for health spending

A wage-based resources system which has increasingly been diversified over the years

The key taxes that raise revenue for health care in France have evolved considerably since the founding of the health care system.

As a social security system that has generally collected revenues for health care through means separate from government revenues at large, it is possible to map the mix of revenues used to finance health care services in France. Mapping the evolution of the form of revenues for health care (as undertaken in Figure 8.14 below) shows that France has made considerable efforts to diversify the sources of health financing over the last two decades. After what was initially a system funded almost entirely from wage-based contributions in 1968, today these contributions account for 47.8% of revenues for health care (primarily levied on employers).

The most profound change to the source of financing for health care has been the introduction of the *Contribution Sociale Généralisée* (CSG), which consists of one single tax with different rates for different types of revenues in a broader range of sources than simply wages. Twenty years after its founding, the CSG today has come to account for some 35.3% of social health insurance revenues. Other earmarked taxes levied on smaller tax bases (including sin taxes) have been the fastest growing source of financing, now accounting for some 13.5% of revenues for health care compared to 4% a decade ago. However, these still remain relatively small in the context of the system's broader financing needs.

The CSG has been the key instrument to broaden the sources of health care financing in France

The CSG levies taxes on a broad range of sources including wage income but also extending to income from financial assets and investments, pensions, unemployment benefits, disability benefits and gambling. At the time of its creation, the CSG rate was low, representing 1.1% of each of these sources of revenue (see Table 8.2). It was solely aimed at financing the family branch of the social security in an effort to mirror the universalisation of the family branch. It was therefore implemented with a complex fiscal arrangement to decrease, at the same time, some wage-based contributions aimed at financing family care. At the time of its founding, the purpose of the CSG was not to create additional funding for social security but to change the overall origins of the revenues. This did not last long and a second extension was made in 1993 to find additional resources for family and pensions branches.

Figure 8.14. **Distribution of CNAMTS resources**

In percentage of total resources by origin

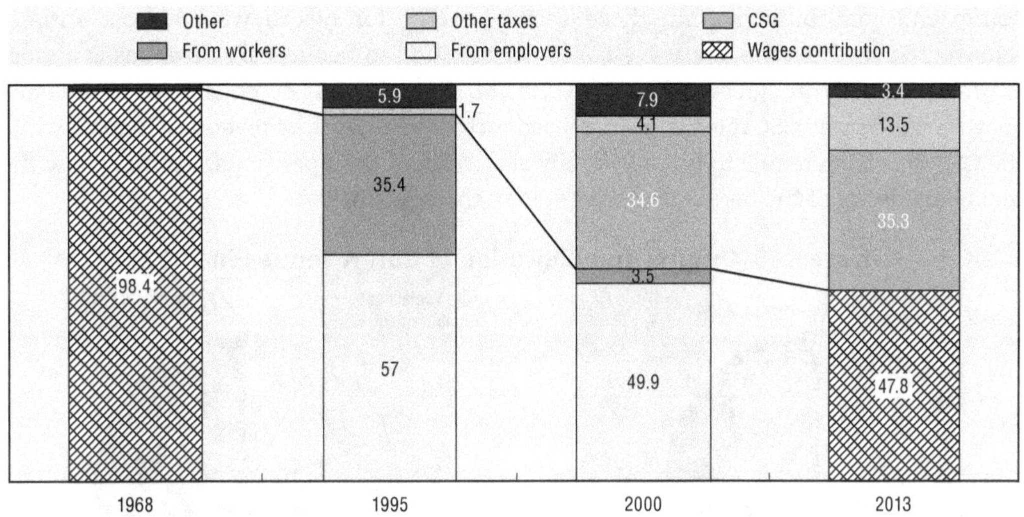

CNAMTS : Caisse nationale de l'assurance maladie des travailleurs salariés.

Source: Bras, P.L. et al. (2014), *Social Security Accounts Commission Report, 2014*, Social Security Directorate, Paris, *www.securite-sociale.fr/Rapports-de-la-CCSS*.

StatLink http://dx.doi.org/10.1787/888933219195

Table 8.2. **Evolution of CSG rates since its creation**

Time of introduction	Earned income	Unemployment benefits (low income people)	Financial assets and investments	Pensions, disability and pre-retirement (low income people)	Gambling (1) depending on the gambling revenue source
1991	1.1%	1.1%	1.1%	1.1%	-
1993	2.4%	2.4%	2.4%	2.4%	-
1997	3.4%	3.4% (1%)	3.4%	3.4% (1%)	3.4%
1998	7.5%	6.2% (3.8%)	7.5%	6.2% (3.8%)	7.5%
2005	7.5%	6.2% (3.8%)	8.2%	6.6% (3.8%)	9.5% / 12%
2010	**7.5%**	**6.2% (3.8%)**	**8.2%**	**6.6% (3.8%)**	**9.5%/12%/6.9%**[1]
Earmarked to health insurance	**5.3%**	**4.0%**	**5.9%**	**4.4%**	**n.a.**

CSG: Contribution Sociale Généralisée.

1. depending on the gambling revenue source.

Source: *Social Security Accounts Commission Report, 2012*, and previous, Social Security Directorate, Paris (*www.securite-sociale.fr/Rapports-de-la-CCSS*).

StatLink http://dx.doi.org/10.1787/888933219500

The appropriation of the CSG to fund social health care insurance began in 1997. Alongside measures to control expenditure (discussed earlier), the Plan Juppé sought to reduce wage-based contributions for health care and replace the lost revenue with an increase in the CSG – i.e., a reduction of 1.3 percentage points on employee wage-based contributions was replaced by an increase of 1 percentage point of CSG rates across its various sources of income. The CSG was also enlarged to include gambling revenues at this time. This began France's process of slowly diversifying revenues for health care away from simply relying on wages and towards a broader definition of income.

However, the major push towards diversifying revenues for health care occurred in 1998. The employee wage-based contribution was reduced by 4.75 percentage points and the CSG on wage income and capital income was increased by 4.1 percentage points. At the same time the CSG on pensions and unemployment benefits was raised by 2 percentage points and contributions from these social benefits for health were almost entirely removed. Since this time, the wage-based contribution to health care revenues is almost entirely financed through contributions levied on employers. As demonstrated in the table above, in 2004 some CSG rates were increased further to raise more revenues. In total, while the CSG was first created to finance family services and then pensions, health is now the main beneficiary of the tax, as demonstrated in the figure below.

Figure 8.15. **Origins and allocation of CSG revenues in 2012**

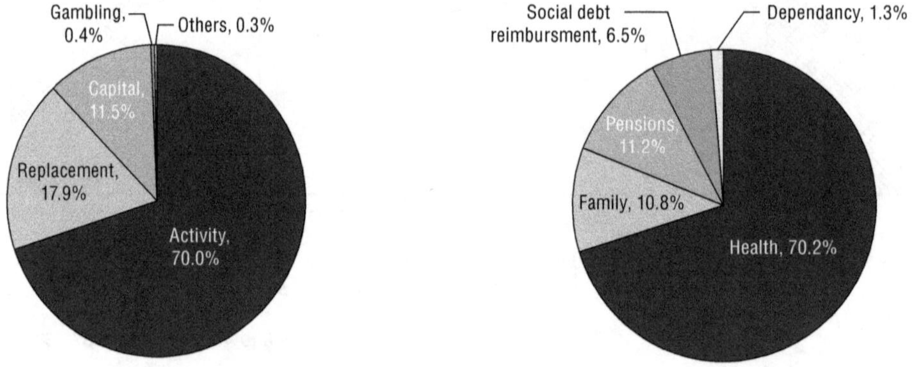

CSG: Contribution Sociale Généralisée.

Source: Social Security Accounts Commission Report, 2013, Social Security Directorate, Paris (*www.securite-sociale.fr/Rapports-de-la-CCSS*).

StatLink http://dx.doi.org/10.1787/888933219202

Other earmarked taxes contribute to health financing in a growing proportion

A wide range of taxes that are each levied on a narrow base have come to form the "third pillar" of revenues for social security, and particularly health care, in France over the past ten years. These taxes are known as the *Impôts et Taxes Affectés* and include more than 20 precise types of taxes.

In 2011, 55% of these earmarked taxes financed social health insurance funds for a total of approximately EUR 27.8 billion (Figure 8.16). These are taxes on enterprises, such as five different taxes on pharmaceutical companies, taxes on company cars and a share of a global tax for all companies above a certain level of net sales. They are also taxes on consumption or behaviour, including a share of the VAT, a tax on personal health insurance and taxes on tobacco and alcohol (Table 8.3).

While these taxes have grown in their share of health care financing, in part this is because the government has replaced employer contributions for the health care of certain low-income workers (especially with salaries below 1.6 times the minimum wage) with a direct payment from the government to social health insurance, as a measure to reduce the cost of labor.

Figure 8.16. **Destinations of earmarked taxes for social security in 2012**

In billion EUR and percentage

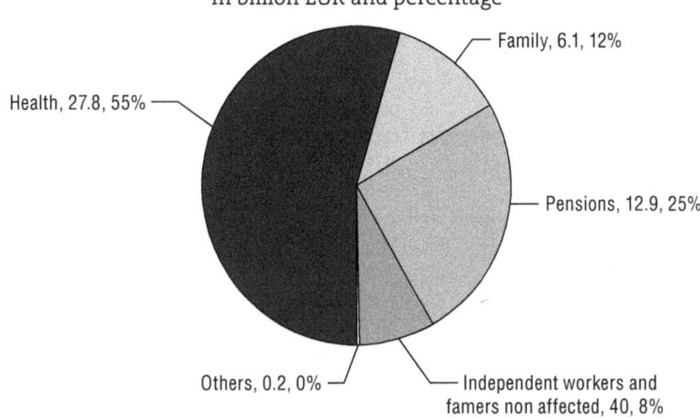

Source: High Council for Social Security Financing report, October 2012, Social Security Directorate, Paris.

StatLink http://dx.doi.org/10.1787/888933219213

Table 8.3. **Presentation of all earmarked taxes related to health in 2012**

In bilion EUR

Portion of VAT	10.6
Tax on tobacco	8.0
Taxes on complementary insurance	2.9
Tax on companies with net sales above EUR 0.76 million	1.4
Pharmaceutical taxes	1.1
Tax on motor insurance	1.1
Tax on alcohol	1.0
Tax on company cars	1.0
Gaming taxes	0.5
Tax on oils and flours	0.2
Total of earmarked taxes affected to health	27.8

Source: High Council for Social Security Financing report, October 2012, Social Security Directorate, Paris.

StatLink http://dx.doi.org/10.1787/888933219516

France's efforts to broaden the sources of revenues for health care to a larger definition of income is a commendable policy response to changing sources of household incomes

The combination of policy efforts over the past two decades has delivered an impressive broadening of the revenues for health care in France. Indeed, this has seen France shift away from a pure model of social insurance financing for health care, which relies predominately on wage based financing. Whereas Germany, Korea and the Netherlands, among others, have taken *ad hoc* contributions from their budgets where revenues from wages have proved insufficient to match health care expenditures, France has proactively sought to expand the base of its sources of financing for health care to lessen the reliance – and therefore the volatility – on simply one key form of revenue.

This represents a sensible policy response to an underlying change in the sources of household income over the past 40 years. As shown in Figure 8.17, the share of labour income (principally wages) in a household's total income in France has decreased from 80% to 71% between 1970 and 2011. At the same time, income from capital and social benefits has come to form a larger share of household incomes, accounting for 29% of total household income by 2011. In this context, the progressive shift away from wage-based income alone to a broader definition of income is also a worthwhile move from the perspective of improving the equity of revenue-raising for health, as wealthier individuals generally demonstrate higher levels of income on capital and financial assets.

Figure 8.17. **Evolution of household income distribution between 1970 and 2011**

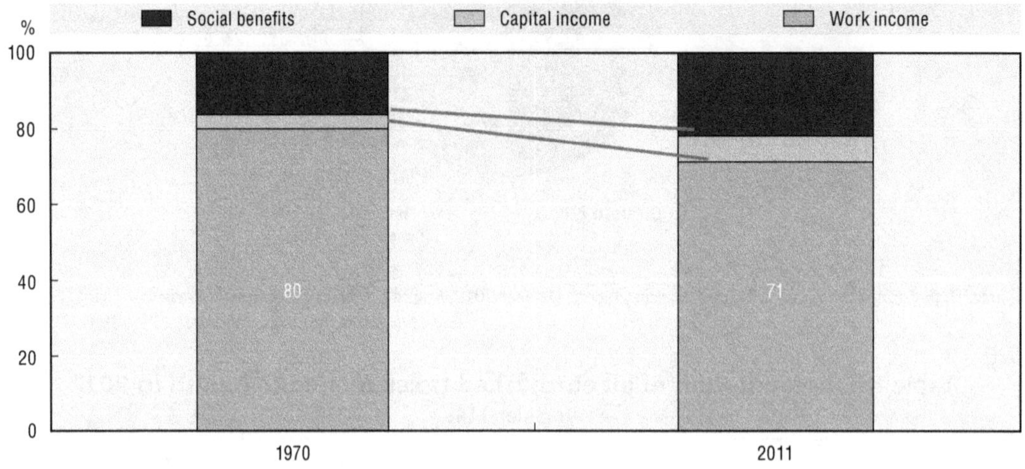

Source: INSEE data with OECD analysis.

StatLink http://dx.doi.org/10.1787/888933219223

Nonetheless, it is worth noting that around two-thirds of revenues for health care still come from wage-based sources. As demonstrated in the graph below, the CSG on wages accounts for around 18% of the revenue for the health care system, which is in addition to the 48% of revenues which come from wage-based contributions. While France has made considerable progress in diversifying its revenue base, it should continue to monitor whether further diversification may be necessary, particularly as workforce participation rates may imply a declining wage share of national income into the future.

Figure 8.18. **Share of CNAMTS revenues by source in 2011**

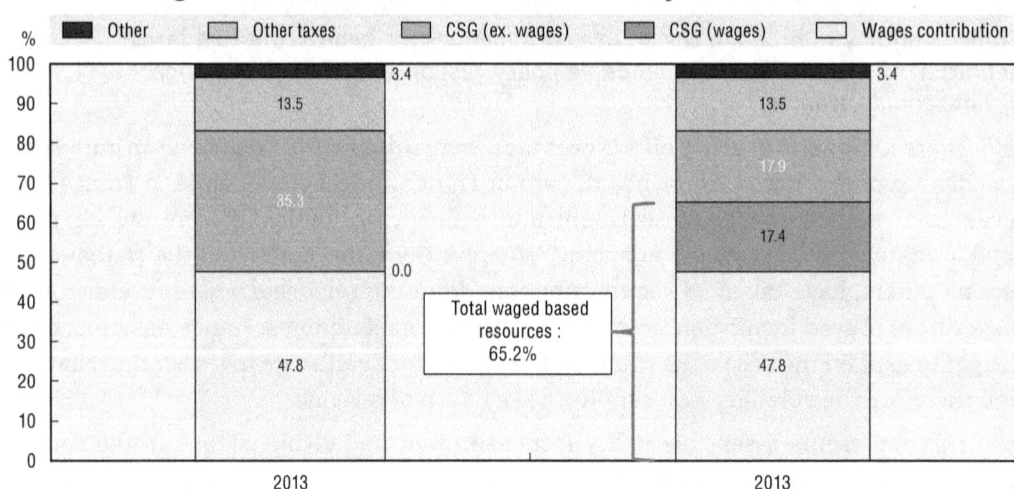

Source: OECD analysis of Social Security Accounts Commission Report, 2014, Social Security Directorate, Paris (*www.securite-sociale.fr/Rapports-de-la-CCSS*).

StatLink http://dx.doi.org/10.1787/888933219234

8.6. Deficit management in France

Social security[1] debt is managed by an independent administration

France currently carries EUR 142 billion in accumulated debts from social security deficits over the past two decades. This debt is held in a public entity, the *Caisse d'Amortissement de la Dette Sociale* (CADES), which can issue bonds in financial markets in order to raise funds to cover deficits in social security from one year to the next.

The CADES was created to help deal with persistent deficits in social security, as social security institutions are not allowed to hold their own debt, though they are entitled to request short-term loans (for less than a year). The three years from 1993 to 1995 saw deficits in social security increase beyond the capacity to be financed by short-term loans. As a result, the government at the time decided to establish the CADES in 1996 as an independent public institution with the ability to raise debt, separate from government debt, to support social security. At the time of its founding, some 13 years of (small) accumulated social security debts were transferred to the CADES, amounting to some FRF 137 billion (more than EUR 20 billion).

The CADES is notionally independent; but in practice, its role and functions are dictated by government

The CADES is a public institution operating under the jurisdictions of the Ministry of Finance and the Ministry of Health and Social Affairs. A Board of Directors steers the organisation, and a Supervisory Committee reviews the agency's operations annually. While the CADES was founded to manage the debt of social security, the Board of Directors did not include representatives from social security institutions until 2010. It was entirely composed of government officials, generally from the Finance and Health and Social Affairs Ministries.

The majority of CADES decisions are of an operational nature and require approval by the ministries which supervise it. As an organisation, the CADES is focused on ensuring that the social security's accumulated debt portfolio is being managed on an active basis and that the term of social security debt facilitate its eventual repayment. When changes to the debt portfolio are sought, the supervising ministries must approve changes to the structure of the debt portfolio and also determine the amount of deficit transfers into the CADES.

Sustained deficits from social security have made the CADES a permanent part of the landscape for financing social security in France

As social security deficits have become persistent, the amount of debt supervised by the CADES has increased substantially. Upon its establishment in 1996, the mandate of the CADES included a target to repay social debt by 2009. By 1997, this end date was pushed back to 2014, when a further EUR 13 billion was transferred into the CADES. The re-emergence of persistent high deficits in social security from 2003 has seen further accumulation of debt in the CADES whose net liability position had grown to EUR 142 billion in 2011 (see Figure 8.19). As the CADES has taken on ever-increasing amounts of social debt, the official "end date" for repaying the debt has continued to be pushed further into the future.

The government seeks new sources of funding to repay the debt accumulated in the CADES

The government created new taxes and redistributed existing taxes to try to repay some of the debt in the CADES over the past two decades. At the time of its founding, the government introduced a new tax called the *contribution pour le remboursement de la dette sociale* (CRDS) which imposed an additional 0.5% on all forms of income. The CRDS was supposed to be a time-limited tax, consistent with the notion that the CADES to be a temporary institution to help manage and eventually repay social security debt.

Figure 8.19. **Evolution of the CADES net liability position**

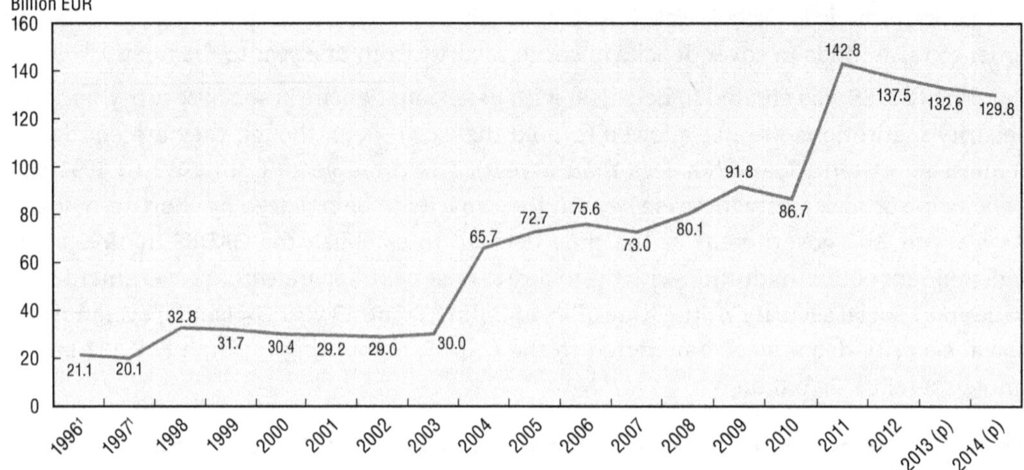

CADES: Caisse d'Amortissement de la Dette Sociale.

1. Indicates that these amounts were denominated in French francs but have been converted to euros for ease of comparison.

Source: CADES, *www.cades.fr/index.php?option=com_content&view=article&id=72&Itemid=159&lang=en.*

StatLink http://dx.doi.org/10.1787/888933219243

However, as social security deficits have persisted and social debt has risen, the government has sought additional sources of revenue. In 2005, a law obliged the government and social security institutions to specify new sources of funding every time further debt was raised by the CADES. By 2009, this led the government to re-allocate to the CADES a portion of the CSG (0.2%) that was formerly earmarked for pensions. Within two years, this portion of the CSG was again raised to 0.48%. Over time, resources devoted to financing the CADES have increased significantly, each of these funded from new or increased taxes (Figure 8.20).

Figure 8.20. **Evolution of the CADES recourses**

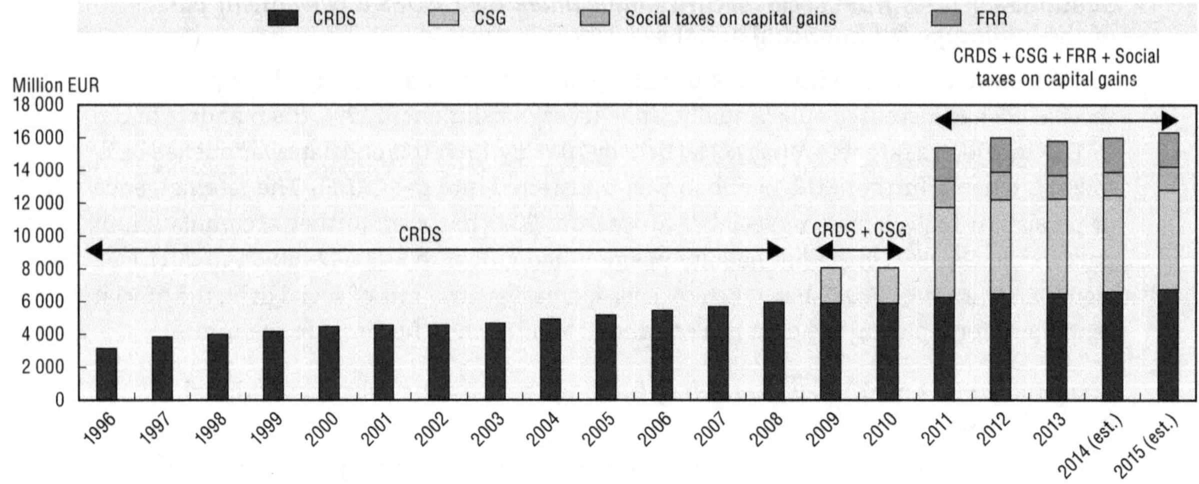

CADES: Caisse d'Amortissement de la Dette Sociale; CRDS : Contribution pour le remboursement de la dette sociale ; CSG : Contribution Sociale Généralisée.

Source: CADES, *www.cades.fr/index.php?option=com_content&view=article&id=72&Itemid=159&lang=en.*

8.7. Conclusion

Facing one of the highest level of health spending in OECD countries, the French challenge was to improve the management of health care expenditure by the progressive introduction of innovative regulatory tools without abandoning the basic principles of the French health insurance system built after the second World War. Change in the management of the French health care system tried to recognize the uniqueness of health insurance expenditure as public spending. Consequently, France gradually implemented a range of regulatory policies, halfway between an "accounting" approach and a medicalised approach. French Government has created institutions in order to ensure the matching of the two approaches (alert Committee on the evolution of health insurance spending, the Steering Committee of the ONDAM). The encouraging success of the changes introduced in France including ONDAM makes the French experience an example for the member countries of the OECD.

Note

1. As described earlier in this chapter, social health insurance for health, pensions, family payments and occupational injuries together form "social security" in France. The relative contribution of health deficits to other forms of social security deficits have been discussed in Section 8.2 of this chapter. As the CADES does not distinguish between debt from different functions of social security, this section discusses social security debt at large, of which health is a significant part.

References

Bras, P.-L. and D. Tabuteau (2012), *Les assurances maladies*, Presses universitaires de France, Paris.

Bras, P.-L., G. de Pouvourville and D. Tabuteau (eds.) (2014), *Traité d'économie et de gestion de la santé*, Presses de Sciences Po, Paris.

Budget Ministry (France) (2012), *Bilan des relations financières entre l'État et la protection sociale*, Paris.

Budget Ministry (France) (2012 and previous years), "Projet de Loi de Financement de la Sécurité Sociale et Annexes 1, 2, 4, 7", Paris.

Chevreul, K., I. Durand-Zaleski and S. Bahrami (eds.) (2011), "Healthcare Systems in Transition - France", European Observatory on Health Systems and Policies, Brussels.

CNAMTS – Caisse Nationale de l'Assurance Maladie des Travailleurs Salariés (2012), "Propositions de l'assurance maladie sur les charges et produits", Paris.

Commission des Comptes de la Sécurité Sociale (France) (2014), "Rapport Juin 2014", Paris.

Cour des Comptes (France) (2012, 2011 and previous years), "Rapport sur l'application des lois de financement de la sécurité sociale", Paris.

Dress – Direction de la recherche, des études, de l'évaluation et des statistiques (France) (2012a), "50 ans d'évolution de la structure de financement de la protection sociale", Ministère des Affaires sociales et de la Santé, Paris.

Dress (2012b), *Les comptes nationaux de la santé*, Ministère des Affaires sociales et de la Santé, Paris.

Dress (2010), *La Protection Sociale en France et Europe*, Ministère des Affaires sociales et de la Santé, Paris.

Fragonard, B. (2012), *Vive la protection sociale!*, Odile Jacob, Paris.

Frotiée, B. (2004), "La fabrique du droit social : L'exemple de la CMU", Groupe d'Analyse des Politiques Publiques, Ecole normale supérieure, Cachan, France.

Haut Conseil pour l'Avenir de l'Assurance Maladie (France) (2011), *Rapport annuel*, Paris.

Haut Conseil pour le Financement de la Protection Sociale (France) (2012), *État des lieux du financement de la protection sociale*, Paris.

INSEE – Institut National de la Statistique et des Études Économiques (2011), *Structure du financement de la dépense courante de soins et de biens médicaux*, Paris.

IRDES – Institut de Recherche et Documentation en Économie de la Santé (2010), "Enquête sur la santé et la protection sociale", Paris.

OECD (2013), *Government at a Glance 2013*, OECD Publishing, Paris, *http://dx.doi.org/10.1787/gov_glance-2013-en*.

OECD (2012a), *Restoring Public Finances, 2012 Update*, OECD Publishing, Paris, *http://dx.doi.org/10.1787/9789264179455-en*.

OECD (2012b), *Health at a Glance Europe 2012*, OECD Publishing, Paris, *http://dx.doi.org/10.1787/9789264183896-en*.

OECD (2011a), *Government at a Glance 2011*, OECD Publishing, Paris, *http://dx.doi.org/10.1787/gov_glance-2011-en*.

OECD (2011b), *Health at a Glance 2011: OECD Indicators*, OECD Publishing, Paris, *http://dx.doi.org/10.1787/health_glance-2011-en*.

Penaud, P., Y.G. Amghar and F. Bourdais (2011), *Politiques sociales*, Presses de Sciences Po and Dalloz, Paris.

Porta, J. (2010), "Le comité d'alerte sur l'évolution des dépenses d'assurance-maladie – Étude de cas", with P.A. Adele, European Commission Sixth Framework Programme – Integrated Project, *Working Paper* REFGOV-SGI-23, Catholic University of Leuven, Belgium, pp. 1-23.

Fiscal Sustainability of Health Systems
Bridging Health and Finance Perspectives

Chapter 9

Health care budgeting in the United Kingdom

by
Anita Charlesworth*

In this chapter, budgeting challenges in the United Kingdom health system are discussed. Health spending trends are presented, followed by a summary of the relevant institutional frameworks for budgeting. Government measures to reduce cost pressures are then assessed, in terms of their ability to make cost savings, their effect on the government's overall structural budget position and their impact on service standards. Evidence on the extent of future funding pressures are then discussed.

* Anita Charlesworth is Chief Economist with the Health Foundation.

9.1. Overview of health in government expenditure

The United Kingdom spent 9.3% of GDP on health in 2012, in line with the OECD average. This is USD 3 289 per capita (adjusted for purchasing power parity), around 5% below the OECD average. Public health spending accounts for an above-average share of total health spending – 84% compared to the OECD average of 72.2% in 2012 (OECD, 2014).

The proportion of UK public spending allocated to the National Health Service (NHS) has risen steadily, from 9.3% in 1949-50 to 18.1% in 2013-14 (Figure 9.1). As a result, almost GBP 1 in every GBP 5 of UK government spending now goes to health care.

Figure 9.1. **NHS spending in the United Kingdom, as a proportion of total public spending**

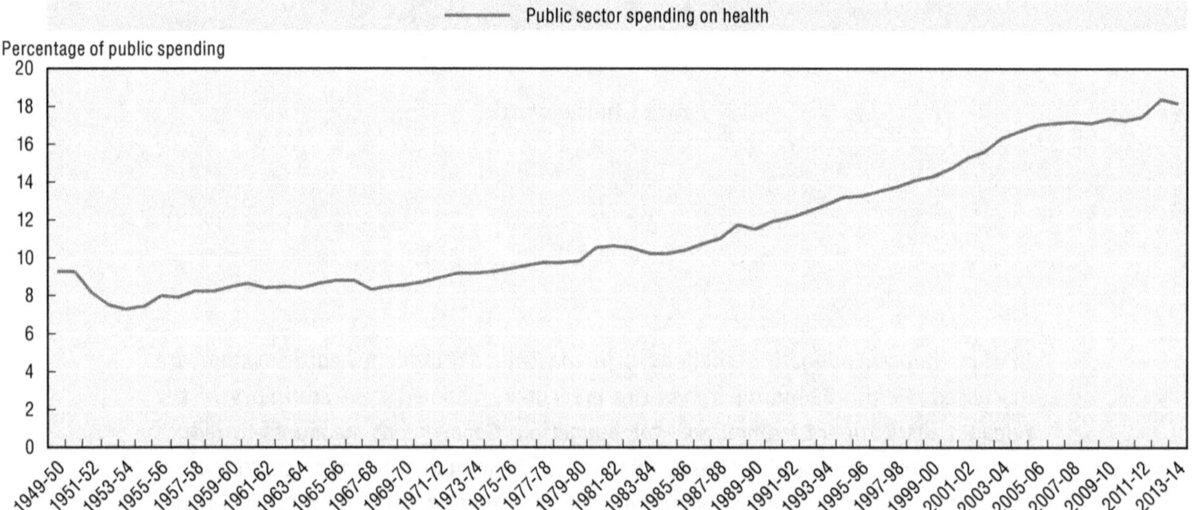

Note: GDP deflators for years 1949/50 to 1954/55 were estimated by applying the same annual change in GDP deflator as for the GDP deflators by calendar year (ONS).

Source: Lloyd, T. (2015), *Funding Overview: Historical trends in the UK*, The Health Foundation, London.

StatLink http://dx.doi.org/10.1787/888933219259

Table 9.1 demonstrates that the rapid growth in health spending has not been accompanied by an increased tax burden. Looking at the three decades preceding the economic crisis, public spending on health increased from 4.3% of GDP in 1978-79 to 6.7% in 2007-08; but over the same period receipts and total government spending both fell as a share of GDP. This was possible as the composition of public spending changed. There has been a significant reduction in the share of GDP spent on other public services and on welfare, and debt interest fell as a share of GDP.

Table 9.1. **Changes in public spending as a share of GDP and tax receipts**

Share of GDP	Total public spending	Health spending	Other public services	Welfare and debt interest	Receipts
1978-79	43.5%	4.3%	25.6%	13.6%	38.6%
2007-08	39.2%	6.7%	20.1%	12.3%	36.6%
Difference	-4.3	2.5	-5.5	-1.2	-2

Source: Author's calculation using data from IFS, OBR and HM Treasury.

StatLink http://dx.doi.org/10.1787/888933219521

This compositional change is clear from a comparison of the main areas of public spending in 1978-79 and 2007-08 (Figure 9.2).

Figure 9.2. **Percentage of public spending in 1978-79 and 2010-11**

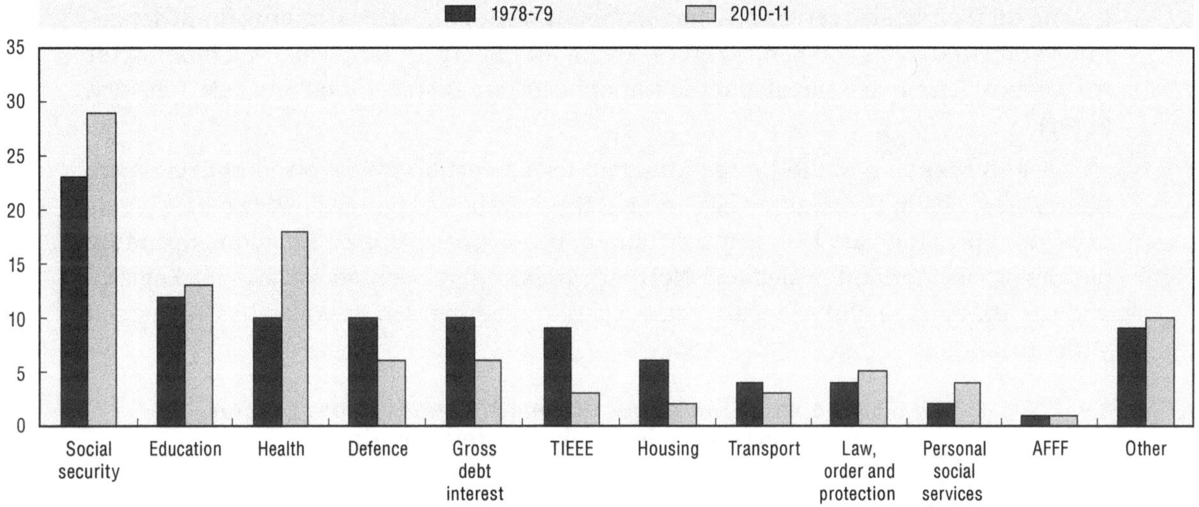

Note: AFFF is spending on agriculture, fisheries, food and forestry. TIEEE is spending on trade, industry, energy, employment and the environment. Other includes overseas spending (including overseas aid), national heritage, miscellaneous expenditure and other accounting adjustments.

Source: Author's calculations using data from Crawford, R. and P. Johnson (2011), "The Changing Composition of Public Spending", *IFS Briefing Note* No. 119, Institute for Fiscal Studies, London.

StatLink http://dx.doi.org/10.1787/888933219264

Trends in health spending

In 2000, spending on health in the United Kingdom was 7% of GDP, below the OECD average of 7.8% (OECD, 2014). In the decade that followed, spending increased rapidly in real terms and as a share of GDP. By 2012, the UK's total spending on health care as a percentage of GDP was 9.3%. This is lower than the EU15 average (ten per cent), but is in line with the OECD average of 9.3%. The United Kingdom spends less than nine other EU15 countries, although that is considerably more than in 2000 when it spent less than 13 of the 15 countries. The increase in health spending as a share of GDP in the United Kingdom in recent years has been driven by increased public spending on health. Public spending on health grew as a share of GDP while private health care spending remained stable.

Government spending on health across the United Kingdom in 2013-14 was GBP 129.4 billion or 7.5% of GDP (HM Treasury, 2014c). Since the formation of the NHS in 1948, this figure has increased by an average of 3.7% in real terms with only seven financial years where there has been a real decrease (The Health Foundation, 2015). Two of these seven years were 2010-11 and 2011-12.

Table 9.2. **Government spending on health in the United Kingdom**

Share of GDP based on UK Office for National Statistics (ONS) GDP figures published on 6 October 2014

Billion GBP	2003-04	2004-05	2005-06	2006-07	2007-08	2008-09	2009-10	2010-11	2011-12	2012-13	2013-14
Cash terms	74.9	82.9	89.8	94.7	101.1	108.7	116.9	119.9	121.3	124.3	129.4
Share of GDP	6.20%	6.50%	6.70%	6.60%	6.70%	7.20%	7.80%	7.60%	7.40%	7.50%	7.50%
Real terms (2014-15)	97.6	104.8	110.4	113.4	117.6	123.3	129.3	129	128.2	129.2	132.1
Real terms % change		7.30%	5.40%	2.70%	3.70%	4.90%	4.80%	-0.20%	-0.60%	0.80%	2.20%

Source: UK Office for National Statistics (ONS) and HM Treasury, London.

StatLink http://dx.doi.org/10.1787/888933219534

A total of 83% of UK government health spending was spent on the NHS in England. The remainder was spent by the devolved governments in Scotland, Wales and Northern Ireland on their health services. A small amount went to the Departments for Business, Innovation and Skills (BIS) and Culture, Media and Sport (DCMS). This was funding for the Medical Research Council and the National Lottery Distribution Fund (HM Treasury, 2014c).

Health spending in the United Kingdom forms part of the devolved budget of the administrations in Scotland, Wales and Northern Ireland. Figure 9.3 shows how levels of health spending vary between the four countries of the United Kingdom. Spending per person in Scotland, Wales and Northern Ireland has been above that for England and the UK average. But in recent years, spending per person in Wales has converged with England.

Figure 9.3. **The variation in public health spending per person in the four countries of the United Kingdom**

2014-15 prices

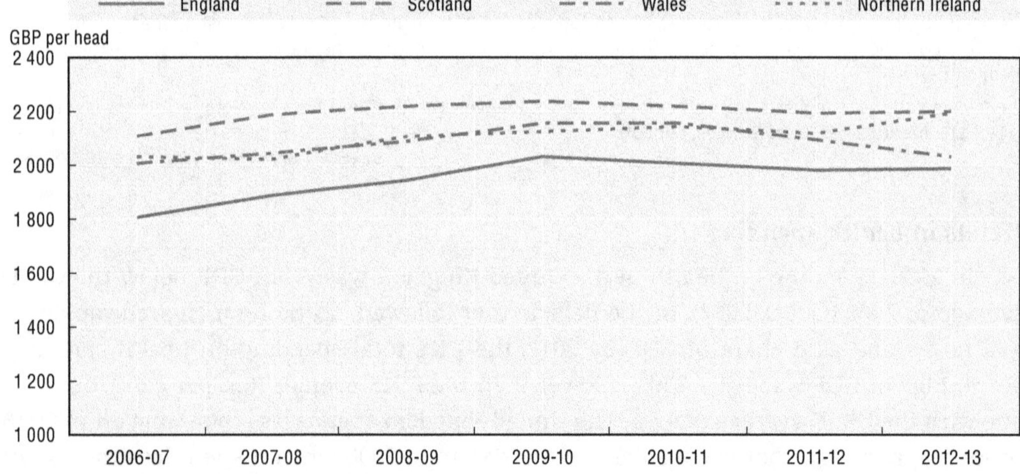

Source: Lloyd, T. (2015), *Funding Overview: Historical Trends in the UK*, The Health Foundation, London.

StatLink http://dx.doi.org/10.1787/888933219276

9.2. Institutional framework and budgeting practices

The NHS is funded by general taxation. General tax policy is the responsibility of Her Majesty's Treasury (HMT) on a UK basis. The administration of the NHS is the responsibility of the administrations of each of the four countries of the United Kingdom. For the English NHS, the budget is set by HMT as part of the periodic, cross-government public spending reviews. This sets a revenue and capital budget for the Department of Health. For Scotland, Wales and Northern Ireland, the UK government sets a population-based allocation of total public spending, comparable to that in England. The UK government does not earmark funding for specific purposes. The devolved administrations determine the allocation of public expenditure between the services under their control, including health.

The current government has undertaken two reviews of public spending in 2010 and 2013 (HM Treasury, 2010, 2013). These set out the government's spending plans for 2011-12 to 2015-16 (Figure 9.4). The English publically funded health budget is currently fixed. However, current financial and service pressures in the NHS have led the government to allocate further funding to the NHS for 2015-16 above the totals planned in the 2013 spending round (HM Treasury, 2014).

Figure 9.4. **English health budget to 2015-16**

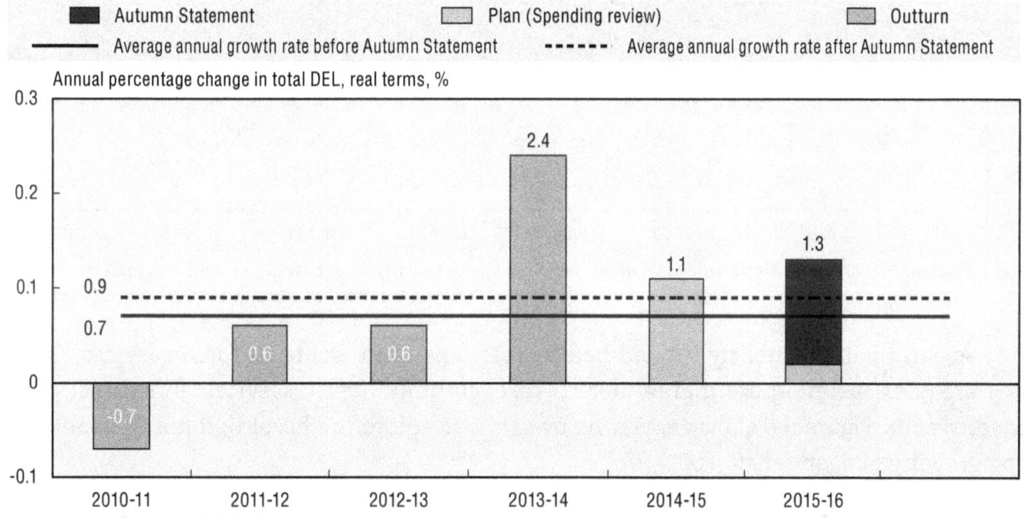

DEL: Departmental expenditure.

Source: LaFond, S. (2015), *Funding Overview: Current NHS Spending in England*, The Health Foundation, London.

StatLink http://dx.doi.org/10.1787/888933219286

The vast majority of the English budget for health care is distributed by the Department of Health to NHS England, the body responsible for commissioning health care across England. NHS England commissions primary care and specialised care services across the country. It allocates around two-thirds of its funding to the local bodies responsible for commissioning routine health care for their local population [211 Clinical Commissioning Groups (CCGs), which largely replaced the functions of Primary Care Trusts following the Health and Social Care Act 2012].

NHS England and the CCGs purchase health care from a mix of NHS and private-sector providers: acute hospitals, mental health hospitals, community nursing services and independent primary care providers (GPs, dentists and pharmacies). Most hospital, mental health and community health services in England are provided by NHS-owned and NHS-managed providers; but there has been a growth in NHS-funded but privately provided care over the last decade (Kelly and Tetlow, 2012; Arora et al., 2013). Figure 9.5 shows the growth in spending on NHS-funded care provided by non-NHS providers over recent years. As a result, the NHS now spends 11% of the budget for commissioners of care on services provided by non-NHS organisations. The use of non-NHS providers varies by health sector – a relatively small proportion of hospital services are delivered by non-NHS providers; but, in community nursing and mental health care, non-NHS providers are responsible for delivering a higher proportion of care (LaFond et al, 2014). In addition, most of the providers of primary care – GPs, dentists and pharmacists – are independent businesses.

Figure 9.5. **Purchase of NHS-funded health care from non-NHS bodies from 2006-07 to 2013-14**

2013-14 prices

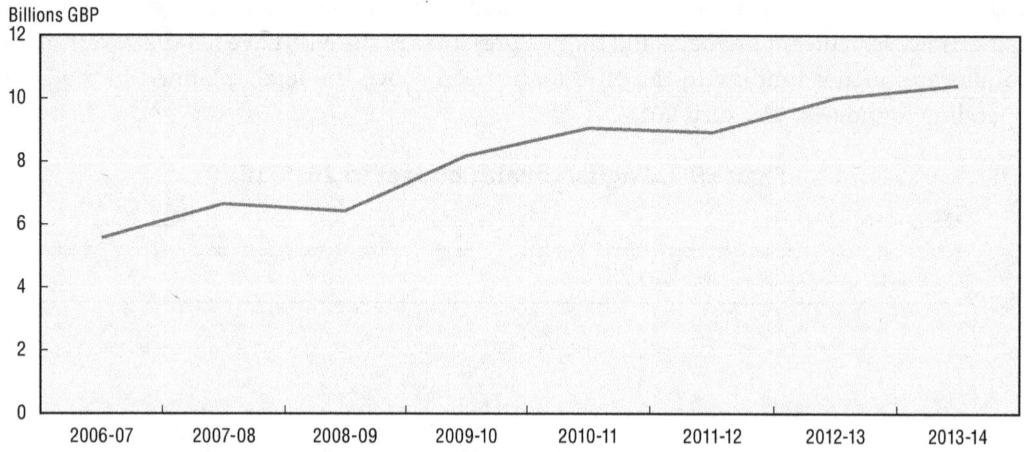

Source: LaFond, S. (2015), *Funding Overview: Current NHS Spending in England*, The Health Foundation, London.

StatLink http://dx.doi.org/10.1787/888933219294

Around half of publicly funded health spending is for acute hospital services. Other key areas of spending are mental health care, community, GP services and prescription medications. Figure 9.6 shows spending by services before the fiscal tightening to address the growing budget deficit (2009-10).

Figure 9.6. **NHS primary care trust expenditures 2009-10 – GBP 97.5 billion**

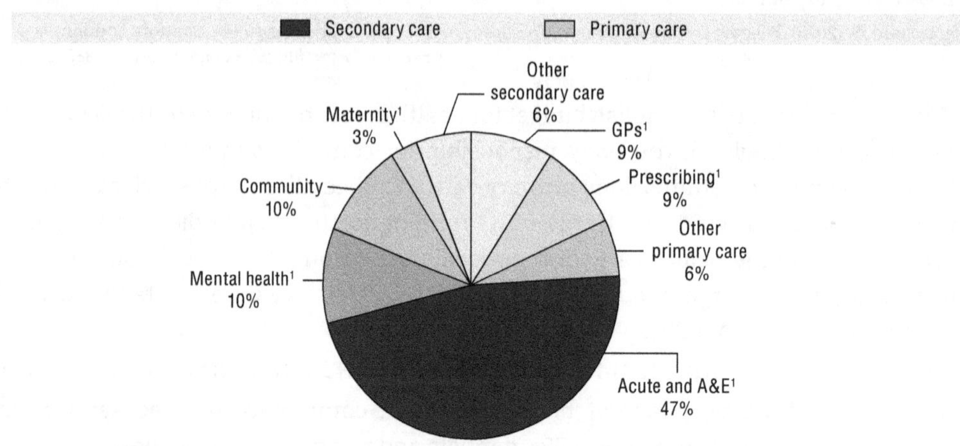

A&E: Accident & emergency.

1. Included in model.

Source: Primary Care Trust (PCT) financial accounts 2009-10.

StatLink http://dx.doi.org/10.1787/888933219302

Figure 9.7. **Percentage change from previous year in English NHS spending by service area**

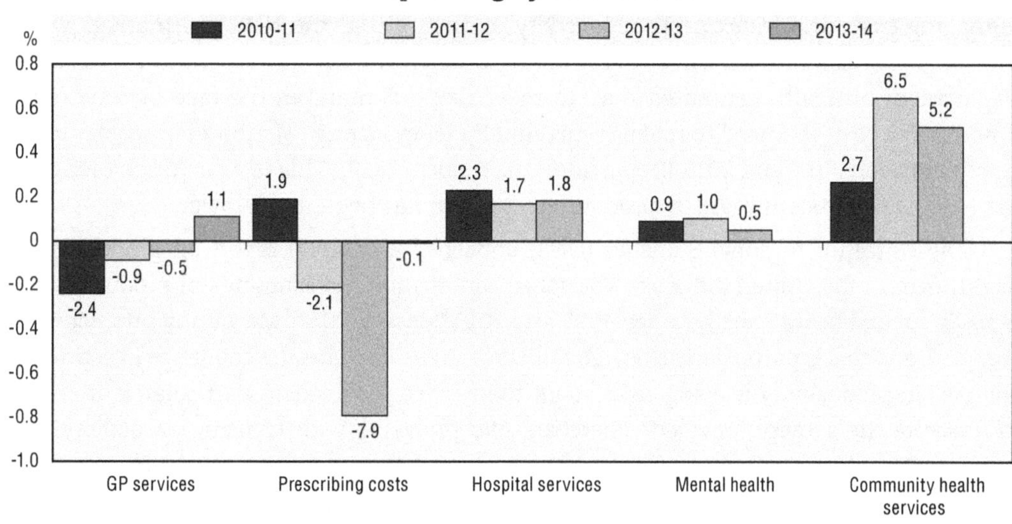

Source: LaFond, S. (2015), *Funding Overview: Current NHS spending in England*. The Health Foundation, London.

StatLink http://dx.doi.org/10.1787/888933219315

Figure 9.7 shows how spending in different service areas has changed since 2010-11.

Direct patient charges make a small contribution to the cost of NHS care. The key areas of charging and co-payments are for prescriptions and services. The bulk of prescription medications are funded by the NHS although there is a small co-pay (GBP 8.05 for item as of April 2014) but with widespread exemptions including all children under age 16, everyone aged over 60 and pregnant women. This means that around 90% of all prescriptions in the NHS are dispensed free of charge (Barker et al., 2014). As a result, the prescription charge system raises a small amount, GBP 471 million in England in 2013-14 (Department of Health, 2014). The exemption regime for dentistry is more complex but also includes children, pregnant women and people on means-tested benefits. For older people, exemptions are more limited than for prescriptions and focused on those on low incomes. In 2013-14, dental charges raised GBP 684 million (Department of Health, 2014). In total across all services, patient fees and charges accounted for around 1.4% of public health spending in the English NHS.

NHS providers are a mix of directly managed hospitals and more autonomous foundation trusts which remain fully public sector bodies but have more freedom to manage their own affairs with risk-based oversight from a national health care regulator (Monitor). These bodies have some flexibility to borrow from the private sector and can earn private income (subject to a cap). The aggregate surplus or deficit of NHS providers forms part of the consolidated financial position of the Department of Health and the UK's government's overall fiscal position.

9.3. Controlling key elements of health expenditures

The government's policy to manage health expenditure since the economic crisis has the following key components:

- a cap on total public health spending
- a reduction in input pressures
- a funding focus on front-line delivery
- improved productivity.

The cap on the health budget since 2010 is the tightest aggregate four-year budget set for the NHS since the 1950s (Crawford and Emmerson, 2012). There is a major focus on managing costs and improving productivity to ensure that the NHS can manage within the tougher fiscal climate whilst maintaining quality of care and access to services. The Department of Health estimated that, to meet rising demand in the face of constrained funding, the NHS will need to make recurrent efficiency savings of around 4% a year in real terms between 2011 and 2015 (Department of Health, 2012). This is a major challenge for the NHS as over recent years its productivity growth has been much lower.

The Office for National Statistics (ONS) publishes an annual report on productivity in health care in the United Kingdom. The latest report provides estimates of productivity for publicly funded health care between 1995 and 2010 (Massey, 2012). Measuring productivity is complex, and this is particularly true in health care. In health care, the challenge in estimating changes in productivity is being clear about the service provided. In particular, is it enough to measure the activity provided? There are two problems with focusing on activity: first, activity alone does not capture changes in quality, yet these are very important outputs of health services; and second, the link between activity and health outcomes is variable. The measurement of productivity of health services is therefore subject to much debate (Black, 2012; Grice, 2012). The ONS measurement attempts to capture quality-adjusted output. The choice and comprehensiveness of quality measures and the relative weight quality is given in the productivity measure will impact on the conclusions that can be drawn.

Figure 9.8. **Health care output, inputs and productivity estimates (nominal terms), 1995-2010, United Kingdom**

Index numbers 1995 = 100

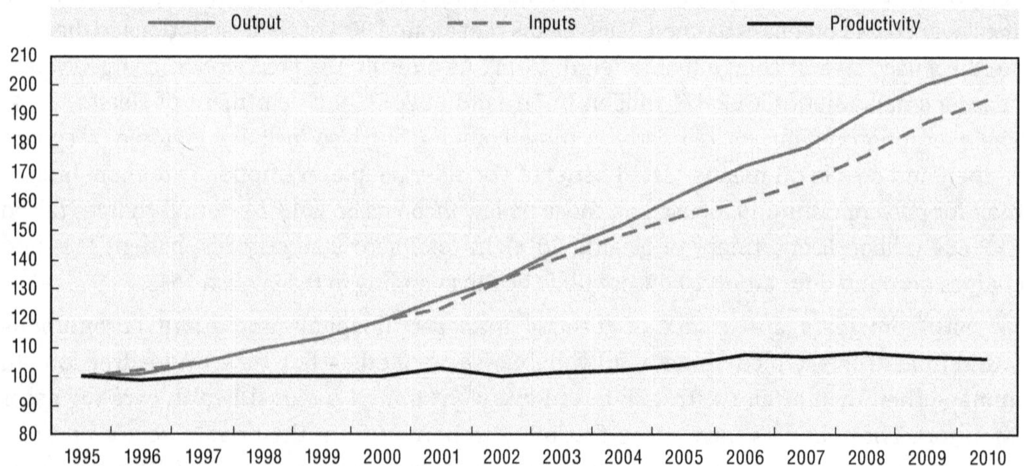

Source: Massey, F. (2012), "Public Service Productivity Estimates: Health Care, 2010", Office for National Statistics, London.

StatLink http://dx.doi.org/10.1787/888933219328

The ONS defines health care productivity as the ratio of quality-adjusted output to the volume of inputs. The outputs are measured as a cost-weighted activity index covering hospital and community health services (hospital inpatient and day cases, outpatient visits and community nursing activity) and primary care (GP and nurse visits, sight tests, prescriptions and dental treatments). These outputs are adjusted for quality, based on the extent to which services succeed in delivering their intended outcomes and the extent to which they were responsive to user needs. The inputs are measured as labour, spending on goods and services, and capital consumption. The ONS produces productivity estimates on data from 1995 onwards for the United Kingdom.[1] Both outputs and inputs have grown continuously during this period, but there was a more rapid increase in outputs than in inputs between 2004 and 2006 (Figure 9.8). The ONS estimates that between 1995 and 2010 the output in the United Kingdom rose by 107% and the input by 95%. This results in an estimated UK productivity growth of 0.4% per year between 1995 and 2010.

Combining the ONS estimates with Cost-Weighted Activity Index (CWAI) estimates[2] for earlier years, it was estimated that productivity in the health care sector has risen on average by about 1% a year between 1979 and 2010 (OBR, 2014a).

The ONS measures of productivity on a UK-wide basis only have data up to 2010, the start of the current period of austerity in the health service. A separate study measures productivity for England only but on a very similar basis to the ONS research. It finds that recent productivity growth has been higher, increasing at a rate of 1.5% a year between 2004-05 and 2011-12. (Bojke et al., 2014).

There are two central government initiatives to help the NHS meet the productivity challenge presented by the tight fiscal settlement. The government introduced a public sector pay policy to reduce input costs. Workforce costs are the single largest element of NHS providers' expenditures. Pay per head for hospital and community health service staff rose by an average of around 2% a year in real terms over the 35 years to 2009-10 (authors' calculations, based on Department of Health, 2011). The government froze pay awards for all public sector workers, including NHS staff, earning basic salaries of more than GBP 21 000 a year in 2011-12 and 2012-13; staff earning less than GBP 21 000 were awarded GBP 250 a year cash uplifts in April 2011 and 2012 (NHS Employers, 2012a). For 2013-14 and 2014-15, the government has set public sector pay awards at an average of 1% a year in cash terms (HM Treasury, 2011).

Despite the two-year pay freeze, overall earnings and aggregate pay costs in the NHS have increased in cash terms due to staff moving up through incremental pay steps, the employment of additional staff and a growing reliance on temporary and agency staff who receive a pay premium. While earnings per head is still rising in cash terms (1.2% a year), in real terms there was a small reduction between 2010-11 and 2013-14 (0.6% a year) (Health Foundation, 2015; see Figure 9.9). Estimates by the Nuffield Trust suggest that the government's pay policy will deliver around 40% of the efficiency savings required between 2011 and 2015 (Roberts et al., 2012).

Figure 9.9. **NHS Staff annual average earnings per person 2010-11 to 2013-14**

2014-15 prices

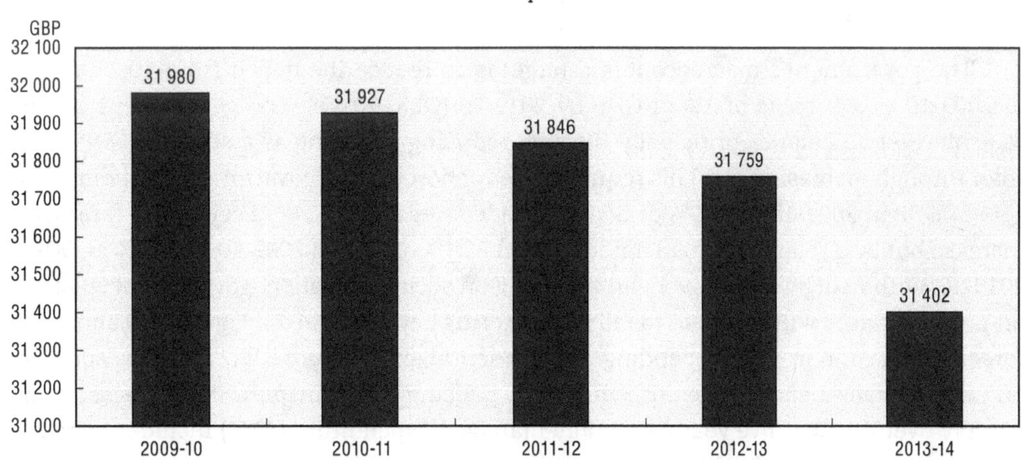

Source: Authors' calculations based on data from the Health and Social Care Information Centre and HM Treasury.

StatLink http://dx.doi.org/10.1787/888933219336

The second area of central government action to support improved productivity is a focus on reducing administrative costs. As part of the 2010 spending review, NHS administrative costs were ring-fenced and reduced in real terms by a third (HM Treasury, 2010). The NHS has been restructured to support this with the abolition of a tier of NHS management (the nine regional Strategic Health Authorities). Administrative costs have fallen from just over 5% at the start of the decade to 2.8% of health spending in England in 2013-14 (HM Treasury, 2014c).

Alongside these national initiatives, the Department of Health and the NHS have a programme to deliver savings and improve efficiency across the NHS, the Quality, Innovation, Production and Prevention (QIPP) programme. Each local commissioning body (PCT/CCG) has a plan to deliver savings, including better medicines management and demand-management measures to reduce growth in the use of hospital care. But a significant component of the savings comes from reducing the price commissioners pay NHS and other providers for care. The national tariff (DRG prices) that commissioners pay NHS providers for care has been reduced by an average of 1.5% in cash terms between 2011-12 and 2014-15 (Marshall et al., 2014). Each NHS provider is then responsible for developing a cost-improvement plan to realise savings. Around 40% of the savings result from nationally-driven initiatives such as the pay policy and reducing the administrative costs of national bodies. A further 40% of the savings are being delivered by health care providers improving their efficiency and reducing cost (through better procurement, a reduction in back-office costs and medicine management). The final 20% is expected to come from more transformative changes in the way services are delivered: shifting care to community rather than hospital settings and more effective management of ambulatory care-sensitive conditions (NAO, 2012). NHS England estimates that over the last four years total savings of GBP 21 billion will have been delivered (2014-15 prices) (Charlesworth, 2015).

Despite the initiatives to reduce input costs and increase productivity, the NHS in England is finding it harder to maintain the quality of care and deliver financial balance. In 2013-14, the NHS had 66 providers in deficit, double the year before. Early indications of NHS financial performance suggest that NHS trust performance deteriorated in 2014-15. The problems are concentrated in acute hospitals. At September 2014, 80% of all NHS acute hospital providers in England were in deficit, amounting to a net deficit of just over GBP 700 million (Charlesworth, 2015).

9.4. The impact of health on the government's structural budget position

The government's macroeconomic target is to reduce the deficit from 10.2% of GDP in 2009-10 to a surplus of 1% of GDP by 2019-20 (OBR, 2014b). The government intends to achieve fiscal balance principally through reducing spending as a share of GDP rather than through increasing tax. This requires a reduction in total government spending from 45% of GDP in 2009-10 to 35.2% of GDP a decade later in 2019-20. Receipts are forecast to increase but by a relatively small amount from 35.1% of GDP in 2009-10 to 36.2% of GDP in 2019-20. With rising debt interest and spending on social protection, government spending on public services will continue to fall in real terms beyond 2014-15. Figure 9.10 shows the forecast reduction in public spending. Departmental expenditure (DEL) includes spending on public services such as health, education, policing and transport. It is forecast to fall sharply over the next five years. Annually managed expenditure (AME) includes spending on social protection and debt interest and is more stable.

Figure 9.10. **DEL and AME components**

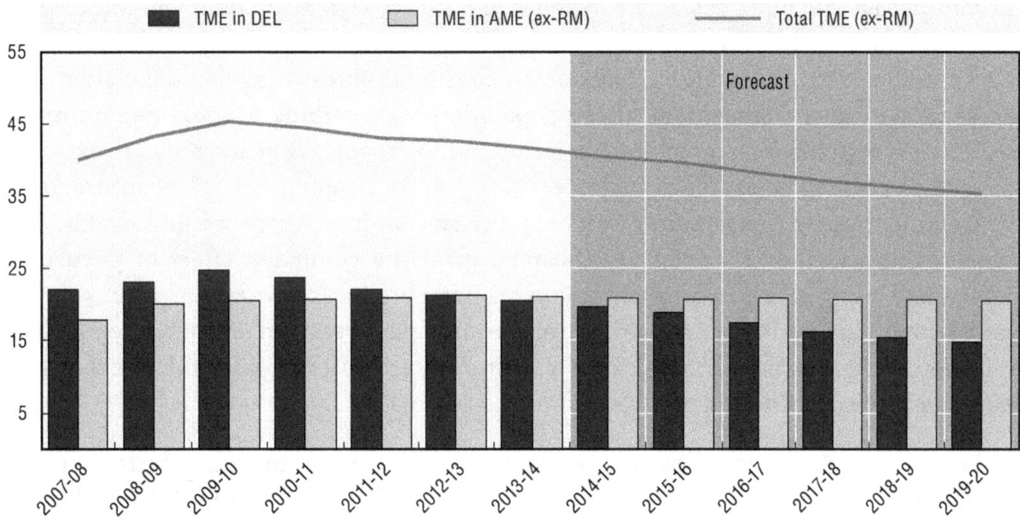

AME: Annually managed expenditure; DEL: Departmental expenditure; RM: Royal Mail; TME: Total Managed Expenditure.

Source: OBR (2014), *Economic and Fiscal Outlook*, Office of Budget Responsibility, The Stationery Office, London.

This puts pressure on the health budget. Work by the Nuffield Trust has examined the impact of demographic changes, rising chronic disease and input costs on health spending pressures. This research shows aggregate funding pressures on the NHS in England continuing to increase by around 4% a year up to 2021-22. If health service funding is held constant in real terms throughout this decade, this would result in a gap between the pressure on the health budget and funding available of around GBP 44 billion in 2010-11 prices (Roberts et al., 2012, see Figure 9.11).

Figure 9.11. **The financial gap by 2021-22, assuming English NHS funding rises as set out in the 2010 Spending Review to 2014-15 and is frozen in real terms**

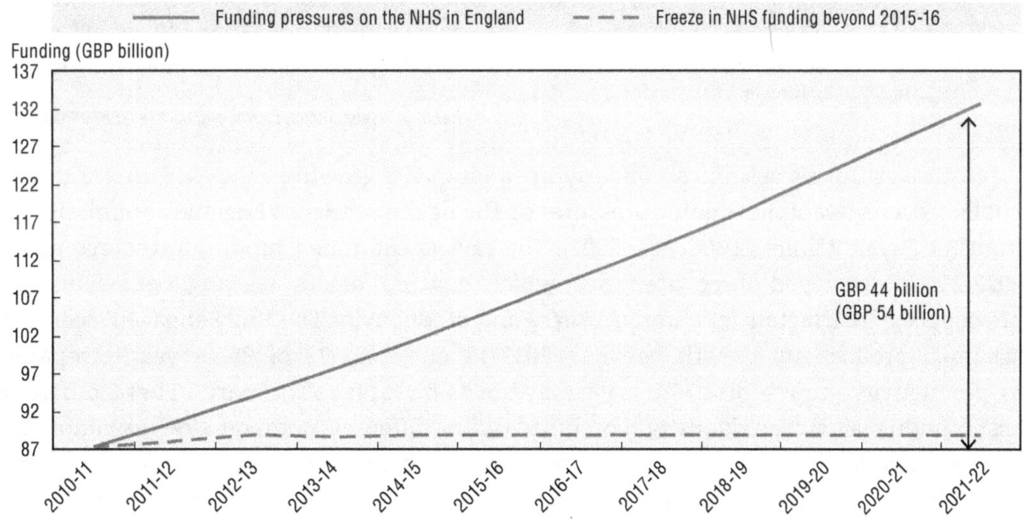

Source: Roberts, A., L. Marshall L and A. Charlesworth (2012), "A Decade of Austerity? The Funding Pressures Facing the NHS from 2011-12 to 2021-22", Nuffield Trust, London.

StatLink http://dx.doi.org/10.1787/888933219352

Within the acute sector we can examine the relative contribution of demography, chronic disease and input costs. The next decade will see significant demographic change. The population of England is projected to increase by 4 million from 52.1 million in 2010 to 56.4 million 2021. In addition, England is expected to have an ageing population over the same period; the percentage of the population over working age will rise from 16% to 19%. Although these changes are significant, during the next decade they are expected to result in funding pressures of just over 1% a year for hospital care. If recent trends in the treatment and management of chronic disease continue, there would be additional pressures of a further 1% a year for hospital care. The combined effect of population change and rising admission for chronic conditions produces demand pressures on the acute services in England of 3% a year in real terms. If pay pressures return to their historic trend before the economic crisis (2% per year in real terms) this would add a further 1% a year to hospital costs (Figure 9.12).

Figure 9.12. **Funding pressures on acute services in England attributable to population change and to the rising probability of admission for chronic conditions**

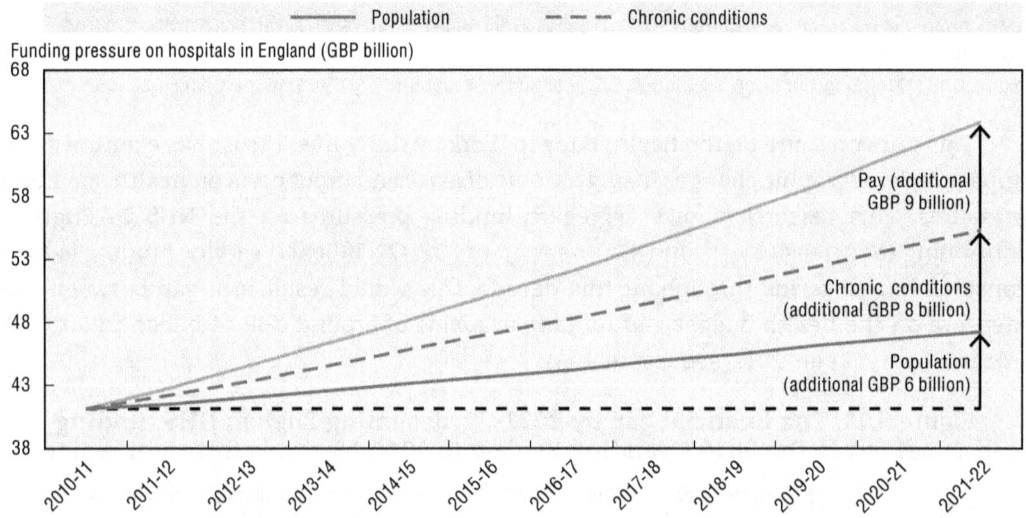

Source: Roberts, A., L. Marshall L and A. Charlesworth (2012), *A Decade of Austerity? The Funding Pressures Facing the NHS from 2011-12 to 2021-22*, Nuffield Trust, London.

StatLink http://dx.doi.org/10.1787/888933219360

These estimates assume no underlying productivity growth in the NHS. In 2002, HMT published a review of the funding pressures on the health service in England commissioned from Sir Derek Wanless (Wanless, 2002). The review examined funding pressures up to 2022-23. It developed three scenarios which covered health seeking behaviour, the prevalence of risk factors for chronic disease and productivity. The "fully engaged" scenario assumed productivity growth between 2012-13 and 2022-23 of 3% a year compared to productivity growth of 1.75% a year in the "slow uptake" scenario. These different assumptions about productivity combined with different demand-side assumptions produce significant differences in the pressures on health funding. Table 9.3 compares the funding pressure projections for the three scenarios from the Wanless Review. The low-productivity, high-demand scenario (slow uptake) results in pressure on health funding which are 2 percentage points of GDP higher in 2022-23 than the high-productivity, low-demand scenario (fully engaged).

Table 9.3. **The 2002 Wanless Review projections of English NHS funding pressures**

	Projections				
	2002-03[1]	2007-08	2012-13	2017-18	2022-23
Total health spending (percent of money GDP)[2]					
Solid progress	7.7	9.4	10.5	10.9	11.1
Slow uptake	7.7	9.5	11	11.9	12.5
Fully engaged	7.7	9.4	10.3	10.6	10.6
Total NHS spending (GBP billion, 2002-03 prices)					
Solid progress	68	96	121	141	161
Slow uptake	68	97	127	155	184
Fully engaged	68	96	119	137	154
Average annual real growth in NHS spending (%)[3]					
Solid progress	6.8	7.1	4.7	3.1	2.7
Slow uptake	6.8	7.3	5.6	4	3.5
Fully engaged	6.8	7.1	4.4	2.8	2.4

1. Estimates.

2. All figures include 1.2% for private sector health spending.

3. Growth figures are annual averages for the five years up to date shown (four years for the period to 2002-03).

Source: Wanless, D. (2002), *Securing our Future Health: Taking a Long-Term View, Final Report*, HM Treasury, London.

StatLink http://dx.doi.org/10.1787/888933219547

NHS England recently published updated estimates of the funding pressures facing the NHS in England for the next five years (2015-16 to 2020-21). They estimate that funding pressures on the NHS will be GBP 30 billion higher at the end of the decade (NHS England, 2014). They then estimate the additional funding requirement above inflation under three scenarios for productivity. These are shown in Table 9.4.

Table 9.4. **NHS England funding pressures facing the NHS by the end of the decade**

Productivity growth assumption	Funding requirement above inflation
0.8% a year	GBP 21 billion
1.5% a year	GBP 16 billion
2-3% a year	GBP 8 billion

Note: NHS England's projections of total spending are in cash terms, allowing them to explore the impact of cost pressures (such as pay) separately to assumptions for GDP deflators. The budget for NHS England is then assumed to rise with inflation.

Source: Charlesworth, A. (2015), "Briefing: NHS Finances – The Challenge All Political Parties Need to Face", The Health Foundation, London.

StatLink http://dx.doi.org/10.1787/888933219557

Recent work by the Health Foundation has used the methodology developed in the Nuffield Trust work to extend the funding projections to 2030. Under the central projection, the NHS in England will continue to achieve productivity close to 1.5% a year, in line with recent trends. Therefore, if a high-quality, comprehensive service is to be maintained, funding will need to rise by around 3% a year, slightly above the expected rate of economic growth of 2.4% a year. If NHS productivity matches the estimate of whole economy trend rate of productivity growth (2.2% a year), public health spending as a share of GDP could remain broadly constant and meet projected pressures. But there is no evidence that productivity at this rate could be sustained in the medium term. Health care provision is relatively labour intensive and it is therefore likely that productivity growth will be slower in this sector than in the economy as a whole. But over the medium term, wages in the sector would still need to rise in line with those in the whole economy. This would lead to what is known as "Baumol's disease" where the cost of the health service rises relative to other sectors of the economy. To maintain an increase in the level of service provided in line with increases in real output across the rest of the economy, government expenditure would have to increase more rapidly than GDP growth.

Table 9.5. **Health Foundation projected funding gap for English NHS in 2030-31 under three assumptions for productivity**

Annual rate of productivity growth	Average annual increase in NHS spending	NHS England estimate 2020/21	Funding gap in 2030-31:		
			Budget stays flat in real terms	Budget rises by 1.6% a year in real terms	Budget rises by 2.4% a year in real terms
0.0%	4.3%	GBP 30 billion	GBP 108 billion	GBP 78 billion	GBP 58 billion
1.5%	2.9%	GBP 16 billion	GBP 65 billion	GBP 34 billion	GBP 15 billion
2.2%	2.2%	GBP 8 billion	GBP 48 billion	GBP 17 billion	GBP 2 billion surplus

Source: The Health Foundation 2015.

StatLink http://dx.doi.org/10.1787/888933219562

Figure 9.13. **Funding pressures on English NHS in 2030-31**

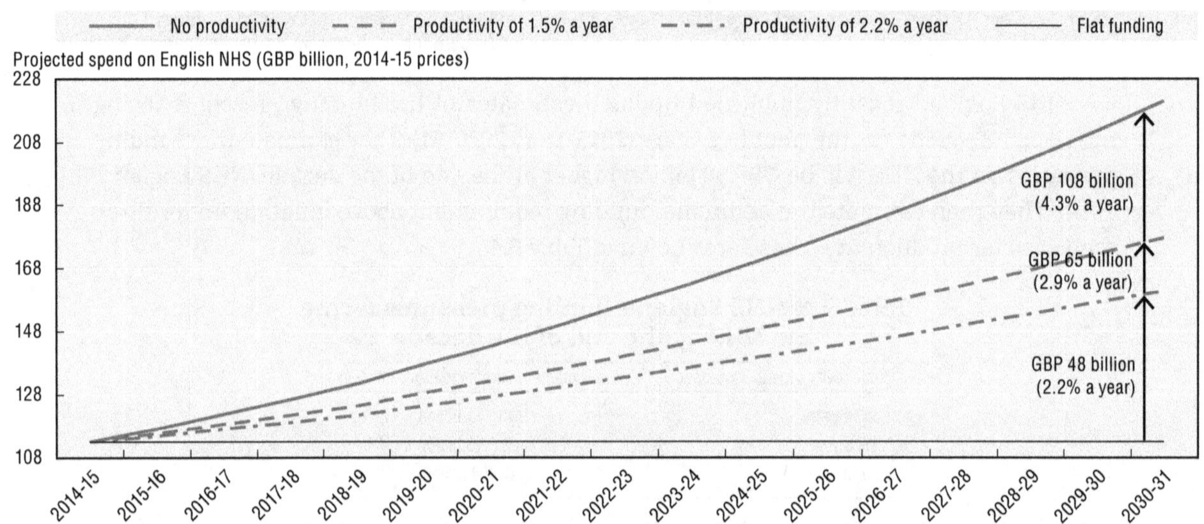

Source: The Health Foundation, 2015.

StatLink http://dx.doi.org/10.1787/888933219376

The work by NHS England, the Nuffield Trust and the Health Foundation looks at the medium-term funding pressures and funding outlook for health (Figure 9.13). For fiscal sustainability we also need to examine the long term. The UK's Office of Budget Responsibility produces long-term fiscal projections over a 50-year horizon (OBR, 2014a). The OBR latest assessment concludes that:

- Public spending other than on debt interest is projected to increase from 34.3% of GDP in 2018-19 to 39.1% of GDP in 2063-64.
- Public health spending is a key contributor to rising spending pressures. It is expected to increase by at least 2.1% of GDP by 2063-64, but this is very sensitive to assumptions about productivity. Long-term care costs are also projected to rise, with public spending increasing by 1.1% of GDP over the projection period.

- Non-interest revenues are projected to be broadly stable. They are projected to rise from 37.3% of GDP in 2018-19 to 37.4% of GDP in 2063-64.
- With spending pressures increasing above projected revenue growth, the overall fiscal position would deteriorate. The primary budget balance is projected to be in deficit of 1.7% of GDP by 2063-64. Public sector net debt is projected to be 74% of GDP in 2015-16. This is projected to fall to 53% of GDP in the mid-2030s but rise rapidly again to reach 84% of GDP in 2063-64.

If productivity growth in the health sector grew in line with recent trends rather than at the rate of the whole economy, real health spending per person would need to rise by 3.4% a year to increase health output by 2.2% a year, in line with real earnings growth. This would see health spending in 2063-64 rise by around 5.9% of GDP and result in a significantly higher path for net debt.

Figure 9.14 shows the difference in productivity estimates between different sectors of the economy. Health and social work productivity is estimated to be around 59% of whole economy productivity.

Figure 9.14. **Change in sectoral job share and level of productivity**

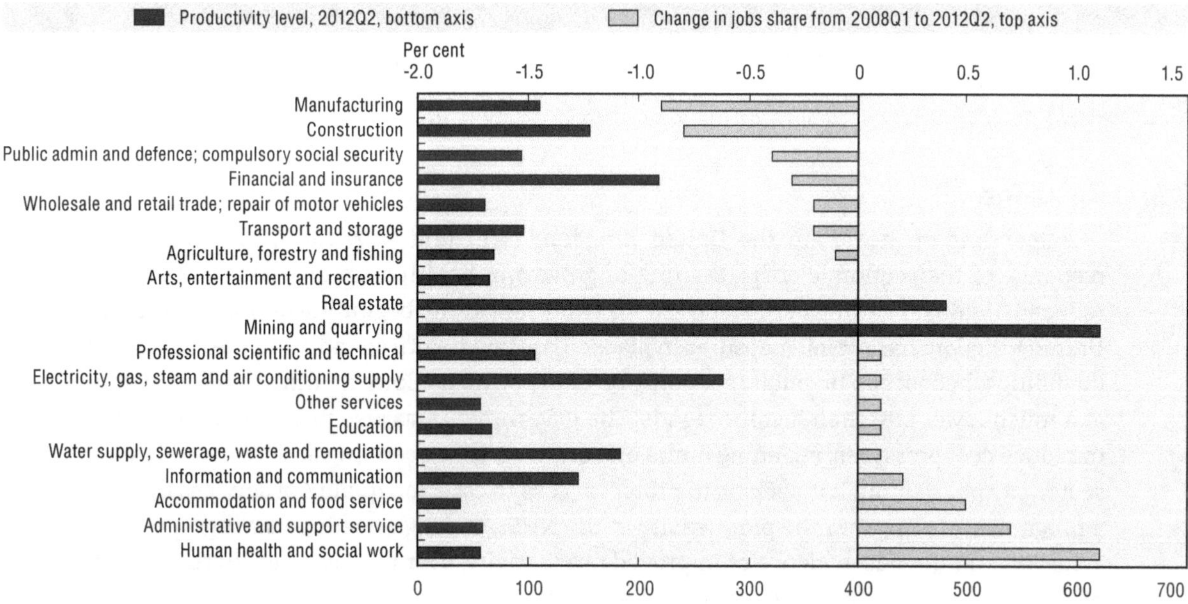

Source: Office for Budget Responsibility (2012), *Fiscal Sustainability Report*, Office of Budget Responsibility, The Stationery Office, London, *http://budgetresponsibility.org.uk/pubs/FSR2012WEB.pdf*.

StatLink http://dx.doi.org/10.1787/888933219387

Research by the Kings Fund has examined the factors which influence health and social care demand over a 50-year period. It reviewed a range of medium-term projections for health (Appleby, 2013). Figure 9.15 from the report compares some of the key projections.

This highlights the uncertainty about the path of spending in the long term. As Appleby notes, for health spending as a share of GDP the OBR's 2012 highest scenario for spending projection suggests that it will have reached 16.6% of GDP by 2061-62. Although this is much higher than current spending it is still lower than US health care spending was in 2010.

Figure 9.15. **A century of health spending: Projections of UK health care expenditure, 1960-2059**

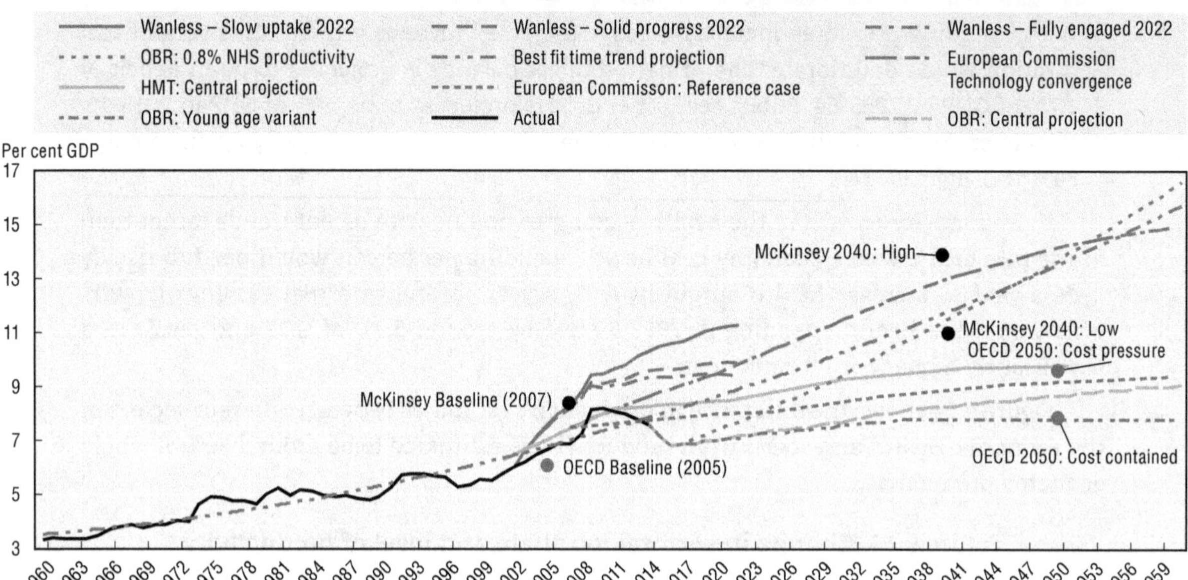

Note: HMT: Her Majesty's Treasury; OBR: Office for Budget Responsibility. All projections are for public health care spending except McKinsey & Co's, which includes private health care expenditure.

Source: Appleby, J. (2013), *Spending on Health and Social Care over the Next 50 Years: Why Think Long Term?*, The King's Fund, London.

9.5. Conclusion

Spending on health in the United Kingdom is in line with the OECD average. In response to the economic crisis, the rate of growth in health spending has been sharply reduced. Health spending per person fell for two years at the beginning of this decade. The United Kingdom has robust measures in place to contain health spending in the short term, including a budget cap on public spending on health which allows health spending to grow at a much lower rate than historic trends. The government has also put in place measures to reduce cost pressures, including limits on administrative spending and a national public sector pay policy limit. It is seeking to protect access to care and quality of services through a programme to improve the productivity of the NHS. Although headline savings are being achieved and there is evidence of improved productivity, over the last year there are signs of pressure on both the budget and service standards. A significant number of NHS acute hospitals are in deficit and national targets for accident and emergency, elective surgery waiting times and cancer care are not being delivered. In December 2014, the government responded by increasing funding for the financial year 2015-16.

Beyond the current economic crisis, however, the United Kingdom faces a fiscal sustainability challenge. Health is an increasing share of total public spending. Health spending (along with pensions) is a major driver of the long-term growth in public spending. At present, health is projected to increase at a faster rate than government receipts. The scale of the potential fiscal gap is very dependent on assumptions about the long-run trend rate of growth in health service productivity.

Notes

1. A change in methodology in 2011 by the ONS means that services provided by non-NHS organisations now count as both an input and an output, while previously these were only counted as an input. This means that estimates produced after 2011 using ONS data are inconsistent with later estimates.
2. Cost-Weighted Activity Index (CWAI) for Hospital and Community Services in England from 1979 to 2000-01 (Oliver, 2005), The English National Health Service: 1979-2005, *Health Economics*, Vol. 14 pp. S75-S99. These estimates do not cover all hospital activities and are not adjusted for quality.

References

Appleby, J. (2013), *Spending on Health and Social Care over the Next 50 Years: Why Think Long Term?*, The King's Fund, London.

Barker, K., G. Alltimes, R. Bichard, S. Greengross and J. LeGrand (2014), *A new Settlement for Health and Social Care: Final Report*, The King's Fund, London, September.

Baumol, W.J., D. de Ferranti, M. Malach, A. Pablos Mendez, H. Tabish and L. Gomory Wu (2012), *The Cost Disease: Why Computers get Cheaper and Health Care Doesn't*, Yale University Press, New Haven, United States.

Black, N. (2012), "Declining Healthcare Productivity in England: The Making of a Myth", *The Lancet* 379(9821), Elsevier, Amsterdam, pp. 1167-1169.

Bojke, C., A. Castelli, K. Grasic and A. Street (2014), *Productivity of the English National Health Service From 2004-5: Updated to 2011-12*, Centre for Health Economics, University of York, United Kingdom.

Charlesworth, A. (2015), "Briefing: NHS Finances – The Challenge All Political Parties Need to Face", The Health Foundation, London.

Crawford, R. and C. Emmerson (2012), *NHS and Social Care Funding: The Outlook to 2021-22*, Nuffield Trust, London.

Crawford, R. and P. Johnson (2011), "The Changing Composition of Public Spending", *IFS Briefing Note* No. 119, Institute for Fiscal Studies, London.

Department of Health (UK) (2012), Quality, Innovation, Productivity and Prevention (QIPP), *www.dh.gov.uk/health/category/policy-areas/nhs/quality/qipp*, accessed 14 November 2012.

Department of Health (UK) (2011), HCHS Pay and Prices Series 2010–11. Hospital and Community Health Services, London, *www.info.doh.gov.uk/doh/finman.nsf/af3d43e36a4c8f8500256722005b77f8/276315c0677bf547802596b00418a4d?OpenDocument*, accessed 14 November 2012.

Grice, J. (2012), "The 'Myth" of Declining Healthcare Productivity in England", *The Lancet*, Vol. 380, No. 9837, Elsevier, Amsterdam.

Harker, R. (2012), "NHS Funding and Expenditure: Social and General Statistics", House of Commons Library, London.

Hawe, E. and L. Cockcroft (2013), *OHE Guide to UK Health and Healthcare Statistics*, second ed., Office of Health Economics, London.

HMT – HM Treasury (2014a), *Autumn Statement* 2014, Cm 8961, HM Treasury, The Stationery Office, *www.gov.uk/government/uploads/system/uploads/attachment_data/file/382327/44695_Accessible.pdf*.

HMT (2014b), "GDP Deflators: September 2014", Quarterly National Accounts: GDP Deflators at Market Prices, and Money GDP, HM Treasury, London, *www.gov.uk/government/uploads/system/uploads/attachment_data/file/362191/GDP_Deflators_Qtrly_National_Accounts_September_2014_update.csv/preview*.

HMT (2014c), *Public Expenditure Statistical Analyses* 2014, Cm 8902, HM Treasury, The Stationery Office, London, *www.gov.uk/government/uploads/system/uploads/attachment_data/file/330717/PESA_2014_-_print.pdf*.

HMT (2014d), "Statistical Bulletin: Public Spending Statistics November 2014", government release, 20 November 2014, HM Treasury, London, *www.gov.uk/government/uploads/system/uploads/attachment_data/file/376816/PSS_November_2014.pdf*.

HMT (2012a), *Budget 2012*, HC1853, HM Treasury, The Stationery Office, London, *http://webarchive.nationalarchives.gov.uk/20130129110402/http://cdn.hm-treasury.gov.uk/budget2012_complete.pdf*, accessed 14 November 2012.

HMT (2012b) *Public Expenditure Statistical Analysis*, Cm 8376, HM Treasury, The Stationery Office, London, *www.gov.uk/government/uploads/system/uploads/attachment_data/file/220623/pesa_complete_2012.pdf*, accessed 10 March 2013.

HMT (2011), *Autumn Statement 2011*, Cm 8231, The Stationery Office, London, *www.gov.uk/government/uploads/system/uploads/attachment_data/file/228671/8231.pdf*, accessed 14 November 2012.

HMT (2010), *Spending Review 2010*, Cm 7942, The Stationery Office, London, *www.gov.uk/government/uploads/system/uploads/attachment_data/file/203826/Spending_review_2010.pdf*, accessed 14 November 2012.

IFS – Institute of Fiscal Studies (2014), "Fiscal Facts: Spending by Function", Excel spreadsheet, Institute of Fiscal Studies, London, *www.ifs.org.uk/uploads/publications/ff/lr_spending_August_14.xls*, accessed December 2014.

IFS (2012), "Fiscal Facts", Institute of Fiscal Studies, London, *www.ifs.org.uk/fiscalFacts*, accessed March 2013.

Jones, N. and A. Charlesworth (2013), *The Anatomy of Health Spending in 2011/12: A Review of the NHS Expenditure and Labour Productivity*, Nuffield Trust, London.

Kelly, E. and G. Tetlow (2012), *Choosing the Place of Care: The Effect of Patient Choice on Treatment Location in England, 2003-2011*, Nuffield Trust, London.

LaFond, S. (2015), *Funding Overview: Current NHS spending in England*, The Health Foundation, London.

LaFond, S., S. Arora, A. Charlesworth and A. Mckeon (2014), *Into the Red? The State of the NHS' Finances*, Nuffield Trust, London.

Lloyd, T. (2015), *Funding Overview: Historical trends in the UK*, The Health Foundation, London.

Marshall, L., A. Charlesworth and J. Hurst (2014), *The NHS Payment System: Evolving Policy and Emerging Evidence*, Nuffield Trust, London.

Massey, F. (2012), *Public Service Productivity Estimates: Health Care, 2010*, Office for National Statistics, London.

National Audit Office (2012), *Progress in Making NHS Efficiency Savings*, report by the Comptroller and Auditor General, HC 686, Session 2012-13, The Stationery Office, London.

NHS Employers (2012a), "The NHS Employers Organisation Submission to the NHS Pay Review Body: 2013-14", NHS Employers, London, *www.gmb-southern.org.uk/download/nhs/pay_&_terms_and_conditions/NHS%20Employers%20submission%20to%20NHS%20Pay%20Review%20body%202013-2014.pdf*, accessed 14 November 2012.

NHS Employers (2012b), "NHS Employers' Submission to the NHS Pay Review Body on Doctors' and Dentists' Remuneration: 2013/14", NHS Employers, London, *www.nhsemployers.org/SiteCollectionDocuments/DDRB%20submission%20final%20version.pdf*, accessed 14 November 2012.

NHS England (2014), "Five Year Forward View", October 2014, NHS England, London, *www.england.nhs.uk/wp-content/uploads/2014/10/5yfv-web.pdf*.

OBR – Office for Budget Responsibility (2014a) *Fiscal Sustainability Report*, Office of Budget Responsibility, The Stationery Office, London, *http://cdn.budgetresponsibility.org.uk/41298-OBR-accessible.pdf*.

OBR (2014b) *Economic and Fiscal Outlook*, Office of Budget Responsibility, The Stationery Office, London, *http://budgetresponsibility.org.uk/pubs/December_2014_EFO-web513.pdf*.

OBR (2012a), *Fiscal Sustainability Report*, Office of Budget Responsibility, The Stationery Office, London, *http://budgetresponsibility.org.uk/pubs/FSR2012WEB.pdf*.

OBR (2012b), *Economic and Fiscal Outlook*, Office of Budget Responsibility, The Stationery Office, London, *http://cdn.budgetresponsibility.independent.gov.uk/December-2012-Economic-and-fiscal-outlook23423423.pdf*.

OECD (2014), "OECD Health Data 2014 – Frequently Requested Data", OECD, Paris, *www.oecd.org/els/health-systems/oecd-health-statistics-2014-frequently-requested-data*, accessed December 2014.

ONS – Office for National Statistics (2014a), "Gross Domestic Product Preliminary Estimate, Q3 2014", Office for National Statistics, London, *www.ons.gov.uk/ons/dcp171778_381573.pdf*.

ONS (2014b), "Quarterly National Accounts – Gross Domestic Product: Expenditure at Current Market Prices", *www.ons.gov.uk/ons/datasets-and-tables/data-selector.html?cdid=BKTL&dataset=qna&table-id=C1*.

Roberts, A. (2015), *Funding Overview: NHS funding projections*, The Health Foundation, London.

Roberts, A., L. Marshall and A. Charlesworth (2012), *A Decade of Austerity? The Funding Pressures Facing the NHS from 2011-12 to 2021-22*, Nuffield Trust, London.

Wanless, D. (2002), *Securing our Future Health: Taking a Long-Term View*, Final Report, HM Treasury, London.

Fiscal Sustainability of Health Systems
Bridging Health and Finance Perspectives

Chapter 10

Health care budgeting in the Netherlands

by
Stefan Thewissen, Patrick Jeurissen and Gijs van der Vlugt*

This chapter describes how the Netherlands implemented a unique system of regulated competition within health care in 2006. It analyses to what extent this system has managed to contain costs, and explores whether three preconditions and two budgeting principles for cost containment in a system of regulated competition are met in the Netherlands. It presents the effects of the 2006 reform on the instruments available to the government to contain costs, and in particular, the effects of the important time-lag between overspending and possible corrective measures. It gives a preliminary assessment of the results of the reform.

* The main authors of this chapter are Stefan Thewissen (Institute for New Economic Thinking at Oxford University), Patrick Jeurissen (Celsus Academy for Sustainable Healthcare, IQ Healthcare and Radboud University Medical Centre in Nijmegen, Netherlands) and Gijs van der Vlugt (Financial and Economic Policy Directorate of the Dutch Ministry of Finance). The authors sincerely thank Camila Vammalle (OECD Budgeting and Public Expenditures Division) and Michael Borowitz (OECD Health Division) for their suggestions and feedback. Much has been gained from conversations with Reinoud Doeschot and Hans van den Hoek (Healthcare Insurance Board CVZ), Laurence Kea (Spaarne hospital), Marco Varkevisser and Erik Schut (Erasmus University Rotterdam), Misja Mikkers and Rein Halbersma (Dutch Healthcare Authority NZa), Esther Mot and Albert van der Horst (CPB Netherlands Bureau for Economic Policy Analysis). An earlier version of this paper was presented at the second OECD Meeting of the Joint Network on Fiscal Sustainability of Health Systems in Paris, 25-26 March 2013. We thank Piet Stam (SiRM) for his permission to use his data on risk bearing by insurers.

10.1. Introduction

Health care in the Netherlands is organised by means of a unique system of regulated competition. As insurers and care providers compete on prices and volumes of care, this system should theoretically be able to contain health care costs by improving productivity. Nonetheless, the Netherlands was the second highest spender, after the United States, on total health care as a percentage of GDP in the OECD area in 2011.

This chapter relates recent trends in expenditures to the changing characteristics of the Dutch institutional system of regulated competition by building on academic literature and expert interviews, as well as policy papers. It illustrates these trends in more detail for hospital care, as hospitals have the highest level of turnover in acute care and were confronted with the most radical changes in their payment structures. Even though the market reforms to Dutch health care have been under way for eight years, empirical evaluations of its effects on cost containment, that is the level of growth of prices and volumes, are still lacking. This chapter contributes to the literature on health care systems and cost containment by examining the Dutch transition to regulated competition and its effects on health care prices and volumes (Marmor and Wendt, 2012). It also contributes to the literature on budgeting and cost containment in health by describing certain constraints for the government to contain costs under a system of regulated competition. This subject has not received much attention but is currently high on the agenda (White, 2013).

This chapter describes the governance system in the Netherlands in Section 10.2. In addition, it describes three preconditions under which regulated competition can effectively contain health care costs, and two budgetary principles to contain costs. Section 10.3 addresses price and volume patterns in the Netherlands and relates the available trends to the system of regulated competition. Sections 10.4 and 10.5 discuss crucial challenges the government faces in controlling and budgeting expenditures under and towards a system of regulated competition. Section 10.6 presents conclusions.

10.2. Reforming towards regulated competition

Reasons for the Dutch shift towards regulated competition

Regulated competition, in which insurers and providers compete, was initially presented and defined by Alain Enthoven (2004) in the late 1970s as a means to organise health care and stimulate both efficiency and equity. The idea was to prevent risk selection by payers through elements such as risk adjustment and community rating. At the same time, competition should be endorsed by open enrolment in insurance companies and selective purchasing on the provider market. In the late 1980s, the Netherlands took up the idea of regulated competition to steer its health care system which at that time was built on public budgeting. Necessary preconditions were implemented gradually in the 1990s. By the end of the 1990s, stiff austerity policies in public budgeting contributed to a "waiting list" crisis which opened up a policy window for the implementation of regulated competition. This was introduced in 2006 when the Health Insurance Act was passed

(Schut and Van De Ven, 2011; Maarse and Paulus, 2011; Okma and Crivelli, 2013). The main goals of the new system were to increase productivity, to create universal coverage and to free providers and payers from many of the strict regulations that existed to steer the costs of the system.[1] Liberalisation was introduced in steps to create competition between payers and providers. Among the most notable achievements are the ending of most certificate-of-need regulations for providers (2008) and central rate settings for most hospitals (2005, 2008, 2011 and 2012). Nevertheless, there is still extensive regulation in many parts of the system. Moreover, oversight mechanisms and anti-trust efforts have stepped up.

Box 10.1 summarises the main elements of the system of regulated competition in the Netherlands.

Box 10.1. **An overview of the Dutch health care system**

Funding health care and pooling risks

The Health Insurance Act is mainly funded through a 50/50 combination of income-related contributions paid through a payroll tax and "nominal" premiums that enrolees pay direct to their health insurer. There are means-tested health care allowances for the majority of households to ensure accessibility. The collected income-related contributions are pooled and distributed amongst insurers to compensate for their enrolees' different risk profiles in order to prevent risk selection. Thus, there is *ex-ante* risk adjustment, which is designed to compensate insurers for predictable higher costs based on characteristics of their population, such as age, labour force status and pharmaceutical consumption. In addition, there exist *ex-post* equalisation formulas that reimburse insurers for higher realised costs above predicted costs as long as these are deemed to lie outside the insurers' sphere of influence. These *ex-post* formulas have been largely terminated since 2012.

Universal coverage

For Dutch citizens, taking out health insurance is mandatory. All persons over 18 are obliged to select a health insurer of their choice. Minors are insured along with their parents. Enrolees can choose their own insurer each year based on the premium which insurers set, the quality of included care and the service. To guarantee near-universal coverage, insurers are not allowed to engage in risk selection by denying applicants for mandatory health insurance (open enrolment). Insurers set their own rate but are obliged to charge equal premiums to all enrolees (community rating). Insurance companies may operate at a loss, but are required to hold reserves that equal 11% of their turnover.

The benefits basket

The treatments covered by the standard benefits package are determined by the central government. Occasionally, there are (marginal) interventions. For instance, the contraceptive pill was included in 2008, and then excluded again in 2011 for women aged above 20. The benefit package has an open character, implying that new treatments more or less automatically become an entitlement, which contributes to the increase of publicly financed care, especially for less severe cases (Ministry of Health Taskforce, 2012, pp. 5-6). Recently there has been a push to manage the package "more stringently". Key concepts of this will be that new entitlements are conditional, guidelines should include value-for-money, and quality-of-care should be more transparent.

Co-payments and supplementary insurance

Out-of-pocket payments mainly consist of a statutory deductible that holds for all services, with the notable exception of general practice. All enrolees face a deductible of EUR 375 a year in 2014. The chronically ill are partly compensated for the deductible. Individuals may decide to increase the deductible by up to EUR 500 voluntarily to obtain premium discounts at the cost of higher financial risk. Individuals also have the choice to expand benefits by taking up supplementary insurance covering, for instance, dental care, physiotherapy and alternative medicine. Around 84% of individuals have supplementary insurance.

Box 10.1. **An overview of the Dutch health care system** *(cont.)*

Health care provision and selective purchasing

Insurers can channel their enrolees towards certain providers by selectively purchasing care. Health care providers "compete" for patients in the provision market (indemnity policies) and by the commissioning of the insurance companies (managed care policies). All patients are allowed to choose their provider, although there can be substantial co-payments for care provided out-of-network. The GP acts as the gatekeeper to refer patients to hospital for further treatment.

10.3. Evolution of health spending under regulated competition

This section discusses the evolution of health spending in the Netherlands at the country level. It then addresses price and volume developments since the introduction of regulated competition. The sections thereafter assess to what extent the price and volume developments can be explained by (imperfect) realisation of the preconditions for regulated competition and cost containment.

Dutch health care spending has exhibited strong growth

The Netherlands has become an above-average spender on health per capita and as a percentage of GDP as shown in Figure 10.1. In 2011, it was the second highest spender on total health care in percentage of GDP in the OECD area, behind only the United States (OECD Health Statistics). The growth rate of total health spending went up considerably in 2000. This was a deliberate political choice, as the Dutch health care system was suffering from decreasing labour productivity, long waiting lists and stagnating life expectancies. Since 2001, waiting lists have decreased (Vijsel et al., 2011; Schut and Varkevisser, 2013), hospital labour productivity has increased to an annual average of 2.2% up to 2006 (Vandermeulen et al. 2012) and life expectancy, in particular for people aged over 65, went up significantly (Mackenbach et al., 2011). In part, rising care costs since 2000 can be seen as a catch-up effect after low growth during the 1980s and 1990s. The increase in spending growth converges with constant long-term expenditure income elasticity (Woordward and Wang, 2012). Nevertheless, the introduction of regulated competition in 2006 has so far not led to a clear deviation from this trend and its continuation will increase the expenditure gap with other countries.

Containment of prices and volume differ under regulated competition

Even though health care spending went up substantially before 2006 when regulated competition was implemented, the transition towards a system of regulated competition may have affected underlying price and volume developments. It seems more appropriate to speak of a transition rather than an implementation, as the government gradually shifted boundaries between the segment of hospital care on which the market players can negotiate prices (the B-segment) and the A-segment for which maximum prices were set centrally. The freely negotiable B-segment increased from 10% of all treatments in 2005 to 20% in 2008, 34% in 2011 and 70% in 2012. For the non-negotiable A-segment, the government sets the rates through the Dutch Health care Authority. As a general rule, the B-segment covers less complex and elective treatments, while the A-segment covers the more complex cases. However, with 70% of all cases now in the B-segment the difference has become somewhat blurred. Due to these expanding segments and changes in product definitions, comparisons in prices and volumes over time should be interpreted with caution.

Figure 10.1. **Evolution of total health expenditure in percentage of GDP and per capita**

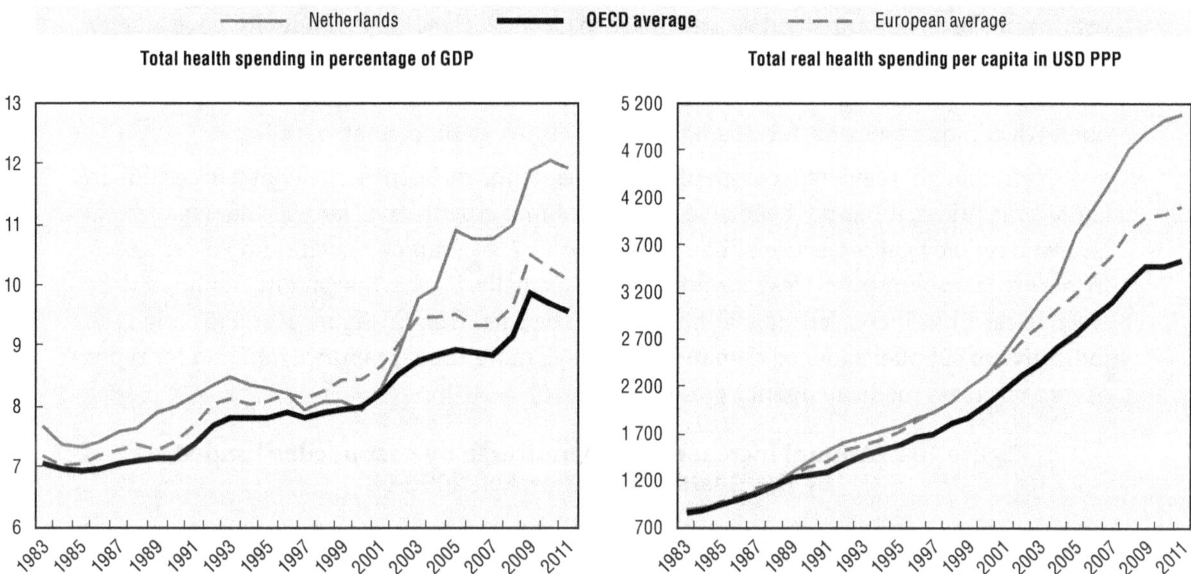

Note: OECD average: all OECD countries except Mexico, Turkey, Chile. European average: all European countries without missing values: Austria, Belgium, Denmark, Finland, Germany, Iceland, Ireland, Netherlands, Norway, Portugal, Spain, Sweden, Switzerland and the United Kingdom. The vertical line indicates the implementation of regulated competition in 2006.

Source: OECD Health Statistics, http://dx.doi.org/10.1787/health-data-en..

StatLink *http://dx.doi.org/10.1787/888933219393*

At first sight, prices show a decreasing trend since the introduction of regulated competition. Administrative costs of insurers decreased from 4.5% in 2006 to 2.9% in 2010 (Vektis, multiple years). Second, insurers seem to be somewhat successful in lowering health care prices, especially in pharmaceutics. Prices of the ten generic drugs with the largest volume fell by between 76% and 93% between 2006 and 2008 as insurers put out to tender high volumes of drugs (Boonen and Schut, 2011).

In addition, hospital prices in the freely negotiable B-segment have increased at a lower rate than the hospital prices still set by the Dutch Healthcare Authority, as shown in Table 10.1.

Table 10.1. **Nominal hospital price developments**

Percentage growth compared to previous year

	2006	2007	2008	2009	2010
Price increase in fixed-price segment A (before budget corrections, see note)	1.5	2.5	3.8	2.9	1.1
Price increase in freely negotiable segment B (tranche 2005, see note)	0.0	2.1	1.1	1.5	-1.8

Note: For the A-segment, the government can apply *ex-post* budget reductions by making price cuts in future years if the total annual health care expenses funded through the Health Insurance Act exceed a certain budget. In 2009 and 2010, tranches have been added to the B-segment. These tranches show price patterns very comparable to the 2005 tranche (NZA, 2011).

Source: NZA (2011), "Marktscan Medisch Specialistische Zorg: Weergave Van De Markt 2006-2010", Government of the Netherlands, Utrecht.

A main reason for the moderate price increases in the B-segment may have been an overestimation of B-segment prices and underestimation of A-segment prices at the start (Vandermeulen and Van Der Kwartel, 2013). Second, there are signs that care providers engage in up-coding, where patients are classified into more expensive diagnosis-treatment combinations (Steinbusch et al., 2007; Tummers and Van De Walle, 2012) Also, a rise in volume has been accompanied by a decrease in caseload, leading to moderate price effects. Indeed, the number of inputs per diagnosis-treatment combination declined rapidly by 4.6% per year (Ikkersheim and Koolman, 2013). It remains to be determined whether this is due to declining caseloads, increasing productivity, up-coding, or all of these.

Even though regulated competition seems to have been somewhat successful in containing prices, it has not been able to keep volume growth on a par with demographical and epidemiological projections that circle around 2.5% (Van Der Lucht and Polder, 2010). In particular, volume for "less severe" care, especially in the B-segment dominated by elective care, has increased substantially, as can be seen from in Figure 10.2. This might be indicative of supplier-induced demand, as there is more room to induce demand for types of care with less medical urgency (Wennberg, 2010).

Figure 10.2. **Annual increase in expenditures by cost deciles funded by the Health Insurance Act, 2006-08**

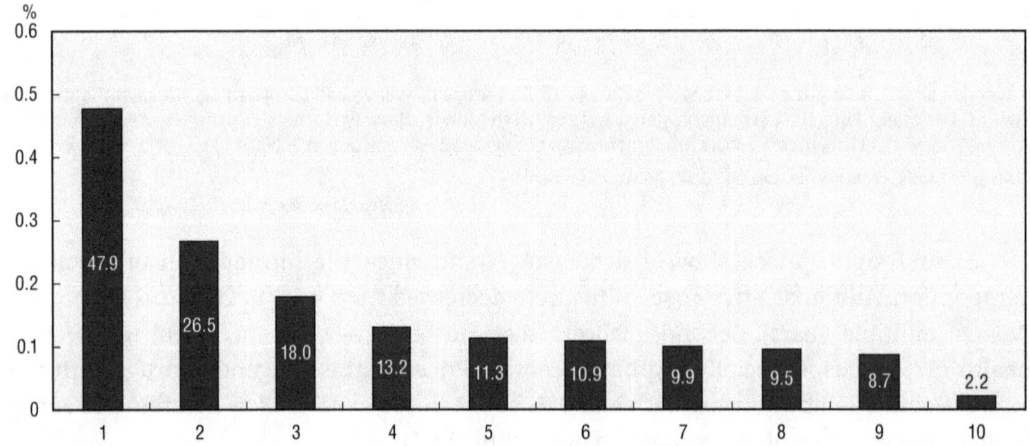

%
0.6
0.5
0.4
0.3
0.2
0.1
0
47.9
26.5
18.0
13.2
11.3
10.9
9.9
9.5
8.7
2.2
1 2 3 4 5 6 7 8 9 10

Note: The figure is sorted along patient cost deciles; for example, annual increases in expenditures went up by 47.9% for the 10% cheapest patients.

Source: APE (2012), *Patiëntprofielen In De Zvw, GGZ, AWBZ*, The Hague.

StatLink http://dx.doi.org/10.1787/888933219406

If we look at the evolution of expenditures within hospital care based on prices and volumes, preliminary figures seem to indicate that the growth has levelled off somewhat in 2012. Figure 10.3 shows this development, which includes the sum of expenditures within the A-segment and the B-segment and the fees for independent medical specialists. Moreover, part of the price increases have been translated into higher provider solvency rates which contributes to the financial resilience of the system. Average hospital solvency levels increased from 9.2 to 16.7% of equity as a percentage of total revenues between 2004 and 2011 (WFZ, 2005; WFZ, 2012). After decreasing solvency rates due to losses in 2006 and 2007, the solvency rates of insurers have remained reasonably stable since 2010 and well above the minimum at roughly 210% of the solvency demands, while solvency demands increased consistently (NZA, 2012a).

Figure 10.3. **Evolution of real hospital care expenditures**
In billion EUR

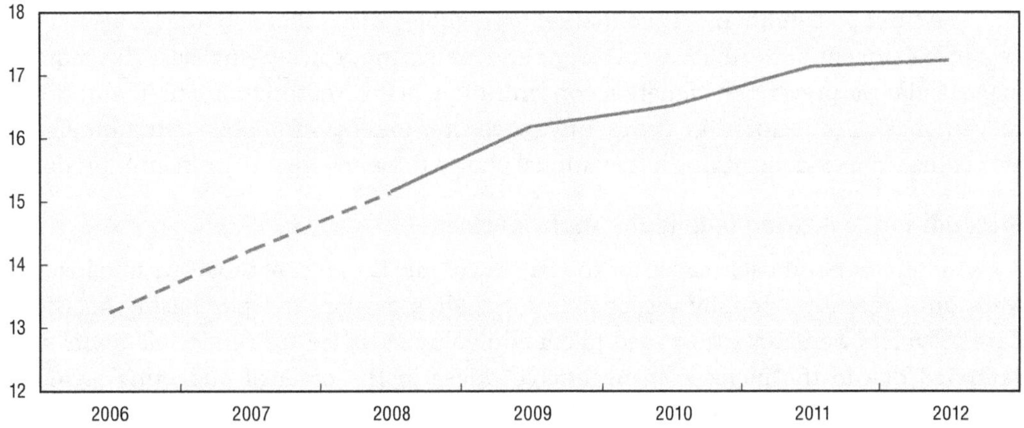

Note: 2008 from the 2012 edition, and the trend in 2006-08 from the 2011 edition adjusted to the level of the overlapping year of 2008 from the 2011 edition. As stated in the text, due to changes in product definitions and expanding segments, comparisons over time should be interpreted with caution.

Source: 2009-12 from NZA (2012), "Marktscan en Beleidsbrief Zorgverzekeringsmarkt: Weergave Van De Markt 2009-2013", Government of the Netherlands, Utrecht.

StatLink http://dx.doi.org/10.1787/888933219416

10.4. Fiscal challenges for regulated competition

Regulated competition lacks the centrally enforced budgetary constraints that were in place in the model it replaced. Due to the devolving of many financial responsibilities to insurers and providers, the fiscal balance needs to be created through an efficiency balance involving competition, fiscal stewardship by the government and restrictive policies regarding entitlements and out-of-pocket payments. This section examines three preconditions and two budgetary principles, and analyses how they have performed in the Netherlands.

Three challenges in making regulated competition work for cost containment

Three preconditions are particularly critical for attaining cost containment by means of regulated competition (Van De Ven et al., 2013). This section discusses the theoretical implementation of these preconditions in the Netherlands and the following two sections explore to what extent these principles have actually been applied.

First, buyers and sellers of care should bear financial risks. Insurers must be individually rather than collectively responsible for their purchasing behaviour and should bear substantial financial responsibility for the prices and volumes of the treatments they reimburse. In the Dutch health insurance market, insurers compete for customers by setting their level of premiums and by the (perceived) quality of covered care.

A second precondition for cost containment is that insurers and care providers need to have discretionary space to engage in contracting. If insurers are individually financially responsible for their purchase of care for their enrolees, this selective contracting should lead to higher value-for-money and cost containment. Providers are at risk from the financial specifications of these contracts such as prices, volumes and recovery formulas. Important elements of this are information and market transparency, insofar as lack of information decreases possibilities to engage in selective contracting. Quality and performance measurement are only discussed briefly here as they have been described extensively elsewhere (Van Der Wees et al., 2013).

The third precondition, for the market as a whole, is that there should be a sufficient degree of competition, so that cost overruns and inefficiency can be penalised. This requires in particular the prevention of market concentration. In the Netherlands, public authorities prevent market concentration. Competitive pressures to offer affordable premiums should also come from citizens having a free annual choice to switch insurer or insurer product.

Precondition 1: Bearing individual financial risks

An important probable cause for the rise in volume is that care providers and insurers were until recently not fully responsible for their provision and purchasing decisions. Care providers were not encouraged to contain volumes as fee-for-service elements were extended due to the increase in negotiable prices in the costs of budgeting elements (Vijsel et al., 2011; Thomson et al., 2013). Approximately half of medical specialists work independently rather than being in salaried service or having some performance contract (Schafer et al., 2010). Using regional variations, Douven et al. (2012) report that a one-percent increase in the number of physicians is associated with an increase of 0.40% in the number of treatments if they were independent physicians, but only an increase of 0.15% if they were salaried physicians.

Until recently, insurers also bore less individual risk for their purchasing behaviour. This was a consequence of "safety nets" implemented alongside regulated competition because of the sheer complexity of the regime shift. *Ex-post* budget corrections, designed to compensate insurers resulting from imperfections of the *ex-ante* equalisation, decreased efficiency incentives as profits and losses were pruned away. In addition, as *ex-post* compensation was mainly used to reduce the losses in hospital care, it decreased incentives to substitute expensive inpatient care for outpatient care. The so-called macroequalisation scheme shifted part of the risk of budgetary overruns to the government (Douven, 2010). Especially since 2012, the macroequalisation scheme and, to a large extent, the *ex-post* equalisation scheme have been cut back.

Figure 10.4 gives an indication of the percentage that an insurer will have to pay from its own funds for costs in excess of the funds received through the risk-adjustment scheme. This percentage went up significantly from around 52% in 2006 to 97% in 2013. The exact percentages should be interpreted with prudence as: the calculations are based on prognoses, net risk percentages are generally lower as a result of compensation for unpredicted high costs (the so-called "threshold adjustment"), there is a limit on the maximum spread of premiums and the macroequalisation scheme (Stam, 2012). Regardless if gross or net percentages are used, risk bearing for insurers went up over time.

Precondition 2: Selective contracting

Selective contracting/purchasing is a key precondition for cost containment. However, enrolees were generally not channelled towards the best performing hospitals as insurers typically contracted almost all providers. Not facing high monetary risks and without clear quality indicators, insurers fear a media and consumer backlash if they restrict provider choice(Van Ginneken and Swartz, 2012). Currently, insight into quality of care and market transparency, a precondition for efficiency under regulated competition, is limited. In particular, public information on medical outcome indicators adjusted for case mix is by and large lacking (Boonen and Schut, 2011; Westert et al., 2009; Boonen et al., 2011). In 2013 around 60 out of the 100 hospitals published their hospital-standardised mortality rates; for 2014 all hospitals are obliged to publish such figures. When transparency is reinforced, insurers may also employ co-payments more often as a mechanism to steer patients to preferred providers. Insurers in such cases may reimburse only part of the costs of treatment at out-of-network providers, and this may increase co-payments considerably.

Figure 10.4. **Risk bearing by insurers went up over time**

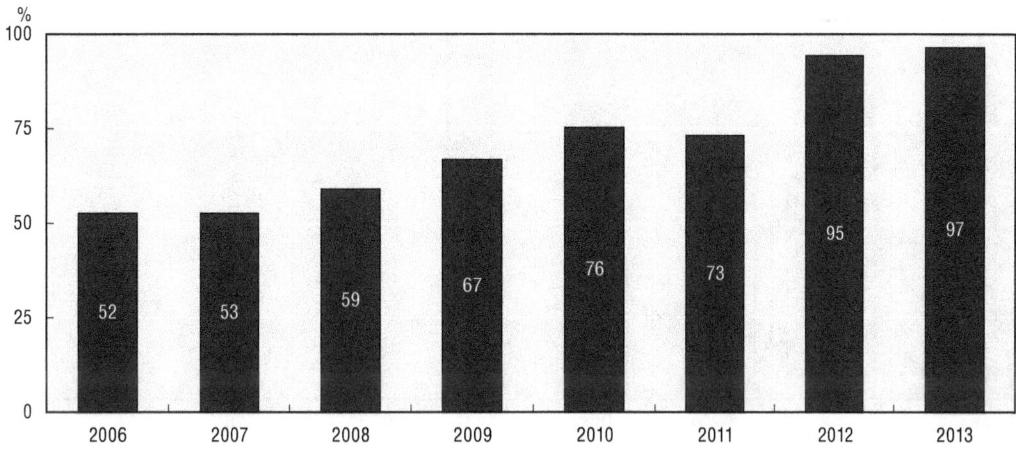

Note: The numbers give an indication of the percentage of risk bearing by insurers in inpatient and outpatient care, excluding mental care, but should be interpreted with prudence (see text); the calculations are based on prognoses and may change over time.

Source: Taken with permission from Stam, P. (2012), "Ontwikkeling Risicodragendheid 1992-2017", Strategies in Regulated Markets, The Hague.

StatLink http://dx.doi.org/10.1787/888933219428

In 2014, for the first time most insurers offered "budget policies" with substantially reduced consumer choice in exchange for significantly lower premiums. Such policies cover only a part of all hospitals and have considerable levels of co-payment for treatment in out-of-network hospitals. Interestingly, these policies have not turned out to be very popular so far. For three of the four largest insurers for which figures are available, between 0.5 and 5% of enrolees chose budget policies (NZA, 2014). It remains to be seen whether these low rates were a consequence of a lack of familiarity or structural low demand.

Precondition 3: Sufficient level of competition

Increased market pressures might have been reduced by the concentration of insurers and care providers, although concentration was already taking place before the market reforms. The number of hospitals decreased from 172 in 1982 to 94 in 2005 (Schafer et al., 2010) and to 92 in 2012. There is at the time of writing renewed interest in mergers with seven applications being filed. Concentration on the provider side may hamper selective contracting when hospitals become regional monopolies, even though it could also increase efficiency and quality of care provision of certain treatments. At the same time, there has been a strong increase in independent treatment centres from 120 in 2007 to 173 in 2010, which may present new competitive pressures (NZA, 2012b).

The insurer side of the market seems a textbook case oligopoly with a small number of insurers to choose from. This may cause strategic behaviour by insurers. However, a certain degree of insurer concentration may also be part of an efficient market to gain economies of scale and bargaining power. In 2013, the four largest insurers had a joint market share of approximately 90%. There is price stability in the market as can be seen by comparing the premiums of the four largest insurers (Figure 10.5). With limited price differences, consumer mobility may be somewhat limited, although 7.2% of enrolees switched in 2013, the highest percentage since 2006 (Vektis, 2013). In addition, the threat of switching may be enough to motivate insurers to set premiums at or close to the competitive level.

Figure 10.5. **Market shares and real monthly premium prices of the four largest health insurers**

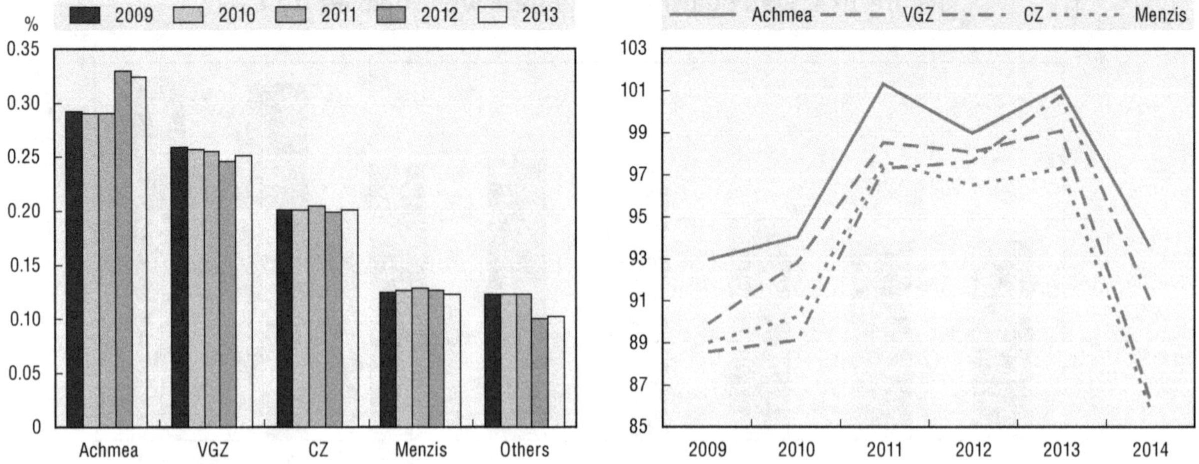

Note: Premium prices: public information, with inflation figures from CBS Statline. Levels of deductible: EUR 255 (2009). EUR 265 (2010), EUR 270 (2011), EUR 320 (2012), EUR 350 (2013), EUR 360 (2014). Selected insurances: Achmea Keuze Zorg Plan, VGZ Zorgverzekering Natura, CZ Zorgkeuzepolis, and Menzis ZorgVerzorgd Natura Polis.

Source: Market shares: NZA (2012), "Marktscan en Beleidsbrief Zorgverzekeringsmarkt: Weergave Van De Markt 2009-2013", Government of the Netherlands, Utrecht.

StatLink http://dx.doi.org/10.1787/888933219434

Nevertheless, the spread in premiums went up, in particular when the aforementioned budget policies were introduced. Around 65% of the population subscribes to an employer-based group contract. These contracts charge a premium of up to ten-per-cent lower than the official rate of the insurance company that provides them (and on which the premiums in Figure 10.5 are based). There are no obvious signs of excessive profits on premiums. In the first years after 2006, the insurers offered steep discounts and many operated at a loss. In 2012, insurers' profits on their standard benefits package policies were an estimated EUR 1.5 billion (DNB, 2013), or roughly 4% of health care expenditures from the Health Insurance Act. In 2014, for the first time in decades insurance premiums decreased significantly, which could be an indication of successful cost containment.

10.5. Role of government in cost containment underregulated competition

Two principles for budgeting and cost containment underregulated competition

Since the implementation of regulated competition, the role of government has changed from direct control of global budgets, volumes and prices to a decentralised system where it is mainly responsible for regulating and supervising. The government no longer allocates the majority of health funding direct, and the limiting of entitlements and increasing out-of-pocket-payments seem difficult to employ.

Also in a system of regulated competition, budgeting practices still are important for containing health care costs as the government defines the size of the health care market by setting coverage and the level of co-payments. This degree of influence and the public nature of the mandatory insurance warrant cost control from the central level. Box 10.2 summarises budgeting practices in the Netherlands.

Box 10.2. **The mid-term expenditure framework and the annual budget cycle in the Netherlands**

Budgeting in the Netherlands takes place in two budget cycles, the large and the small budget cycle. In the first large budget cycle, the incoming government lays down its overall budget policy proposals and spending caps for five years as stated in the governing parties' coalition agreement. In the Netherlands there is a rather rigid demarcation between spending and revenues. Tax revenues are projected over a five-year period and a corresponding expenditure framework is set. Over the years, deviations in revenue from the business cycle are accommodated through "automatic stabilisation". Therefore, budgetary ceilings and tax rates are in general not altered to realise expected annual revenue levels. This ensures pro-cyclical effects are countered since there is no direct relation between spending and revenue raised. An exception on the revenue side is health care where spending is covered by cost-based premiums. Insurers in addition may use the nominal premium to offset higher than expected spending. The expenditure side is divided into three separate sectors, one of which is the health care sector. Thus, irrespective of the system of "regulated competition", public expenditure caps affect spending levels within the health care sector.

The health care sector budget is subdivided into different care sectors, such as long-term care, hospital treatments and spending on GPs. Policy priorities can be set by shifting budgets between different sub-sectors, or by choosing which care will be collectively funded by fine-tuning the standard benefits package and the level of statutory out-of-pocket payments.

The second phase in health care budgeting is the annual budget cycle in which the coalition implements the plans laid down in the coalition agreement and in which it addresses unforeseen overruns. This process starts at the beginning of the preceding year when the Ministry of Finance updates its expenditure projections and receives spending proposals from ministries. After intensive negotiations between the different ministries and the Ministry of Finance, the coalition agrees on revenues and budget cuts around August. On the third Tuesday of September the annual budget is presented to parliament. During the year the central budgeting arm of the Ministry of Finance monitors possible overruns that in principle need to be redressed if they occur. The Ministry of Health can compensate with underspending in other areas if applicable, reducing benefits or putting pressures on set fees and budgets.

Little has been written so far on budgeting and cost containment in health under regulated competition. For this reason, this chapter speaks of principles rather than preconditions. Generally, pressure to increase public spending on health care is likely to be very strong. This may come from the fact that care is widely seen as a necessity and that being sick is something to which the public at large can relate (White, 2013). Public support for egalitarian access and equality in the Netherlands is high, even when compared to primary needs such as food and habitation. Because of this, public support to stretch the coverage of collective care is strong. In addition, in health there is substantial discretionary pressure to increase public spending, for example as a result of ageing, technological advances and supplier-induced demand resulting from information asymmetries.

A first budgetary principle to contain costs would be that budgeting policies should be designed to dampen increased public demand, for example by stringently defining coverage. This can be seen as an *ex-ante* cost-containment principle. A more gradual instrument to reduce public spending and consumer demand is the use of co-payments.

As a second budgetary principle, governments should be able to prevent or redress overruns as quickly as possible. This requires timely information on spending levels and rapid implementation and realisation of measures taken.

Budgetary principle 1: Stringent coverage and sufficient co-payments

Cutting specific health services is seen in the budgeting literature as a more unpopular strategy than reducing spending in general – this fits with a blame-avoidance strategy in which policy makers choose not to deny people direct treatment by taking away entitlements (White, 2013). The benefit package in the Netherlands is open, implying that new treatments more or less automatically become an entitlement, which contributes to the increase of publicly financed care, especially for less severe cases. Occasionally there are financially marginal interventions, for instance, the contraceptive pill was included in 2008, and then excluded again in 2011 for women aged above 20. The Netherlands is just behind Italy and Germany, but before 22 other OECD countries, in the degree of generosity with which 11 expensive medicines with disputable results are publicly financed (Böhm et al., 2014).

In the Netherlands, the government defines the coverage for the standard benefits package and sets the level of out-of-pocket payments for these entitlements. Increasing co-payments might be a more gradual instrument to reduce public spending and consumer demand. Before 2013, citizens were scarcely encouraged to contain demand, as the share of co-payments in the Netherlands was relatively low compared to other countries (OECD Health Expenditure and Financing). In addition, important parts of care are exempted from co-payments, such as GP visits and maternity and children's health care, because the government does not want to place a financial barrier in the way of their consumption. In 2013, the deductible went up significantly from EUR 220 to EUR 350 for every person aged over 18.[2] The rise in out-of-pocket payments in 2013 might have contributed to the declining trend in recent health care growth depending on the price elasticity of the services at stake.

Budgetary principle 2: Timely information

In order to contain costs by taking corrective public measures, timely information is key. Yet, there is a substantial time gap of up to two and often three years between overspending and the moment government interventions can take effect, as shown in Table 10.2. Apart from the regular spending assessments, there are no formal early-warning systems. The time lags can to a certain extent be attributed to the decentralised nature of the system of regulated competition. It takes time before the Ministry of Health receives the actual spending figures from the insurers. Providers claim their expenses from insurers by means of a complex system of 4 000 diagnosis treatment combinations (Thomson et al., 2013), which can be open for a maximum of a year from the moment a treatment for a patient starts. To reduce this delay, the government plans to curb the length of a diagnosis treatment combination to 120 days.

Table 10.2. **Time lags between realisation of spending and implementation of measures**

T	t+1	t+2	t+3
Overspending takes place	Preliminary figures are known For quickly available indications measures can be taken that will take effect in *t+2*	Definitive figures are known Measures can be announced that will take effect in *t+3*	Implementation of the measures

There is an implementation lag of almost a year. After April, the budget discussions between the Ministries of Finance and Health end and dependable final figures are needed to motivate possible cuts. Spending overruns that become apparent after April generally cannot be amended in the next year's budget. In addition, insurers have to present their policy conditions for next year's policies before 19 November, as enrolees are entitled to know which providers are included and what the level of premiums will be. Thus, well before this date the exact public policies that apply next year need to be specified, including the coverage of the standard benefits package, deductibles, co-payments and prices of treatments.

Time lags also hamper the purchasing process. Opportunities for selective contracting suffer from substantial transaction costs as a result of the long lags between the start of treatment and the invoice, and parties have difficulty in finalising negotiations on price and volume before the financial year begins. For example, at the end of December 2010, around 10% of the care for that year was still not contracted. The general default option is that it will be reimbursed on a case-by-case basis. Recently, contracting has been moved forward in time under pressure from the government as the supervisor. However, the Netherlands Institute of Chartered Accountants has stated that to date accountants are not able to test the soundness of forecasts and results for 2013 accountants in order to validate the annual financial reports of the Dutch hospitals.

Budgeted versus realised spending

Considering the difficulties in limiting entitlements or increasing out-of-pocket payments and the lack of timely information, it may come as no surprise that the Netherlands has witnessed significant overruns in health care. Despite significant budget increases, spending has consistently exceeded the health care budget, not only from the introduction of managed competition in 2006 onwards but in 15 out of the last 16 years. This illustrates that spending projections are poorly aligned with actual spending. Moreover, financial forecasts are largely based on the average increases in health expenditure since 2000, which implies spending growth is on a relatively high baseline already. The high baseline may also imply an anchor effect on health care spending, as expectations are anchored to previous high-growth paths. As regulated competition has thus far not solved the problems of budget containment, new instruments have been implemented.

New instruments for cost containment and a reintroduction of corporatism

The government has implemented new instruments to control total health care spending now that the *ex-ante* setting of global budgets for care providers has largely been eroded. Since 2012, the government made an effort to regain direct influence on provider overspending beyond the predetermined macro level. All providers (hospitals, mental health institutions and primary care providers) need to refund the percentage overrun of their own sub-sector, standardised by their own market share (the "macro-controlling instrument", or MCI). For example if the hospital budget has an overrun of five per cent, each individual hospital has to pay back according to its share in the market. Providers as a group are thus encouraged to contain costs; however, efficient hospitals are required to refund as well, which makes the instrument rather blunt (Schut et al., 2013). Hospitals might be hurt disproportionately if they have low margins due to competitive price-setting that increases their market share.

As the government was limited in its direct ability to contain health care expenditure, in 2011 it chose to shift back to corporatist agreements with various stakeholders. This model of consultation and co-ordination does not fit naturally with the competitive structure of a market. Nevertheless, it can be seen as a way to share risks and it does fit with the neo-corporatist traditions in the Netherlands (Tuohy, 2012). The parties have agreed that real expenditures (excluding indexation) in hospitals and clinics will rise only 2.5% annually for the period 2012-15, just above half of the growth path up to 2012. Comparable ceilings have been set for mental health (2013-14), and for GPs (2012-13). New negotiations have led to a growth path of 1% for hospitals and mental health institutions and 2.5% for primary-care providers (2015-17). Due to the time lags and the complex payment transitions, it is still not fully clear if overruns have come to the fore. If an overrun exists, the only thing the government can do to recoup these funds is to use the macro-controlling instrument or implement new budgetary cuts. However, it seems that these agreements might contribute to purchasing contracts that take the lower agreed numbers as the default option, thus leading to a lower growth path.

10.6. Conclusion

The Dutch health system is characterised both by its unique institutional system of regulated competition and by its high and, for a long time, rapidly rising expenditures. An obvious but important question is whether the system of regulated competition is one of the causes of these high spending levels. Rising health care costs can partly be seen as a catch-up effect as major investments were made to shorten waiting lists and improve labour productivity well before the introduction of regulated competition. Nevertheless, the introduction of competitive elements in 2006 did not put a halt to this upward trend. Although unit prices have declined since then in certain parts of the health care sector such as generics, the volume of less-severe cases in particular went up considerably. In addition, health care providers and insurers have strengthened their solvency positions, which can be seen as a direct consequence of the new competitive landscape.

For regulated competition to lead to contained costs, certain preconditions have to be met which were imperfectly implemented, at least initially. First, insurers and care providers did not bear the financial consequences of their provision and purchasing decisions individually. Fee-for-service elements for care providers in combination with *ex-post* budget corrections pruned away losses for health care insurers and decreased cost-containment incentives for both parties. Second, enrolees were generally not channelled towards the best performing hospitals as insurers typically signed contracts with almost all providers as insights into quality of care were lacking. A third precondition is that there should be a sufficient degree of competition amongst both care providers and health insurers so that cost overruns can be penalised. Although the insurer side is an oligopoly, there are no signs of rents on the premiums.

Proper incentives for health insurers, care providers and citizens to contain costs are necessary but insufficient conditions for regulated competition to lead to cost containment. Also, the budgeting side is important. Budgeting should be designed to dampen increased public demand by stringently defining coverage to high-value services or by setting co-payments. Yet, cutting health services is seen as a very unpopular strategy as it essentially entails taking away entitlements. The benefit package in the Netherlands is open so that new – though not necessarily better – treatments become an entitlement more or less automatically. The share of co-payments is still moderate. A second budgetary principle is that the government should be able to redress overruns as quickly as possible. However, there are substantial time lags of up to three years between when overspending takes place, when it is noted and when corrective measures can be implemented. Interestingly, because of its reduced toolbox the government has chosen to shift back to corporatist agreements to share risks with the different stakeholders.

There are preliminary signs that from 2012 onwards the rise in health expenditure seems to have flattened. Given the challenges all actors face from continuous reform efforts, any structural breaking point from the introduction of regulated competition may well only been found many years after its 2006 introduction. The growth in real hospital care expenditures seems to have levelled out in 2012 and average real monthly premium prices even went down considerably in 2014. It could be that these first signs of containment are a consequence of fiscal consolidation in response to rising deficits resulting from the financial crisis. Yet, it also coincides with the further implementation of elements of regulated competition as described here. In 2012, the B-segment for which prices are freely negotiable went up from 34% to 70% of all treatments. *Ex-post* budget correction mechanisms have been decreased so that health insurers are encouraged to contain costs individually. The level of co-payments for citizens increased as the deductible went up considerably in 2013. The shift back to corporatist agreements with budget ceilings could have a cost-containing function as well.

In conclusion, it seems too early to tell whether regulated competition had a role in this recent incidence of cost containment. Regardless, the Dutch health care system now appears to have moved closer to satisfying the preconditions and seems therefore much better prepared to bend the cost curve in the coming years.

Notes

1. Dutch health care was divided along income lines between coverage by sickness funds (bottom 65%) and coverage by private indemnity insurers (top 35%). It was a long-sought goal to merge both schemes in one universal health care insurance system.
2. Note that the deductibles are not taken into account by the OECD's health statistics as out-of-pocket payments due to the absence of a direct payment relation between patients and providers in the Dutch case.

Bibliography

APE (2012), *Patiëntprofielen In De Zvw, GGZ, AWBZ*, The Hague.

Böhm, K., C. Landwehr and N. Steiner (2014), "What Explains 'Generosity' in the Public Financing of High-Tech Drugs? An Empirical Investigation of 25 OECD Countries and 11 Controversial Drugs", *Journal of European Social Policy*, Vol. 24, No. 1, Sage Publications, London, pp. 39-55.

Boonen, L. and F. Schut (2011), "Preferred Providers and the Credible Commitment Problem in Health Insurance: First Experiences with the Implementation of Managed Competition in the Dutch Healthcare System", Health Economics, Policy and Law, Vol. 6, No. 2, Cambridge University Press, United Kingdom, pp. 219-235.

Boonen, L., B. Donkers and F. Schut (2011), Channelling Consumers to Preferred Providers and the Impact of Status Quo Bias: Does Type of Provider Matter?", Health Services Research, Vol. 46, No. 2, AcademyHealth, Blackwell Publishing, Chicago, pp. 510-530.

DNB – De Nederlandsche Bank (2013), « Central Bank Data Individual Insurers », accessed 9 August.

Douven, R. (2010), "Ex-Post Correctiemechanismen In De Zorgverzekeringswet: Hoe Nu Verder?", *CPB Document* No. 212.

Douven, R., R. Mocking and I. Mosca (2012), "The Effect of Physician Fees and Density Differences on Regional Variation in Hospital Treatments", *IBMG Working Paper* W2012.01, Institute of Health Policy and Management, Erasmus University, Rotterdam.

Enthoven, A. (2004), "Market Forces and Efficient Healthcare Systems". *Health Affairs*, Vol. 23, No. 2, Project HOPE: The People-to-People Health Foundation, Bathesda, United States, pp. 25-27.

Ikkersheim, D. and X. Koolman (2013), "The First Effects of Dutch Healthcare Reform on Hospitals", D. Ikkersheim (ed.), *The Dutch Health System Reform: Creating Value*, Free University, Amsterdam.

Maarse, H. and A. Paulus (2011), "The Politics of Healthcare Reform in the Netherlands since 2006", *Health Economics, Policy And Law*, Vol. 6, No. 1, Cambridge University Press, United Kingdom, pp. 125-134.

Mackenbach, J. et al. (2011), "Sharp Upturn of Life Expectancy in the Netherlands: Effect of More Health Care for the Elderly?", *European Journal of Epidemiology*, Vol. 26, No. 12, Springer, London, pp. 903-914.

Marmor, T. and C. Wendt (2012), "Conceptual Frameworks for Comparing Healthcare Politics and Policy", *Health Policy*, Vol. 2012, No. 107, Elsevier, Amsterdam, pp. 11-20.

NZA – Dutch Healthcare Authority (2014), "Monitor en Beleidsbrief Zorginkoop", Government of the Netherlands, Utrecht.

NZA (2012a), "Marktscan en Beleidsbrief Zorgverzekeringsmarkt: Weergave Van De Markt 2009-2013", Government of the Netherlands, Utrecht.

NZA (2012b), "Monitor Zelfstandige Behandelcentra", Government of the Netherlands, Utrecht.

NZA (2011), "Marktscan Medisch Specialistische Zorg: Weergave Van De Markt 2006-2010", Government of the Netherlands, Utrecht.

OECD, "Health Expenditure and Financing", database last updated June 2013, OECD, Paris.

Okma, K. and L. Crivelli (2013), "Swiss and Dutch 'Consumer-Driven Health Care': Ideal Model or Reality?", *Health Policy*, Vol. 109, No. 2, Elsevier, Amsterdam, pp. 105-112.

Schafer, W. et al. (2010), "The Netherlands: Health System Review", *Health Systems In Transition*, Vol. 12, No. 1, European Observatory on Health Systems and Policies, Copenhagen.

Schut, F. and W. Van De Ven (2011), "Effects of Purchaser Competition in the Dutch Health System: Is the Glass Half Full or Half Empty?", *Health Economics, Policy and Law*, Vol. 6, No. 1, Cambridge University Press, United Kingdom, pp. 109-123.

Schut, F. and M. Varkevisser (2013), "Tackling Hospital Waiting Times: The Impact of Past and Current Policies in the Netherlands", *Health Policy*, Vol. 113, No. 1-2, Elsevier, Amsterdam, pp. 127-133.

Schut, F., S. Sorbe and J. Hoj (2013), "Health Care Reform and Long-Term Care in the Netherlands", *OECD Economics Department Working Paper* No. 1010, OECD, Paris.

Stam, P. (2012), "Ontwikkeling Risicodragendheid 1992-2017", Strategies in Regulated Markets, The Hague.

Steinbusch, P. et al. (2007), "The Risk of Upcoding in Casemix Systems: A Comparative Study", Health Policy, Vol. 81, No. 2-3, Elsevier, Amsterdam, pp. 289-299.

Thomson, S. et al. (2013), "Statutory Health Insurance Competition in Europe: A Four-Country Comparison", *Health Policy*, Vol. 109, No. 3, Elsevier, Amsterdam, pp. 209-225.

Tummers, L. and S. Van De Walle (2012), "Explaining Health Care Professionals' Resistance to Implement Diagnosis Related Groups: (No) Benefits for Society, Patients and Professionals", *Health Policy*, Vol. 108, No. 2-3, Elsevier, Amsterdam, pp. 158-166.

Tuohy, C. (2012), "Reform and the Politics of Hybridization in Mature Healthcare States", *Journal of Health Politics, Policy and Law*, Vol. 37, No. 4, pp. 611-632, Duke University Press, Durham, United States.

Vandermeulen, L. and A. Van Der Kwartel (2013), "Sturen Op Doelmatigheid", Kiwa Prismant, Utrecht.

Vandermeulen, L., A. Beldman and A. Van Der Kwartel (2012), "Productiviteitswinst In De Zorg: Who Gets What, When And How?", Kiwa Prismant, Utrecht Tackling Hospital Waiting Times: The Impact of Past and Current Policies in the Netherlands.

Van De Ven, W. et al. (2013), "Preconditions for Efficiency and Affordability in Competitive Healthcare Markets: Are They Fulfilled in Belgium, Germany, Israel, The Netherlands and Switzerland?", *Health Policy*, Vol. 109, No. 3, Elsevier, Amsterdam, pp. 225-245.

Van Der Lucht, F. and J. Polder (2010), *Van Gezond Naar Beter*, RIVM Bilthoven.

Van Der Wees, P. et al. (2013), "Governing Healthcare through Performance Measurement in Massachusetts and the Netherlands", *Health Policy*, Vol. 116, No. 1, Elsevier, Amsterdam, pp. 18-26.

Van Ginneken, E. and K. Swartz (2012), "Implementing Insurance Exchanges: Lessons from Europe", *New England Journal of Medicine*, Vol. 367, No. 8, Massachusetts Medical Society, Waltham, United States, pp. 691-693.

Vektis (2013), "Zorgthermometer: Verzekerden In Beweging 2013", Zeist, Netherlands.

Vektis (multiple years), Zorgmonitor, Zeist, Netherlands.Vijsel, A., P. Engelfriet and G. Westert (2011), "Rendering Hospital Budgets Volume-Based and Open-Ended to Reduce Waiting Lists: Does It Work?", *Health Policy*, Vol. 100, No. 1, Elsevier, Amsterdam, pp. 60-70.

Vijsel, A., P. Engelfriet and G. Westert (2011), "Rendering Hospital Budgets Volume-Based and Open-Ended to Reduce Waiting Lists: Does It Work?", *Health Policy*, Vol. 100, No. 1, Elsevier, Amsterdam, pp. 60-70.

Wennberg, J. (2010), "Tracking Medicine: A Researcher's Quest to Understand Health Care", Oxford University Press, Oxford.

Westert, G., J. Burgers and H. Verkleij (2009), "The Netherlands: Regulated Competition Behind The Dykes?", *British Medical Journal*, Vol. 339, British Medical Association, London, pp. 839-842.

WFZ – Waarborgfonds voor de Zorgsector (2012), Jaarverslag 2012. Waarborgfonds voor de Zorgsector, Utrecht.

WFZ (2005), Jaarverslag 2005, Waarborgfonds voor de Zorgsector, Utrecht.White, J. (2013), "Budget-makers and Healthcare Systems", *Health Policy*, Vol. 112, No. 3, Elsevier, Amsterdam, pp. 163-171.

White, J. (2013), "Budget-makers and Healthcare Systems", *Health Policy*, Vol. 112, No. 3, Elsevier, Amsterdam, pp. 163-171.

Woordward, R. and L. Wang (2012), "The Oh-So Straight and Narrow Path: Can the Health Care Expenditure Curve Be Bent?", *Health Economics*, Vol. 21, No. 8, John Wiley and Sons, pp. 1023-1029.

ORGANISATION FOR ECONOMIC CO-OPERATION AND DEVELOPMENT

The OECD is a unique forum where governments work together to address the economic, social and environmental challenges of globalisation. The OECD is also at the forefront of efforts to understand and to help governments respond to new developments and concerns, such as corporate governance, the information economy and the challenges of an ageing population. The Organisation provides a setting where governments can compare policy experiences, seek answers to common problems, identify good practice and work to co-ordinate domestic and international policies.

The OECD member countries are: Australia, Austria, Belgium, Canada, Chile, the Czech Republic, Denmark, Estonia, Finland, France, Germany, Greece, Hungary, Iceland, Ireland, Israel, Italy, Japan, Korea, Luxembourg, Mexico, the Netherlands, New Zealand, Norway, Poland, Portugal, the Slovak Republic, Slovenia, Spain, Sweden, Switzerland, Turkey, the United Kingdom and the United States. The European Union takes part in the work of the OECD.

OECD Publishing disseminates widely the results of the Organisation's statistics gathering and research on economic, social and environmental issues, as well as the conventions, guidelines and standards agreed by its members.

OECD PUBLISHING, 2, rue André-Pascal, 75775 PARIS CEDEX 16
(81 2015 111 P1) ISBN 978-92-64-23337-9 – 2015-17

www.ingramcontent.com/pod-product-compliance
Lightning Source LLC
LaVergne TN
LVHW081402110826
845149LV00010B/1637

* 9 7 8 9 2 6 4 2 3 3 3 7 9 *